THE CLINICAL MANAGEMENT
OF
BASIC MAXILLOFACIAL ORTHOPEDIC APPLIANCES

VOLUME I: MECHANICS

Terrance J. Spahl, DDS

in collaboration with
and presenting the case studies of

John W. Witzig, DDS

PSG PUBLISHING COMPANY, INC.
LITTLETON, MASSACHUSETTS

Library of Congress Cataloging in Publication Data
Spahl, Terrance J.
    The clinical management of basic maxillo-facial
orthopedic appliances.

    Includes index.
    Contents: v. 1. Mechanics.
    1. Orthodontic appliances. I. Witzig, John W.
II. Title. [DNLM: 1. Orthodontic Appliances.
WU 400 S733c]
RK527.S63 1986   617.6'43   86-91476
ISBN 0-88416-558-2 (v. 1)

Published by:
PSG PUBLISHING COMPANY, INC.
545 Great Road
Littleton, Massachusetts 01460

Printed in Hong Kong.

International Standard Book Number: 0-88416-558-2

Library of Congress Catalog Card Number: 86-91476

Last digit is print number: 9 8 7 6 5 4 3 2

To the children, EmmaLee, Teddy, and Joey Spahl and their devoted mother, Susan, for all the sacrifices of time such a young and growing family had to make to allow this book to come into being.

ABOUT THE AUTHORS

Terrance J. Spahl, D.D.S. has been in private practice in St. Paul, Minnesota since 1971. He is a dental products consultant for the 3M Company and Ohlendorf Company Orthodontic Laboratory, and a clinical consultant for Ortho-Diagnostics Ltd.

Dr. Spahl has lectured widely to dental and medical groups on the subject of the temporomandibular joint and co-developed the Witzig-Spahl Analysis, the first computerized method for analyzing TMJ x-rays.

A clinician with extensive orthodontic experience, Dr. Spahl has studied under noted experts in the United States and abroad. He is a member of the American Equilibration Society, the American Endodontic Society, the American Dental Association, the American Academy of General Dentistry, and the American Association of Functional Orthodontics.

John W. Witzig, D.D.S. maintains a private practice devoted exclusively to orthodontics and TMJ pain patients, in Minneapolis, Minnesota. He is regional editor of *The Journal of Cranio–Mandibular Practice* and contributing editor to *The Functional Orthodontist*.

Dr. Witzig is author of *Orthodontic and Orthopedic Appliances* and co-author of *Orthodontics and Its Effect on the TMJ* and *Clinical Management of TMJ Pain*. He developed and patented the Orthopedic Corrector I Appliance and the Orthopedic Corrector II Appliance and is co-holder of the U.S. patent on the Sagittal III Appliance. Dr. Witzig is a member of the American Equilibration Society, the American Association of Functional Orthodontics, the European Orthodontic Society, the International Association of Orthodontics, and the American Dental Association.

An experienced clinician who has studied in the United States and Europe, he was honored as "Man of the Year" in 1984 by the American Association of Functional Orthodontics. Since 1972, Dr. Witzig has conducted dental education courses for more than 15,000 doctors in North America.

CONTENTS

FOREWORD

When I first introduced the Bionator appliance to the United States in 1973, the American orthodontic world was dominated almost exclusively by the use of fixed appliances. At first a great deal of controversy and rejection prevailed concerning the use of functional appliances. After making some design modifications to the original Bionator of Dr. Wilhelm Balters of Germany, I developed the Orthopedic Corrector appliances. As I toured the country giving many courses over the early years of my lecturing career on the principles of Functional Jaw Orthopedics, many clinicians began using these techniques and obtained superior results. The refinement of the functional appliance, active plate, and second molar replacement techniques in conjunction with the development of more manageable modern-day fixed appliances has greatly changed the manner in which we may now treat problems of both the malocclusion of the teeth and jaws, and the pain and dysfunction of the temporomandibular joint. The combined use of removable maxillofacial orthopedic and fixed orthodontic appliance techniques allows the modern practitioner to obtain the highest quality results for not only the occlusion but also the face and temporomandibular joints. These results are often difficult if not impossible to achieve by using a single appliance system alone.

Since the approach of Functional Jaw Orthopedics in conjunction with fixed appliances gives a much more superior result than the use of a single appliance type, and since there is such an enormous demand for knowledge of the clinical usage of these techniques, I felt a text covering as much of the subject as possible would greatly aid the clinician. It was also felt that due to the demands of time necessary to maintain a busy lecture schedule as well as a private practice, I could not produce such a text on my own. A co-author would be needed who could work with me and accurately and competently record my ideas and teachings, and skillfully organize them into readable book form. He would have to be an experienced clinician familiar with both removable and fixed appliance techniques. He would also have to be familiar with the entire spectrum of treatment in vogue for problems of the temporomandibular joint. He would have to be free of any prejudiced opinions or favoritisms of one technique over another, and it was hoped that he would be free of any of the constraints imposed by affiliation with an academic institution. Although academia has a very respectable place, this book should be written *by* a clinician *for* clinicians. Since I would be delegating a great deal of responsibility to him to produce the text, he would have to possess not only fortitude and perseverance but also a sense of humor. Lastly, he would have to be able to write. I was most pleased and happy to engage for this project the services of a man with excellent qualifications, Terrance J. Spahl, D.D.S., of St. Paul, Minnesota. Dr. Spahl has a great talent at writing, and he has an uncanny knack for condensing and interpreting large volumes of information into a clear easy-to-read style that is direct and to the point. This is important for busy practitioners. We have spent many long hours together preparing material for this text. Dr. Spahl has taken this vast body of information and made it into more than a guide through modern combined orthodontic techniques. He has fashioned it into something that will help the clinician on many levels. This book will greatly aid practicing clinicians in obtaining the best and most stable treatment results for their patients. It will also help them find their way out of the maze of confusion and discord that accompanies such a sweeping change in treatment technique and philosophy. I firmly believe that this is the finest and most important book on this subject available today. It is hoped that the knowledge represented in its pages will serve both the practitioners, and as a result their patients, and point the way for further development to even greater heights of orthodontic health care in the future.

John Witzig, D.D.S.
Minneapolis, Minnesota

PREFACE

Upon being approached by certain members of the profession with the proposal to write a book concerning the techniques and teachings of John Witzig, D.D.S., this author soon realized that such an endeavor would require more than a mere polemic on modernized European orthodontic methodologies. Several of the parties concerned quickly and clearly pointed out that although the orthodontic principles espoused by Dr. Witzig in his numerous lectures and seminars over the years were clear, simple, forward-looking, and well organized; the orthodontic world in which they were promulgated was not! Not only would the main subject matter of Dr. Witzig's methods of appliance usage have to be clearly defined and explained, but also a broad range of auxiliary and supportive techniques would have to be discussed in an effort to give insight to a more complete picture of therapeutic approach that represents on the broadest of scales an entire philosophy, the philosophy of Functional Jaw Orthopedics. This would, of course, necessitate the inclusion of the Witzig techniques and those appliances and methods developed by many of the other great contributors to the orthodontic field from across the decades and across the continents. This led to something that might be somewhat unique for this text; an identity crisis!

This particular treatise has been written for the practicing clinician and therefore assumes a certain working knowledge of the basic biological, anatomical, and physiological entities concerned in the growth and development of the dentition in particular and the entire maxillofacial complex in general. Such information of the level necessary to qualify this text is common and familiar territory to all practicing clinicians, and its details have been clearly and adequately covered in numerous books on the subject. This text is devoted to the discussion of the design, purpose, management, and common usage of appliances and methodologies inherent in the overall FJO system of treating malocclusions on the most basic of levels. Due to the limitless variety of possible malocclusions, this, of course, becomes a necessity. Unless a basic understanding is first established, meaningful consideration of the individual variations of specific cases and their significance becomes difficult if not impossible.

Yet in a project such as this, due to the revolutionary nature of many of its basic tenets, the discussion of appliance usage—the how—must be matched by a supportive and complementary discussion of the philosophical and theoretical approaches of the system—the why. The most basic components of the system, both philosophical and mechanical, are radically different from anything that has preceded it. And of course with such a divergent embarkation from traditionally held values and beliefs, one must accept the appearance of one of the cardinal signs of such departures from the status quo—controversy! This will no doubt be the fate of this particular volume because one of the overall goals it has set for itself is to change not only what the orthodontic discipline does but also what the discipline thinks about what it does. Though some may consider this novel or dynamic, unfortunately, others may consider it threatening. It is meant only to be enlightening.

Thus from the onset, we realized this project would be faced with at least two missions. The first was to clarify and expand upon the clinical aspects of the various appliance usages of the system. The second would be to challenge the traditionally held values with a newer, and what is believed to be a far superior overall treatment philosophy. Neither could be given preference, for both are equally important, and a serious effort at discussing either would be a major undertaking in its own right. However, it was also soon determined that yet a third mission would be necessary for this text, that of assisting the clinician with the human element involved in expanding oneself into the relatively uncharted and radical areas of combined American and European orthodontics and orthopedics. This would require the consolidation of a wide variety of techniques into a unified whole, the aggregate of which would be greater than the sums of its parts. The effort to seriously address these separate missions while at the same time keeping each in appropriate balance is reflected in one of the more uncommon aspects of the work, its style. Rather than conform to the conventional, esoteric, and somewhat distant style common to most scientific writings, a form of delivery was selected that would hopefully make the assimilation of these various levels of thought and information easier and perhaps even enjoyable for the reader. We felt that indeed a great deal was at stake and we had an important story to relate. With consideration for the disposition of the type of clinician who would be reading this text, the style selected may be seen to approach that of a narrative. It is simple, straightforward, serially organized, and at times potently concentrated. And as if in a form of scientific "poetic justice," this is the same style, natural and personal, used in lecturing by the system's champion proponent, Dr. John Witzig.

For these reasons the text may take on the aspects of a casual conversation between the author and the reader. Yet after considering the circumstances of its purpose, what other choice would be appropriate? It will at times be somewhat strongly weighted in history, for it is strongly felt that we cannot clearly understand where we are at present and where we will be going in the future if we are not aware of what has come to us out of the past. This also helps serve to remind us of how common we are in our interdependence on our fellow members of the profession, and of how much effort of yesterday has gone into getting us where we are today.

In another vein, the text at times may also appear to be a report of the general views and practices of the profession on a given subject or technique, offering the reader the choice of position in the matter as per his or her own personal preferences. In other instances it will steadfastly assume an impregnable and unalterable position to which it fondly hopes all will subscribe. Due to the profundity of the premises involved in those particular areas, no doubt, all eventually will.

The appliances and techniques of many great clinicians, men who may be considered as true founding fathers of the orthodontic discipline, are represented in this text. They have been purposefully selected for their respective places in the overall scheme of things. They have been garnered from a wide variety of times and places. It is hoped that not too much was lost concerning them in the condensation and organization process, but the mere logistics of such an effort as represeneted by this text required that this consolidating approach be taken. The simple style in which the appliances, techniques, and treatment approaches are at times discussed may belie the profound meaning and far-reaching implications of the very words used to describe them. This caused no undue difficulty on occasion during the production of this text. At certain times, whole paragraphs or even entire pages on the subject concerned could be easily dispatched with reasonable effort, usually due to the very nature of the subject matter itself. Yet at other times, weeks or even months were required for the selection of a single word or phrase. Both when used properly and improperly, words can be powerful. Sometimes many are needed to describe a simple notion, while ironically at other times a complex idea may only require the use of one or two to stand alone.

Considering its starting point, its multiple missions, and its upstart position in modern orthodontic thinking, it was clear that this text could only serve the office of a primary introduction to the treatment of malocclusions on the most basic of levels, "garden variety" discussion if you will. But then, most malocclusions are of a garden variety nature. It would be impossible to discuss every ramification of every treatment problem of every type of malocclusion, as these are as numerous and varied as the patients that present for treatment on a daily basis. Yet a certain common thread runs through all classes of malocclusions to which certain common treatment principles and techniques may be applied. For the sake of preserving the clarity of the overall therapeutic concept, it was determined that relevance and simplicity had to remain paramount. Further refinement of individualized detail and extension beyond the most basic of levels will come easily for the clinician in due time once the fundamentals of the procedures are adequately understood and placed under control. It is hoped that this text will provide the essential ideas upon which the clinician's thought can reflect and build. Though it does not presume to think for the clinician, neither is it a dictatorial manual of rote procedures. Thinking will be a definite part of the process of engaging this text, but this will be a pleasant and positive experience. With all the exciting ideas and concepts defined herein, there will be plenty of good things to think about, if only the reader's interest will not become lost along the way before our story is completed. There is so much to tell and it is all so important!

It may now be seen why this text was written in the fashion in which it now appears. An unusual style is required for an unusual book. Its goal is to set forth, as straightforwardly as possible, the complex tapestry of design and thought, of technique and therapeutic approach, of movement and management in the broad spectrum of the most recently evolved sequential treatments of today's new orthodontics. It is hoped this will allow the clinician to see, learn, and understand the significance and importance of the scene before him. It is truly a scene of inspiring grandeur composed of many threads; no single one of which is as potent or revealing as all are when woven together. Out of many, truly one.

The patient's problems of malocclusion are seldom, if ever, singular; therefore, neither should be the treatment approach used to help them. The multiplicity of techniques for directly addressing the component problems of teeth, bone, and muscle now made available to the modern practitioner by the FJO system of therapeutics, opens up vast new treatment possibilities never before possible under more restricted regimens of fixed or removable appliances alone. Now a list of the patient's needs may be determined, and specific techniques may be drawn upon to directly address each of those needs. The days of doubling over and forcing one technique or methodology to do the work for which it was not originally intended are over. Now more than ever, each player may be called upon for its part.

The purpose of this text is not to divide but to bring together, not to limit but to extend, not to disjoin but to heal. As might be surmised from the above, it is felt that the limitations of a single regimen, fixed-appliance therapeutic technique until the present have been so demanding that the preoccupation with overcoming the difficulties of complex therapeutic administrations may have overshadowed a little of the human element involved. The return to humanism represented by this text also reminds us that possibly some of us might have temporarily followed the beat of the wrong drummer. No one is to blame. No doubt this was a product of the profession's never having had a complete armamentarium of therapeutic technique available and fully at the disposal of the treating clinicians. The profession had to plow its own furrows and do the best it could with what it had, regardless of how incomplete its powers might have been at a given point in its development. It was truly a sincere, honorable, and noble effort. Since its approach to therapeutics was sometimes by necessity incomplete and somewhat distorted, its therapeutic results were on occasion somewhat incomplete and distorted. This was a position given little credence in the age of orthodontics. But now we live in the age of orthopedics. We see with a broader vision and from a greater distance. Orthodontics can no longer stand alone. In the future we will be held responsible for more.

But now the armamentarium has been expanded. Sequential treatment has its assigned place. Teeth, bone, temporomandibular joints, and muscle each may now be directly addressed with appliances and techniques specifically designed for them. Now, more so than ever, it becomes a matter of recognition, identification, clarification, organization, and implementation in the modern clinician's approach to treating the patient's malocclusion. A combined orthodontic and orthopedic approach to treating a true combination of clinical problems is the only philosophy that makes true advancement possible. Though some of the ideas and even appliances we will discuss are old, by virtue of the manner in which they may be orchestrated with more modern techniques, the directions they will take us will be new. This will force us to think about things differently. Some things will take on different meanings or a new significance. This may at first seem foreign or even intimidating to us. Growth always does. Due to the appearance of these ideas on the scene, whether we like it or not, in a way we are all starting over.

Terrance J. Spahl, D.D.S.
St. Paul, Minnesota

ACKNOWLEDGMENTS

"I am part of all that I have met"

Ulysses
Alfred Lord Tennyson
1809–1892

"And now I would like to thank . . . " is usually a signal to the reader to skip to the opening page of the first chapter. However, in this instance it not only signals the just acknowledgment of those who have generously contributed so greatly of their time to the production of this text, but it also gives the reader an insight to the expansive scale of areas and issues condensed within its pages. Such revelations as this help stress the notion of a common, universal bond between the efforts of the reader in attempting to confront the challenges of maxillofacial and orthodontic therapeutics, and those brothers of the healing arts who represent the long line of professionals who have gone before. It is this heritage of universality, of common bond, that helps break down the walls of isolation and insecurity and makes us feel as one with another, or at least reminds us that we should be.

As for our European colleagues, I should like to start first with the Germans! Being of direct German heritage myself, it was a great thrill and honor for me to travel to "the old country" to study there. I owe an enormous debt of gratitude to the eminent German orthodontist Dr. Hans Peter Bimler of Wiesbaden, West Germany, for his most gracious assistance with some of the historical passages of the text. I am also extremely grateful for his invaluable assistance over the years in unraveling some of the mysteries and seeming contradictions in the interpretation of the science of cephalometrics, both European and American methods. I am also thankful to Dr. Anna Barbara Bimler for her gracious assistance in obtaining rare photographic materials and other important reference material for the text. Special thanks should also be afforded to Professor Dr. E. Hausser and the staff at the library of the University of Hamburg, and also to Professor Dr. C. W. Schwarze of the University of Cologne.

In England we are grateful to Dr. H. E. Wilson of London for his gracious assistance and also to Dr. Hans Eirew of Manchester for his most generous contributions of some of the most dramatic case photographs of the text, the now famous Eirew twins.

The list of American colleagues who have assisted us is both long and prestigious. The contributions of Dr. Merle Bean of Des Moines; Dr. Lloyd Truax of Rochester, Minnesota; Dr. Jay Gerber of St Mary's, West Virginia; and Dr. James Krygier of Wilmington, Delaware are greatly appreciated. Dr. Samuel Higdon of Portland, Oregon contributed a truly spectacular series of illustrations of TMJ function and dysfunction. Dr. Jerry Barns of St Paul, and Dr. Robert Smyth of New Orleans, provided photographic help and Dr. Jack Hockel of Walnut Creek, California assisted with both photographic and editorial help for the section on Crozat appliances. The most gracious Dr. William L. Wilson and his son Dr. Robert E. Wilson of Winchester, Massachusetts provided both photographic and editorial assistance of enormous value for the section on "Wilson" appliances. Dr. Waldemar Brehm of Encinetas, California provided generous personal assistance with the section on the Brehm Utility Arch. Further historical material was provided through the kindness of Dr. H. C. Pollock of Denver, and Dr. George Albu of Brookfield, Ohio.

A great deal of effort was expended in the physical production of this text. We are deeply indebted to Mr. Howard Ohlendorf and Mark Ohlendorf for their invaluable assistance in the production of many of the appliance photographs used in this text. Many other technical and liaison services were also provided through the kindness of Ohlendorf Company. Additional photographs were provided by Jack Skay of Dynaflex and Don Neuschwander of Johns Dental Laboratories. Additional material was provided by Arnie Newman of Unitek Corporation, Derek Evans of "A"-Company, Inc. and of course the most generous contributions of Martin Brusse and Rocky Mountain/Orthodontics are deeply appreciated. A note of gratitude is also due to Bob Cooley, Julie Jackson, and the staff at European Orthodontic Products for their technical assistance. We are also very appreciative of the superb original artwork provided by Jan Bilek.

For their assistance with the library research necessary for this project, we are grateful to Carol Murray, Jeanny Chan, and Dr. George Selfridge and the library of Washington University of St Louis, and also to Jolene Baker, Joan Freeman and Diane Dickson of the BioMedical Library of the University of Minnesota.

The secretarial staff that has served us from the onset of the project has given tireless effort and their constancy is deeply appreciated. They are Denise Dege, Marilyn Weidell, Jodi England, Grace Theisen, Caroline Nentwig, and Judy Cloutier.

Personal support was also provided at critical points throughout the five-year production of this text by Dr. D. D. Smith of Corning, New York and the noted dental author Dr. Joe Dunlap of Clearwater, Florida. I would also like to extend special thanks to Dr. Steven P. Kulenkamp and Dr. James M. Gayes for their continued support and sustenance throughout the entire length of this project, as well as to Stan and Nancy Weaver of Big Sandy, Montana.

Of course last but certainly not least, I would like to thank my friend and colleague, Dr. John Witzig for all his guidance and patience. He provided counsel and direction to me during the writing of this text and allowed me the honor of working with him in an atmosphere of mutual respect. His kind consideration for myself along with the support of my family generated the inspiration and sustaining element that no other source could have provided. I hope this humble effort will prove worthy of their faith as well as that of the reader.

TJS

To believe in your own thought,
to believe what is true for you
in your private heart is true for all men:
that is genius.

Ralph Waldo Emerson
Essay II, Self-Reliance

*"Error of opinion may be tolerated
when reason is left free to combat it."*

Thomas Jefferson

CHAPTER 1
Why Start?

THE ORTHODONTIC DICHOTOMY OF OUR TROUBLED TIMES

Were one to survey the general history of the development of the status of present-day orthodontic thinking, it would soon be discovered that there are two major philosophical schools of thought on dealing with malocclusions. The first is basically the American school which has been chiefly concerned with the pure orthodontic movement, repositioning and alignment of teeth through bone.[1-4] This has been, for the most part, traditionally carried out in the last century by numerous series of fixed appliances which employ an external mechanically produced force system of some sort and usually impart this force directly to the teeth through a system of individually cemented bands and brackets. This approach is predicated on the belief that certain bony dimensions are essentially immutable,[5-12] such as the length of the mandible for instance; and that if the jaws in which the teeth reside are too small for the volume of teeth that occupy that space the clinician has the choice of either attempting to "shoehorn fit" the teeth into the size jawbones Nature has given both him and the patient to work with,[13] or alternatively sacrifice certain teeth by means of extraction in order to gain the sorely needed extra space in the dental arch required for the uncrowded realignment of the remaining teeth.[14] This approach in certain instances forces the practitioner to position teeth in the arch-shaped manner in jaw-bones that are less than adequately arch-shaped in their apical bases, or that in turn may not be properly aligned on an interarch basis according to commonly accepted norms of orthopedic anteroposterior or vertical balance. It also has other far-reaching orthopedic ramifications relative to the structural integrity of the temporomandibular joints.

A second general school of thought founded in Europe hypothesized that the reason orthopedic malalignment of the apical bases and dental crowding of the individual arches exists in the first place is due to improper muscle function inhibiting the growth and development of the jaws themselves.[15-18] This philosophy also theorizes that changing the function of those muscles and the direction of forces they impart to the teeth and basal bone about which they exist could, in fact, change the shape of the bones back to their normal interarch alignment and size once again: a size large enough to accomodate all of the naturally existing teeth. This would be ideal in the example of treating a retruded skeletal Class II mandible with its resultant Class II dental arrangement. Rather than taking out upper bicuspids and retracting the anterior teeth into the extration spaces in order to couple the upper anterior teeth with the lower anterior teeth, the mandible in turn could be "stretched" forward to meet the nonextracted, nonshortened upper arch, which would be far better for the face and allow for more favorable orthopedic considerations. This system was known by various names such as the "European method" or the "Norwegian system" before it eventually

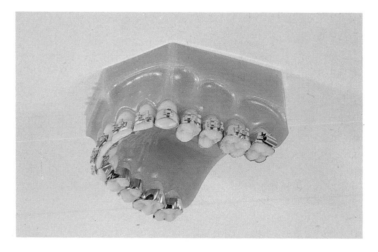

(A)

Figure 1-1 Fixed appliances in the orthodontic approach to malocclusion treatment. **(A)** Edgewise. **(B)** Perfect arch. **(C)** Johnson twin-tie extraction. **(D)** Twin-wire arch. (*Courtesy of Ohlendorf Co., St. Louis, MO.*)

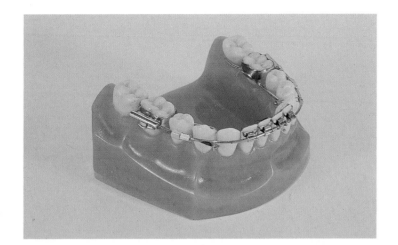

(B)

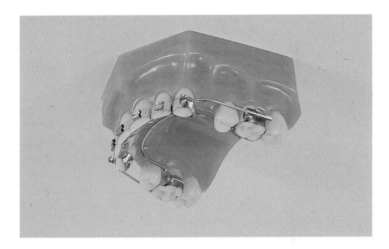

(C)

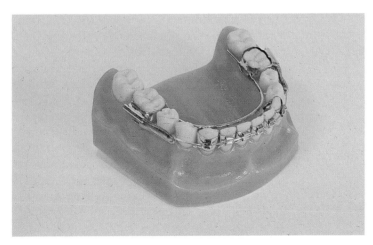

(D)

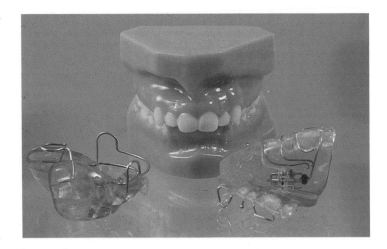

Figure 1-2 Most commonly used removable appliances in clinical practice are the Bionator functional appliance (left) and Sagittal active plate (right). They form the mainstay of conventional Class II deep bite mandibular retrusion treatment. (*Courtesy of Ohlendorf Co., St. Louis, MO.*)

became known as functional jaw orthopedics. As might be guessed, a huge controversy arose between the two schools of thought and even among certain European authorities themselves that persists to this day as to whether the theories of the orthopedically oriented concept were, in fact, clinically producable.[19] Progress was at first slow in this area and riddled with inconsistency. Furthermore, the fact that the therapeutic techniques the European system developed in order to clinically implement its ideas centered around removable and nonfixed appliances did nothing to help the levels of skepticism with which they were initially viewed. Of course, the preceding represents an overly simplified version of the evolutionary history of the entire spectrum of orthodontic therapy, but the basic delineations it proposes are handy for an orderly approach to understanding basic trends in the development of treatment philosophies.

The idea of functional appliance therapy as we know it today originated in Europe over the past half century or so. It has gained slow acceptance on the American side of the Atlantic for several reasons. Misunderstanding, prejudice, and conservatism are chiefly to blame. However, in the past decade a ground swell of popularity for the "new" orthopedically oriented technique has suddenly arisen as its revolutionary ideas have suddenly blossomed forth among the American orthodontic community. Some of the most pivotal figures responsible for bringing about this broad and wholesale change in thinking in America have been men like Dr J. McNamara and Dr John Witzig. Legions of followers now faithfully reside in the new camp. But there was a time, not too long ago, when it wasn't so. In the decade of the 1970s, when this movement began to take hold in America, these men stood alone "like a voice crying in the wilderness" extolling the virtues of functional appliance therapy. How lucky for us they did.

The resistance of the conservative establishment of the main body of orthodontic practitioners was at first exceedingly intense. Ridicule and rejection on occasion sometimes replaced what should have been objective consideration of the facts. But there were those among that body of practitioners who listened, learned, and subsequently initiated a new direction of orthodontic care in America.

Now numerous lecturers and groups have sprung up all over the nation expounding the benefits of FJOs (functional jaw orthopedics). Numerous opportunities exist for doctors to learn the newer methods and apply them to their practices. But who among them cannot but owe a debt of gratitude to the aforementioned pioneering men who championed their cause before it became accepted by the multitudes? The courage and vision of Drs Witzig and McNamara are all the more enhanced when one realizes that they began their teachings during a time when no one wanted to listen. Yet, these courageous men, and others like them, steadfastly persisted in their efforts to elucidate the truth, thus paving the way ahead for those who in ever-increasing droves would follow.

Upon entering the world of FJOs, the first thing a practitioner must do is try to sort out all the information with which he will most likely become deluged, ie, try to make order out of chaos. At first glance, the vast numbers of appliances and gadgets, bite plates and activators, screws and wires seem a veritable jumble of techniques all rolled into one. Confusion and uncertainty can soon easily replace excitement and inspiration in the minds of the uninitiated if some orderly approach is not given to the scene.

Yet, with a step-by-step organized study of both diagnostic and clinical treatment methods, a clearer picture begins to take shape in the mind of the practitioner. One must learn first to separate the malocclusion into its component parts of orthodontic and orthopedic considerations and then in treatment planning select the best appliances that are specifically designed for each particular phase. Our goal should be to put the bones in the right place as well as the teeth in the right place and also readapt the errant musculature[20-24] with every effort to keep simplicity the order of the day. If this is done, the concept of functional orthodontic treatment will emerge as a manageable and practical modality, which will willingly serve as a faithful friend to both the patient and the doctor. Humans are fragile.

The purpose of this text is to serve as an initial bridge in the gap between an idea and a reality. It is a *clinically* oriented manual concerned with the practical application of *how* functional jaw orthopedics works in the treatment of dental and skeletal malocclusions and is less concerned with the scholastic aspect of *why* the system works. The system has been found to produce successful results clinically and has occasionally outstripped research on the subject in some aspects. However, this slight imbalance between research data and clinical observation will, no doubt, soon right itself. For scientific research will presently complement direct clinical findings since the researcher cannot help but soon discover the truths Nature reflects in what the practitioner has already repeatedly accomplished. That is why at this point, the inability to support each and every minute aspect of functional appliance therapy with documented experimental, scientific data only acts as a deterrent to the overall comprehension of the entire program in the mind of the student-doctor wishing to master its techniques. The ultimate documentation is the successfully treated, happy, healthy patient. There are thousands!

This text is not intended to serve the office of a comprehensive resource material covering all aspects of functional appliance therapy, but rather acts as an introduction to the most important, basic, and often-used appliances, both removable and fixed, employed today.

The methodology of functional jaw orthopedics is not a discipline totally devoted to one sole appliance or technique but is truly a *system* incorporating the use of: removable functional appliances; their nearest neighbors, the active plates; and their most distant neighbors, the fixed appliances. The smelting of these various approaches forms an alloy which gives the orthodontist, pedodontist, and general practitioner a new metal with which to cast a double-edged sword enabling him to deliver the absolute best possible orthodontic care to his patients. Forged in the furnace of careful diagnosis, this team of tandem regimens produces a formidable weapon which the practitioner may use in the daily battle against the improperly functioning, facially deforming malocclusion. Though active plates and/or fixed appliances are important in obtaining proper arch form, proper interarch alignment is the official *domain* of the functional appliance. And to date, the one functional appliance that towers above all others in this respect, and as a result forms the cornerstone of modern-day functional jaw orthopedic therapy, is the Bionator![25]

THE NEED FOR MORE THAN ORTHODONTICS

As the discerning diagnostic eye of orthodontics has seasoned over the last half century, it has been generally determined that something more was needed to facilitate the delivery of orthodontic care other than the mere straightening of teeth. For some patients the purely tooth-oriented techniques of conventional fixed orthodontic appliances provided an adequate standard of care. But for a large percentage it did not, for there were a goodly number of patients whose malocclusions entailed more than the mere malpositioning of teeth alone. It was determined that not only were there orthodontic problems to deal with but also orthopedic discrepancies and muscular dysfunctions as well. The three major components of the maxillofacial stomatognathic system—the teeth, the bones, and the musculature—could all contribute in their own way and to varying degrees to the development

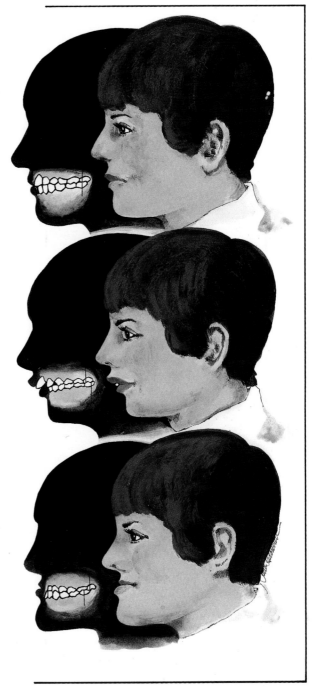

NORMAL FACE
The NORMAL FACE is characterized by a NORMAL and HARMONIOUS RE-LATIONSHIP of the TEETH and JAWS.

CLASS II MALOCCLUSION
A Class II malocclusion is characterized by what is commonly considered a receding lower jaw, with protruding upper front teeth.
A Class II malocclusion with a receding lower jaw and with the upper front teeth tipped back is called a Division II.
66% of all malocclusions are Class II malocclusions.

CLASS III MALOCCLUSION
A Class III malocclusion is characterized by the under development of the upper jaw and a protruding lower jaw.

RECOMMENDATION:
Disfiguring facial conditions can be corrected by proper treatment.

European Ortho Products P.O. Box 4142 St. Paul, MN 55104 (612) 646-5950

Figure 1-3 How irregularities of the teeth affect the face. (*Courtesy of European Orthodontic Products, St. Paul, MN.*)

CHART #1

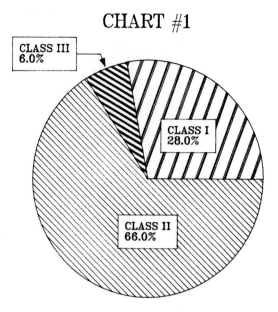

CLASS III
6.0%

CLASS I
28.0%

CLASS II
66.0%

INCIDENCE OF THE VARIOUS TYPES OF
MALOCCLUSIONS. CHART SHOWING APPROX-
IMATELY 2/3 OF ALL MALOCCLUSIONS ARE
OF THE CLASS II VARIETY.

Figure 1-4

of a malocclusion. Such being the case, each in turn should be addressed
by techniques specifically designed to confront the particular problems they
represent in order to deliver the most complete orthodontic/orthopedic/
muscular rehabilitative care possible. Since the evolution of the fixed metal
appliances at the turn of the century, much was quickly learned about moving teeth, but advancements in the other two areas took some time. Early
orthodontists had to do the best they could with what they had. What they
had was precise, definitive, and controllable fixed appliance methodology
which received the lion's share of the attention such that its development

Figure 1-5 Classic skeletal Class II large overjet, deep overbite facial
appearance with **(A)** pathognomonic retrusive facial outline in profile
and **(B)** curled lower lip tucked under overhanging upper lip due to
mandibular insufficiency. **(C)** Cephalometric view showing dental Class
II molar relationship and deep overbite, large overjet relationship of
anteriors.

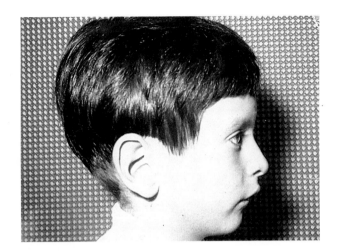

(A)

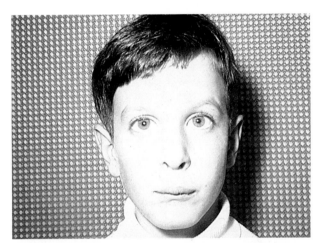

(B)

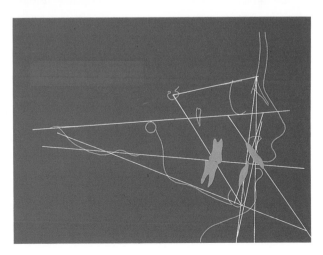

(C)

was brought to extremely high levels of sophistication, while orthopedics and myofunctional considerations were thought of somewhat as "children of a lesser god." They were acknowledged but considered not to be in full capacity. Things are different now.

It is in the sheer broadness of the system that the appeal of FJO methodology exists. It corrects not only the malposed teeth but also corrects the malposed bones and readapts musculature,[26-33] thus giving the recipient the benefit of total patient care. All orthodontic techniques are concerned with the realignment of teeth, but no technique is more facially oriented than that of FJOs. By properly applying the correct appliance at the correct time during therapy, the patient benefits from a broad beautiful smile, excellent functional occlusion, a full face with a beautiful jaw line and lateral profile, and maybe most importantly, a sound, stable, and healthy temporomandibular joint!

A perceptive eye cannot help but observe, in a certain percentage of cases, the shortcomings of the more conventional bicuspid extraction–type therapy used in conjunction with fixed appliances and head gear for the treatment of certain Class II-type malocclusions. Sometimes the list of untoward "sequelae" of such types of treatment can be formidable.

The lack of support for the corners of the mouth, the loss of vertical dimension, the weak and unassuming chin and profile, the often poorly occluded and tilted molars, and most importantly, the strained temporomandibular joints (TMJs) are all side effects of this type of treatment for many, not all to be sure, but nevertheless many a patient who has received four bicuspid extraction tooth-oriented orthodontics. Retracting the usually correctly positioned premaxilla[34] to meet the retruded skeletal Class II mandible does nothing to correct the retrusive mandibular situation, but merely perpetuates the "natural mistake" of the original malocclusion. Is this necessary? Should retrusive jaws, faces, and potentially compressed TMJ's be left uncorrected or even worsened? When other forms of therapy evolve

---

Figure 1-6 Case study illustrating some problems resulting from treatment of Class II, Division 1 deep bite malocclusions with accompanying mandibular retrusion by means of conventional fixed appliance technique, four bicuspid extraction, and headgear. **(A)** Pretreatment profile. Note retrusive mandible, accentuated mentonian groove, pronounced curl to the lower lip, and general weak appearance of the chin. **(B)** Models reveal large overjet, deep overbite, and severely retruded mandibular arch. **(C)** Posttreatment facial view. Note that retrusive lower facial profile remains. **(D)** Posttreatment view of teeth reveals steep interincisal angle of over retracted anteriors, shortened posterior quadrants due to missing bicuspids, and retained deep bite all of which contribute to retrusive mandibular condition. Contrast with Figure 1-7.

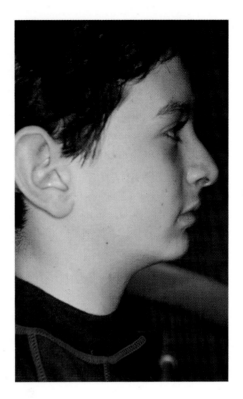

(A)

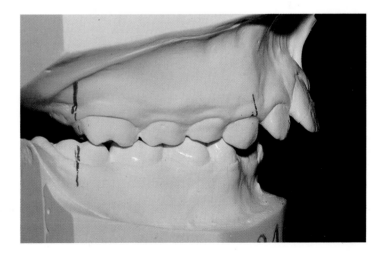

(B)

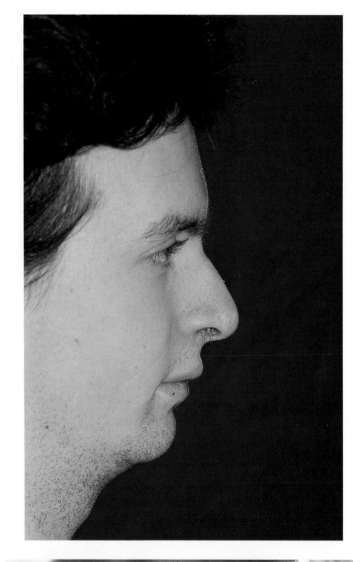

(C)

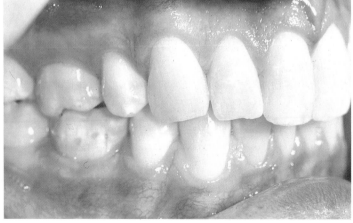

(D)

12

that avoid these pitfalls and have been acclaimed by many to be superior, why do we continue in persisting in such methods? Do we owe some sort of religious loyalty to one technique over another simply because "that is the way it has always been done"? The most fundamental cornerstone of science is its unemotional and nonjudgmental objectivity. It desires the pursuit of the truth in its purest form through the direct unbiased observation of the physical world by means of our senses.

"You see but you don't observe."
Sherlock Holmes to Dr. Watson

"Scandal in Bohemia"
Sir Arthur Conan Doyle
1859–1930

The amount of controversy associated with FJO technique is well known and in some circles still passionately debated,[35-37] although less so now than in the past. When the technique was first brought to this country from Europe it was replete with criticisms from the American orthodontic community and its detractors were legion. However, quiet and steady change has begun and is gaining strength in its movement throughout the many who have now seen the advantage and superiority of this newer method for treating those cases for which FJOs are intended.

Of all the components of FJO therapy, those which are most highly contested are the principles of second molar extraction, and artificially induced mandibular growth and advancement. For years orthodontists have thought nothing of extracting four bicuspids in order to gain space when necessary only to have no room in the arches for erupting third molars. Thus, in addition to the extraction of four premolars, they subject their patients to the arduous ritual of impacted third molar surgery (in a patient whose TMJs may be already compromised!). The end result: 24 teeth, all-around smaller dental arches; less facial support; usually some degree of instability along with a fervent hope of no postsurgical mandibular paresthesia or TMJ damage. The second molar extraction principle, where indicated, avoids these problems and leaves the patient with 28 teeth, stability (because the gigantic forward thrust of second molars is gone), healthy TMJs, and a nice full face. Other than that it's no different! But the fear of extracting a second molar to some clinicians seems insurmountable. It is as if they have been endowed with some sort of reverence for a molar over a bicuspid requiring incense to be offered to the stately molar and enmity offered the lowly bicuspid. Nonsense! No one tooth is any more favored over another in nature. It is merely the artificial standards created in the recesses of man's mind that place such values on teeth. The real culprit in arch-crowding problems often *is* the second molar; and its removal, where indicated, can only help the patient, and never harm him. After their removal the third molars actually do come in with little effort or worry. Rarely, one will "stick" against the distal of a first molar. In the event of such an unlikely occurence, uprighting it orthodontically is "child's play." In the meantime tremendous strides are accomplished in the treatment of the patient's malocclusion. When properly applied, second molar extraction principles avoid all of the pitfalls of bicuspid technique. Yet this principle of removing second molars and allowing thirds to erupt in their place is met with surprisingly emotional resistance among many clinically experienced, and it might be added in their defense, well-meaning practitioners today.

The concept of mandibular advancement at first also met with staunch resistance. Many believed that the mandible could not be artificially stimulated to increase in size, or overall diagonal length from the condylar head to pogonion. But recent unbiased computerized serial cephalometric radiographic analysis of patients treated with various types of functional appliances has shown that the mandible can, in fact, be stimulated to increase its length by the use of these appliances and the greatest area of increased (or "unlocked natural" if you will) growth is in the condylar head and neck.[38-41] But confusion and controversy still exist on this issue among those unfamiliar with modern-day scientific findings concerning appliance initiated mandibular growth.

THE "PRIDE AND THE PREJUDICE"

Why does such rejection to such plainly observable phenomena occur? Is it a product of our modern age? Hardly. Resistance to change is, of course, not without precedent in the history of scientific endeavors. Many of the great advancements in scientific thought have been violently opposed by the existing establishment. The works of Louis Pasteur are well known. Many

---

Figure 1-7 Case study illustrating results of treatment with active plates and functional appliances. **(A)** Pretreatment facial view and **(B) (C)** study models divulge the classic Class II, Division 2 malocclusion with deep bite and concomitant mandibular retrusion. Advancement of the maxillary anteriors by means of active plates was followed by functional appliance treatment (Bionator) to advance the mandible and increase the vertical dimension of occlusion. **(D)** Note improved, advanced, nonretracted posttreatment profile. **(E)** Improved overbite. **(F)** Longer posterior quadrants due to the presence of both sets of upper and lower bicuspids.

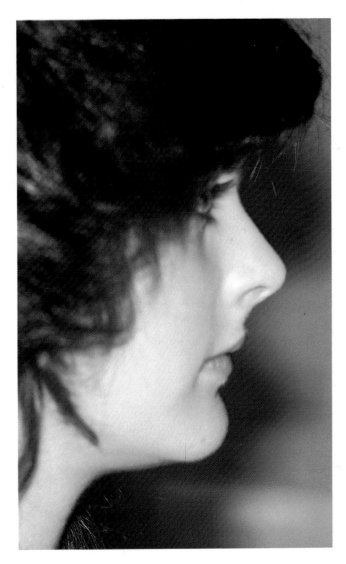

(A)

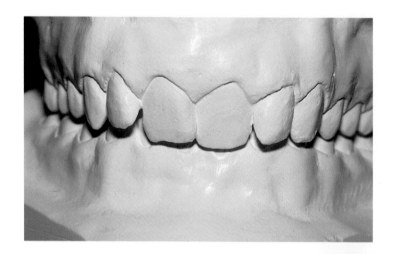

(B)

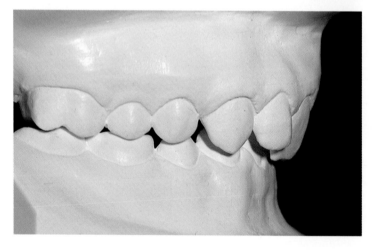

(C)

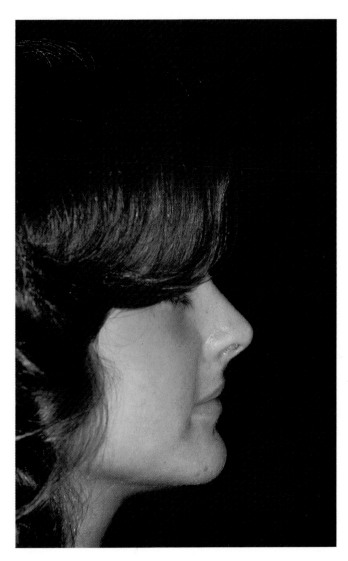

(D)

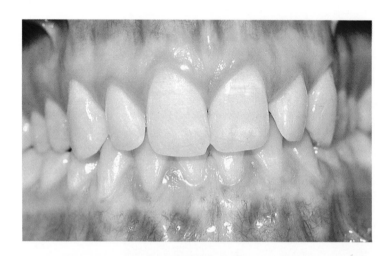

(E)

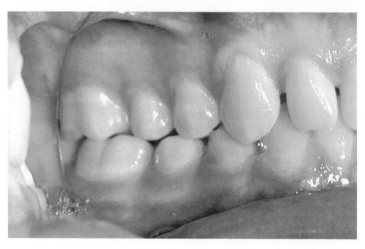

(F)

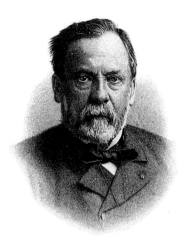

Figure 1-8 Louis Pasteur

times he had to devise elaborate experiments to support his efforts on debunking the theories of spontaneous generation. One time he had to perform an experiment 100 times in a row to prove the hypothesis concerned. The experiment worked perfectly each and every time. Some of his samples of culture media still exist to this day in various museums and institutions in France. They are still unspoiled by bacterial contamination, though not hermetically sealed. As of yet no organisms have "spontaneously arisen!"

A more tragic example exists in the life of the Hungarian physician Ignaz P. Semmelweis. As an instructor in a medical school at Vienna General Hospital in 1848, he discovered the rate of fatalities from the then prevalent puerperal fever (septicemia) could be reduced in his maternity wards by a great percentage by merely having his students wash their hands thoroughly between their studies in the pathology laboratories (ie, of severely infected cadavers) and their efforts in the delivery rooms. He theorized the students were transferring minute pathogens from the infected specimens to the delivering mothers. This, and even rudiments of aseptic surgery, predated the famous work of England's legendary Lord Lister by some 15 years!

In 1861 in Budapest he published a great paper to this effect entitled "The Etiology, Concept and Prophylaxis of Puerperal Fever." He also wrote open letters to the heads of the various medical centers in Europe criticizing the rejection of his new ideas. That was his mistake. This brought down upon him years of opposition, controversy, and discord. It finally led him to suffer a serious mental breakdown. Ironically, he died in 1865 from a septicemia resulting from a cut finger received while performing an autopsy before a group of students.

In 1842 Dr Horace Wells, a young dentist from Hartford, Connecticut, teamed up with Dr William Morton of Charlton, Massachusetts, to develop

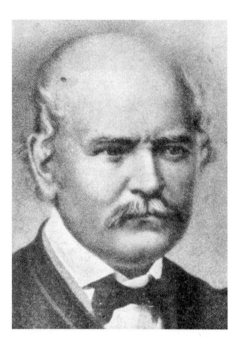

Figure 1-9   Ignaz P. Semmelweiss

and promote the initial use of nitrous oxide as an anesthetic. During a demonstration at the Harvard Medical School, where he tried to extract a tooth on a patient being administered N_2O, something went amiss and the patient cried out in pain. The demonstration was a failure and Morton and Wells were laughed and booed out of the auditorium. (Later it was discovered the patient had been bribed to act as if he felt the pain of the extraction forceps.) In similar experiments later on, another patient was administered an overdose of the gas and subsequently died. Despondent over these failures, Wells broke up his partnership with Morton, and after several years of unsuccessful ventures in other areas, died in the slums of New York City, the victim of suicide.

The young Dr Morton fared only a little better. He continued his search for an anesthetic and finally developed the use of ether. Yet tragically he only lived to see the patent he tried so desperately to obtain for his discovery annulled by a court of law. He suffered a stroke in 1868. To this day October 16 is still celebrated at the Harvard Medical School as "Etherday."

But the medical sciences are not the only victims of entrenched and narrow-minded resistance to changing ideas and new discoveries. For seven centuries, peasant and scholar, beggar and king subscribed to the teachings of the second-century astronomer Ptolemy, who said that all the celestial bodies, including the sun and the stars, revolved around a stationary Earth.

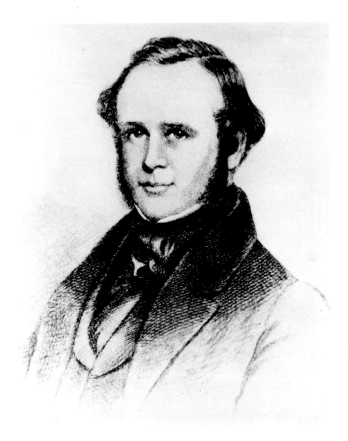

Figure 1-10 Horace Wells

But in 1543 a Polish Catholic cleric named Nicolas Copernicus, after making many careful calculations and observations, thrust his heliocentric theories of the solar system upon a laughing world. How brave he must have been.

All people in all times generally react negatively to change. They simply don't like anything that upsets the status quo. Great changes require an equally great amount of courage.

NEW DIRECTIONS IN ORTHODONTICS

This brings us to the main question of this chapter—Why start? As an orthodontist, why change a discipline and mode of thinking it has taken a lifetime to cultivate? As a general practitioner, why expand into a field

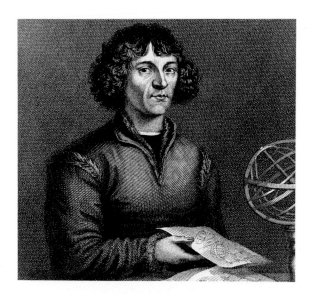

Figure 1-11   Nicolas Copernicus

full of new ideas and gremlins of unfamiliarity? As a pedodontist, why subject a carefully constructed treatment regimen to change?

A ground swell of converts to this type of treatment is growing across the nation.

When lecturers nationally known in the field give seminars on the subject, they always speak before packed houses (and command the highest lecture fees, I might add). The practitioners who gather at these conclaves bubble with enthusiasm over their results obtained with FJOs and are eager for any tidbit of new knowledge on the subject. The grounds of the premises are replete with nationally known dental laboratories all displaying their wares and encouraging individual doctors to sample their work. Something is going on!

In an era of excellent preventive measures, ie, high rates of municipally flouridated water and low rates of caries; in a time when there is a plethora of young graduates streaming out of dental schools across the country; in a time when third party systems, franchise dentistry, and ever-increasing government regulation, taxation, and intervention causes ever-mounting pressures in the daily practice of dentistry, it becomes increasingly more difficult for a young practitioner to manage a practice into a healthy, growing, and profitable business.

The stresses associated with building a practice in this day and age are well known to any dentist who has been working during the last 10 years.[42-45] Totally unprepared for this by their respective academic institutions, the graduating young (or in many cases graduating middle-aged) prac-

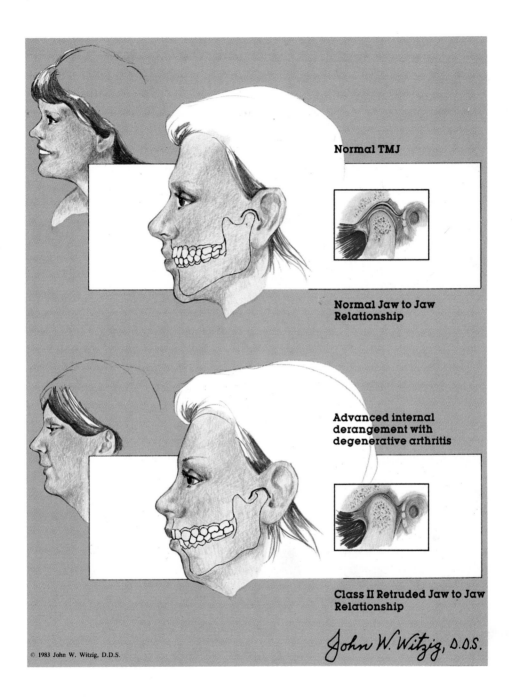

Normal TMJ

Normal Jaw to Jaw Relationship

Advanced internal derangement with degenerative arthritis

Class II Retruded Jaw to Jaw Relationship

© 1983 John W. Witzig, D.D.S.

John W. Witzig, D.D.S.

Figure 1-12

titioner is forced to confront these problems head on and shift for himself, learning by costly experience as he jostles for a position in the race to success. Stress is a key factor in the displeasure of many dentists with their profession. As a man approaches his mid-career, often after pulling himself up by his own bootstraps, there is often an emotional letdown as he reflects upon his situation; he is a long way from the beginning to be sure and yet still a long way from the end. Bogged down in the daily routine of his practice, he questions whether he will be happy in the future if he continues grinding out his present pace. He craves renewal, stimulation, a new challenge to inspire and excite him again. But this time, one with not quite so much of a stress load associated with it. It should be something he can study, learn, master, and enjoy at his own pace; something that brings satisfying and excellent results, something that brings the fun back into being a dentist again. After all, when he was conferred a doctor's degree upon graduating from dental school, he wasn't required to turn in his membership card to the human race!

Also, it is important to remain with the future in a profession as dynamic as dentistry. One can't live in the past. One has a hard enough time living in the present. One must always anticipate and attempt to live for the future, for it universally lies before all of us. And no single movement in the treatment of malocclusions is ever going to sweep the general thinking of a professional community as that of FJOs.

Patients come into the office seeking out this form of therapy, having compared and seen results on friends and relatives. Due to the convenience and comfort associated with the technique, the patients are happy to have it. Parents and children who are extremely gratified with the excellent results act as excellent referral sources for new patients. Enthusiasm is contagious.

Also the satisfaction for the doctor as he sees the results of his handiwork transform a harmful and disfiguring malocclusion into a beautiful broad smile in a beautiful young face is overwhelming. What is also pleasing to the doctor is that this is accomplished with a minimum of stress to both the patient and himself in an elegant and humane treatment methodology. The practitioner also has the satisfaction of knowing he is giving his patient the absolute best form of treatment available. The technique carries with

---

Figure 1-13   Case study. **(A)** Pretreatment upper maxillary arch shows crowding and 6.4 mm shortage of arch length. **(B)** Frontal view shows crowding and 80% overbite. **(C)** Mandibular view of crowding. **(D) (E) (F) (G) (H)** Posttreatment occlusion shows proper interdigitation and correction of crowding by means of active plate, functional appliance, and second molar replacement techniques. **(I)** Full normal profile, no mandibular retrusion. **(J)** Full smile line frontally balanced to rest of face.

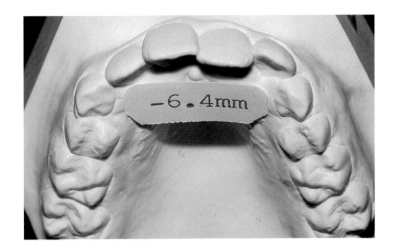

(A)

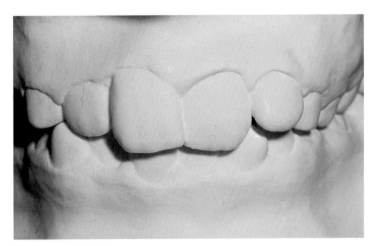

(B)

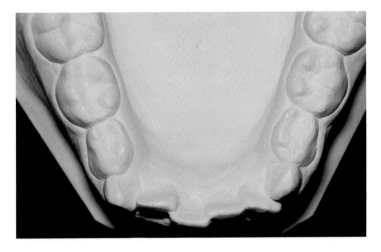

(C)

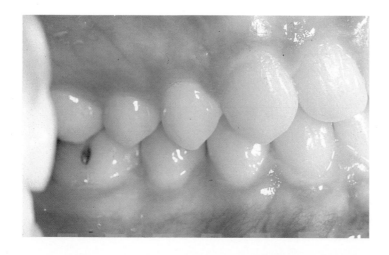

(D)

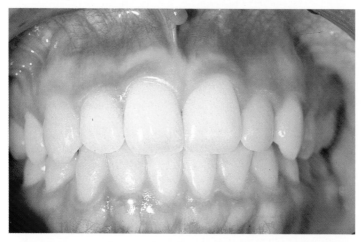

(E)

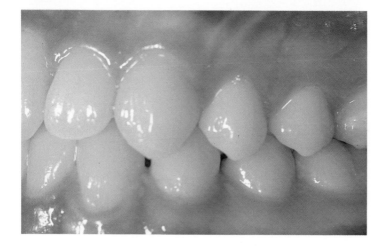

(F)

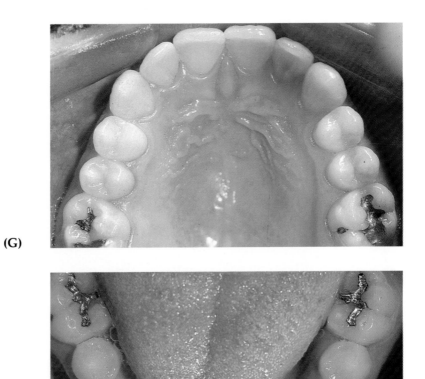

(G)

(H)

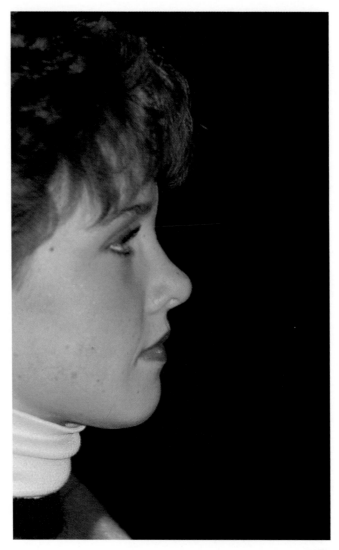

(I)

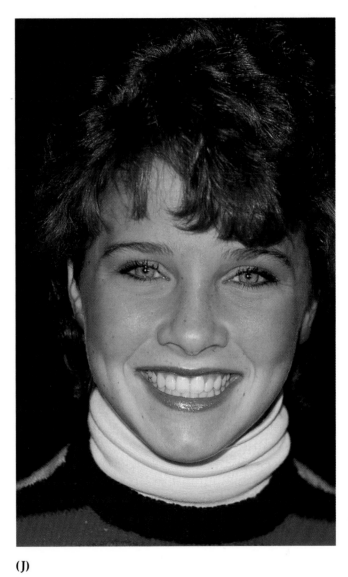

(J)

it a blessing of peace of mind in knowing that the state-of-the-art technology is being delivered through the doctor's care. He is building, not destroying; he is shaping, not crippling; he is helping, not hindering his patient. And he can sense this as he feels within himself his talents growing and perceives his own individual participation in becoming one of what Dr John Austin refers to as "the facial architects of the future!"

So to address our initial question, we might state that in order to expand and build a practice, to increase income and establish inflation-proof aspects into a practice; in order to reduce stress and rejuvenate the doctor's interest and enthusiasm for his work; in order to give patients broad full smiles, functional occlusion, healthy, sound temporomandibular joints, full even faces and profiles, dimensionable stability and improved self-image; in order to do all these things and still have fun knowing one is giving patients the absolute best—this is why we start.

"Our doubts are traitors
and make us lose the good we oft
might win by fearing to attempt."

Measure for Measure
William Shakespeare

Figure 1-14 RMDS serialized computer analysis of cases treated with fixed appliances *v* functional appliances reveals dramatic results. One hundred cases of fixed appliance treatment show that, on average, the mandible finishes 2 mm behind the predicted untreated (natural) position; 20 cases using FJO methods show the mandible finishes 2 mm ahead of the predicted untreated position.

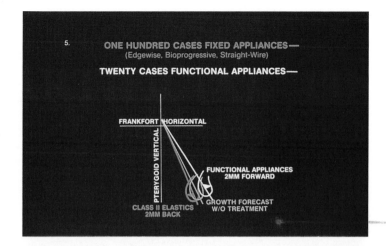

Figure 1-14

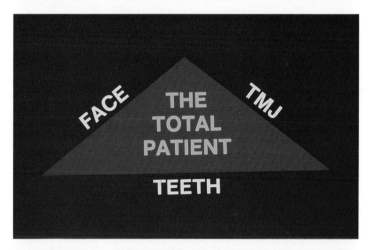

ORTHODONTIC PRINCIPLE   NUMBER ONE

The patient has a <u>much happier attitude</u> with removable appliances rather than fixed appliances

This <u>happier patient attitude</u> makes the day better for the doctor <u>and</u> his staff

---

ORTHODONTIC PRINCIPLE   NUMBER TWO

The patient demand for removable appliances is far greater than the patient demand for fixed appliances.

Despite this, many more doctors are treating with fixed appliances where the patient demand is the least

---

ORTHODONTIC PRINCIPLE   NUMBER THREE

It requires 3 seconds to take a removable appliance from the mouth and 3 seconds to replace it in the mouth

It takes 5 minutes to remove wires from the mouth and 10 minutes to replace wires in the mouth

Three times as many patients can be seen in the same amount of time

---

ORTHODONTIC PRINCIPLE   NUMBER FOUR

95% of the sagittal appliances and 80% of the transverse appliances should be made

INCONSPICUOUS APPLIANCES

You will find excellent patient cooperation and tremendous patient demand with INCONSPICUOUS REMOVABLE APPLIANCES

ORTHODONTIC PRINCIPLE   NUMBER FIVE

The patient should experience no pain with removable appliances.

EXTREMELY IMPORTANT FOR SUCCESS:

If pain occurs, patient should call the doctor before removing appliance from the mouth

---

ORTHODONTIC PRINCIPLE   NUMBER SIX

The finest orthodontic and orthopedic results:

1. Beautiful facial esthetics
2. Full, complete smile
3. Healthiest TMJs
4. Best stability

Are achieved with removable appliances.

If rotations remain, or more alignment is needed, bonded brackets will do this best.

REFERENCES

1. Angle EH: *Treatment of Malocclusion of the Teeth,* ed 7. Philadelphia, SS White, 1907.
2. Angle EH: The latest and best orthodontic mechanism, *Dent Cosmos* 1928;70: 1143–1158.
3. Angle EH: A message bearing on the treatment of Class II, division 1 malocclusion. *Angle Orthod* 1932;2:121–123.
4. Oppenheim A: Tissue changes, particularly of the bone, incident to tooth movement. *Eur Orthod Soc Trans* 1911, pp 303–359.
5. Sicher H: *Oral Anatomy,* St Louis, CV Mosby Co, 1952.
6. Hixon E, Klein P: Simplified mechanics: A means of treatment based on available scientific information, *Am J Orthod* 1972;62:113–141.
7. Odegard J: Mandibular rotation studied with the aid of metal implants. *Am J Orthod* 1970;58:448–454.
8. Cross JJ: Facial growth: Before, during and following orthodontic treatment. *Am J Orthod* 1977;71:68–78.
9. Horowitz SL, Hixon EH: An approach to diagnosis and implications for treatment, in *The Nature of Orthodontic Diagnosis.* St Louis, CV Mosby Co, pp 344–378.
10. Bennett DT: Reinforced occipito-mental traction and its effect on the incisor teeth in Class III malocclusions. *Tran Br Soc Stud Orthod* 1967;54:59–67.
11. Hawley CA: Treatment of Class II or distocclusion. *Int J Orthod* 1930;16:127.
12. Hellman M: Cusps and occlusion. *Dent Cosmos* 1923;65:503–518.
13. Grimm FM: Bone bending as a feature of orthodontic tooth movement. *Am J Orthod* 1972;62:384–393.
14. Tweed CH: Indications for extraction of teeth in orthodontic procedure. *Am J Orthod Oral Surg* 1944;30:405–428.
15. Andresen V, Haupl K: *Functions-Kiefer Orthopädie.* Berlin, Hermann Meusser, 1936.
16. Andresen V: The Norwegian system of gnathological functional orthopedics. *Acta Gnathol* 1939;4:5–36.
17. Häupl K, Grossman WJ, Clarkson P: *Textbook on Functional Jaw Orthopaedics.* London, Henry Kimpton, 1952.
18. Graber T, Neumann B: *Removable Orthodontic Appliances,* ed 2. Philadelphia, WB Saunders Co, 1984.
19. Jakobsson S: Cephalometric evaluation of treatment effect on Class II, division 1 malocclusions. *Am J Orthod* 1967;53:446–457.
20. Subtelny D: Malocclusions, orthodontic corrections and orofacial muscle adaptation. *Angle Orthod* 1970;40:170–201.
21. Straub WJ: Malfunction of the tongue: pt I. *Am J Orthod* 1960;46:404–424.
22. Straub WJ: Malfunction of the tongue. pt II. *Am J Orthod* 1961;47:596–617.
23. Blyth P: The relationship between speech, tongue behavior and occlusal abnormalities. *Dent Pract* 1959;10:11–22.
24. Tulley WJ: A critical appraisal of tongue thrusting. *Am J Orthodont* 1969;55: 640–650.
25. Schulhof RJ, Engle GA: Results of Class II functional appliance treatment. *JCO* 1982;16:587–599.
26. Simoes WA: Some oral neurophysiological resources applied in the use of functional orthopaedic techniques. *J Jpn Orthod Soc* 1979;38:40–48.

27. Baume LT, Haupl K, Stellach R: Growth and transformation of the tempo-romandibular joint in an orthopedically treated case of Pierre Robin's syndrome. *Am J Orthod* 1959;45:901–916.

28. Elgoyhen JC, Moyers RE, McNamara JA Jr, et al: Craniofacial adaptations to protrusive function in young rhesus monkeys. *Am J Orthod* 1972;62:469–480.

29. McNamara JA Jr: Neuromuscular and skeletal adaptations to altered function in the orofacial region. *Am J Orthod* 1973;64:578–606.

30. McNamara JA Jr, Connely TG, McBride HC: Histological studies of tempo-romandibular adaptations, in McNamara JA Jr: *Determinants of Mandibular Form and Growth.* No. 4 in Craniofacial Growth Series. Ann Arbor, Center for Human Growth and Development, University of Michigan, 1975, pp 209–227.

31. McNamara JA Jr, Carlson DS: Quantitative analysis of temporomandibular joint adaptations to protrusive function. *Am J Orthod* 1979;76:593–611.

32. Wieslander L, Lagerstrom L: The effect of activator treatment on Class II malocclusion. *Am J Orthod* 1979;75:20–26.

33. Freeland TD: Muscle function during treatment with functional regulator. *Angle Orthod* 1979;49:247–258.

34. Luzi V: CV value in analysis of sagittal malocclusions. *Am J Orthod* 1982;8:478.

35. Hotz RP: Application and appliance manipulation of functional forces. *Am J Orthod* 1970;58:459–478.

36. Weinberger TW: Extra-oral traction and functional appliances – a cephalometric comparison. *Br J Orthod* 1973;1:35–39.

37. Moss JP: Cephalometric changes during functional appliance therapy. *Trans Eur Orthod Soc* 1962;327–341.

38. Meikle MC: The role of the condyle in postnatal growth of the mandible. *Am J Orthod* 1973;64:50–62.

39. Enlow DH, Harris DB: A study of postnatal growth of the human mandible. *Am J Orthod* 1964;50:25–59.

40. Charles SW: The temporomandibular joint and its influence on the growth of the mandible. *J Br Dent Assoc* 1925;46:845–855.

41. Brodie AG: On the growth pattern of the human head. *Am J Anat* 1941;68:209–262.

42. Dunlap JE: *Stress, Change and Related Pains for Dentists and Those Nearby.* Tulsa, PennWell Books, 1981.

43. Dunlap JE: *Surviving in Dentistry.* Tulsa, The Petroleum Publishing Co, 1977.

44. Rose KD, Rosow I: Physicians who kill themselves. *Arch Gen Psychiatry* 1973;29:802.

45. Blachly PH, Osterud HT, Josslin R: Suicide in professional groups. *N Engl J Med* 1963;268:1278–1282.

CHAPTER 2
The Bionator

OVERVIEW

The Bionator is an *arch-aligning* appliance. The Bionator, and its nearly identical first-born offspring, the Orthopedic Corrector I, are the best appliances available today for the purposes of correcting a skeletal Class II malocclusion to a Class I molar relationship, increasing the vertical dimension of occlusion, and bringing the mandible down and forward when needed, thus developing the entire lower face.[1] With simple modifications, these appliances can be used to increase the vertical dimension of occlusion only; advance the mandible from a Class II molar relationship to a Class I relationship only without increasing the vertical, or in combination with either one or both actions also moderately widen the maxillary and mandibular dental arches, especially in the lower anterior area. After their use has been mastered by the clinician, they can even be used to accomplish minor individual tooth movements.

This is all accomplished in a gentle and effective manner by means of an easily removable appliance that fits loosely in the mouth and is well tolerated by the patient. Children and adults accomodate in a very short time to wearing this appliance and have little difficulty with speech or swallowing functions. By virtue of its light weight and low porosity acrylic, the appliance is extremely hygienic for the mouth. This helps eliminate one of the troublesome postorthodontic problems of caries, a frequent result of the difficulty of proper oral hygiene for a patient with fixed appliances. By virtue of being a removable appliance, it is comfortable to the soft tissues of the mouth, since the cheeks and tongue are not required to rub constantly against rough irregular metallic surfaces as with conventional orthodontic bands and wires. Since only the labial wire across the maxillary teeth and a small clear acrylic cap on the lower teeth are apparent to the eye when the patient is wearing the appliance, it is much more esthetic than the more standard fixed appliances. And of course, for entirely human reasons, such as special social events, photographic sessions, etc, its removable aspect can for a short period of time make it instantly extremely esthetic!

Though intended for the treatment of reasonably normal dental arches that are merely malaligned either horizontally or vertically, the appliance can be constructed in such a way as to accomodate arches that are slightly irregular or crowded and correct them to the more standard "Roman arch form" we desire, by means of proper adjustments. But the more irregularities in arch form that are taken care of before the insertion of the appliance, and the more "arch-shaped" the maxillary and mandibular dentitions are, the better.

Many orthodontic treatment regimens are capable of correcting Class II relationships to Class I, but the Bionator's big advantage is that it moves the mandible as a *whole* and unlocks what might possibly be strained temporomandibular joints in the process. This temporomandibular joint condition, or malarthrosis, often accompanies the loss of vertical dimension and the retruded mandibular position of a Class II malocclusion. By bringing the mandible down and forward and developing the lower face, it gives the male patient a masculine, square jaw and rugged appearance. It gives the female patient a full facial profile and a pleasing and attractive lower face. It eliminates the weak and unassuming chin associated with Class II maloc-

---

Figure 2-1 **(A) (B) (C)** Basic Bionator, cornerstone of skeletal Class II treatment, used to advance mandibles from skeletal Class II to skeletal Class I, increase vertical dimension of occlusion, correct deep overbite, and relieve possible compressed temporomandibular joints. **(D)** Bionator compared with Orthopedic Corrector I. Note expansion screws for advancement in mandibular bicuspid area of Orthopedic Corrector I. (*Courtesy of Ohlendorf Co., St. Louis, MO.*) **(E)** There is no acrylic over occlusal surfaces of posterior teeth in Bionator I appliance except for acrylic covering of lower incisors of the cap area. (*Courtesy of DynaFlex, St. Louis, MO.*)

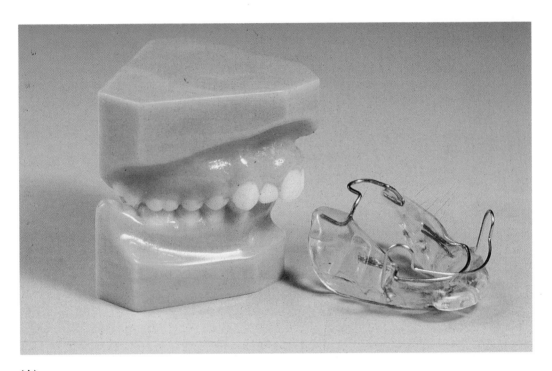

(A)

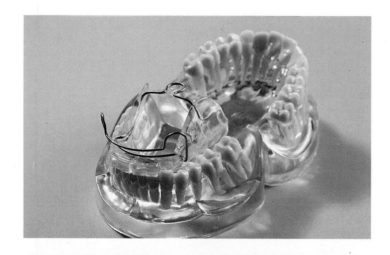

(B)

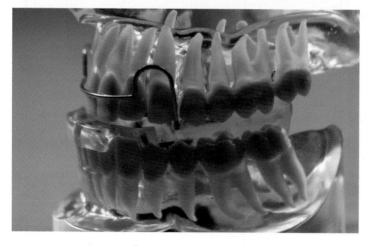

(C)

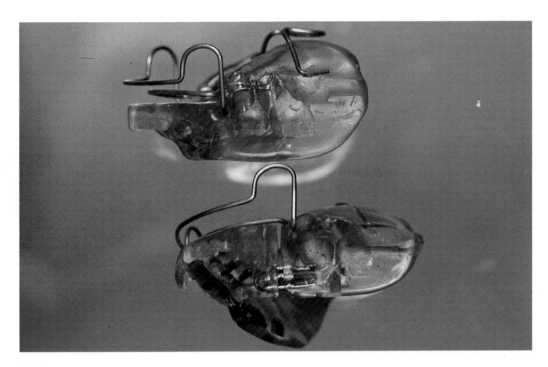

(D)

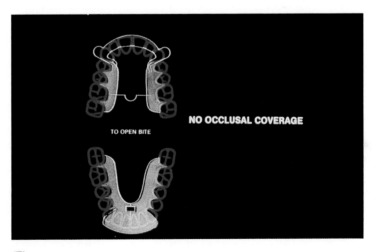

(E)

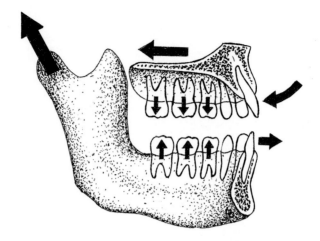

Figure 2-1 **(F)** Demonstration of action of the Bionator. Downward and forward displacement of mandible results in stimulation of condylar development while tension placed on appliance by mastication muscle stretch cause headgear effect on maxillary denture base and distal drift to maxillary posterior teeth, especially first molar. Maxillary anteriors can be brought inward while lower anteriors have a tendency to be "dumped" forward if not restrained by the cap lip. Increased vertical distance which is direct function of cap thickness stimulates eruption of posterior teeth and vertical alveolar development.

clusions exhibiting concomitant deep overbite and excessive overjet. Thus the Bionator is a "facemaker" as well as a "mouthmaker." It also gives great stability in its final treatment position by virtue of stimulating condylar growth, which is impossible to obtain with the use of Class II elastics.[2-3] The latter often produces a dual or "Sunday" bite.[4]

So, Bionators do indeed give a pleasing, full face, a balanced profile, and an attractive smile. They produce a full functional occlusion, correcting a Class II retruded mandible to a full Class I molar relationship. They in-

Figure 2-2 Classic example of Bionator capabilities. **(A)** Note large overjet, deep overbite of typical skeletal Class II case, most common malocclusion and one of most difficult to treat with conventional fixed appliance technique, usually requiring extraction of at least one pair of bicuspids to correct excessive overjet. **(B)** After 18 months of Bionator treatment. Note reduction of overjet, advancement of entire mandibular denture, correction of occlusion from dental Class II to Class I without extraction of bicuspids, and correction of excessive overbite.

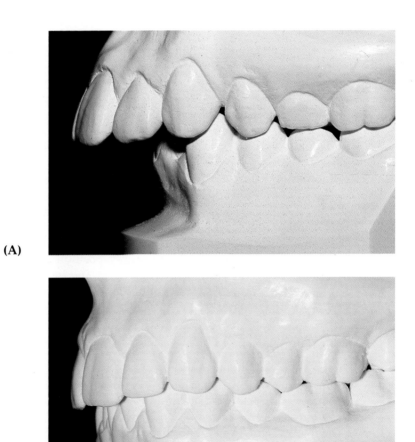

(A)

(B)

crease the vertical dimension of occlusion and eliminate deep overbites, thus relieving strained temporomandibular joints. By virtue of taking the condyle out of a superior posterior retruded position in the temporomandibular joint, they eliminate the pain and discomfort, and even dysfunction, which are often associated with extreme examples of this condition. They can widen moderately narrow maxillary and mandibular arches and correct protruding maxillary anterior teeth by rotating the premaxilla downward and distally, thereby correcting excessive overjet problems. They can also be used to flare lower anterior teeth forward that have become lingually inclined in the lower arches. In the labial area, they can eliminate the lip trap and liberate the curled lower lip and strained orbicularis oris muscle often associated with excessive overjet. They help enable the patient to obtain a proper lip seal and correct improper upper and lower lip relationships. They also are capable of eliminating the severe periodontal and mucosal damage done to the palate and gingivae by excessive deep overbite problems. By virtue of correcting severe mandibular retrusion, they also correct the malpositioning of the tongue and thereby the resultant deviant swallowing pattern which complicates so much of present-day orthodontic therapy. By acting as a screening device, they also prevent the tongue from widening out over the occlusal surfaces of the posterior teeth, thus expediting the correction of vertical problems and assisting in attainment of the correct occlusal plane. These appliances bring the tongue back into proper position against the soft palate, eliminate tongue thrust during swallowing, and help retrain the tongue to a more correct and proper function. By holding the mandible in an inferior and protruded position, these appliances also allow for the tongue and cer-

---

Figure 2-3 Dental and Skeletal Class II correction. **(A)** Frontal and **(B)** lateral pretreatment facial views. Note lip incompetency, mandibular retrusion, and lack of adequate lower face height, a direct result of deep bite problems intraorally. **(C) (D) (E)** Study models reveal classic Class II, Division 1 deep bite malocclusion with narrowed maxillary arch, flared forward maxillary incisors, large overjet, deep overbite and severe skeletal Class II mandibular retrusion. **(F) (G) (H)** After proper application of FJO techniques of mandibular advancement with Bionator appliances, note improved arch form (due to proper use of mid-line expansion screw of Bionator), the retraction of the labially-flared maxillary incisors (due to proper use of labial bow of Bionator), increased vertical dimension of occlusion (due to proper adjustment of interproximal acrylic of Bionator), and complete correction of Class II occlusion to full Class I (due to proper registration of construction bite for appliance). Two appliances were used over approximately a 15 month period to complete the case. No other appliances, fixed or removable were needed. **(I) (J)** Final facial views five years after treatment, no retention.

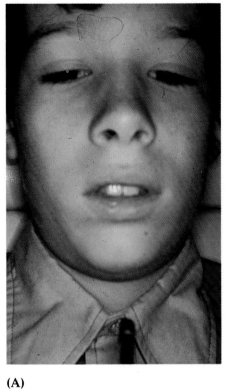

(A)

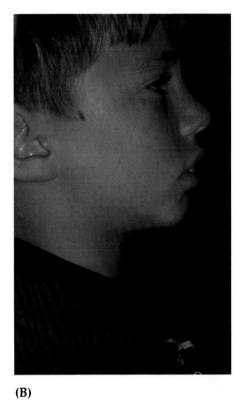

(B)

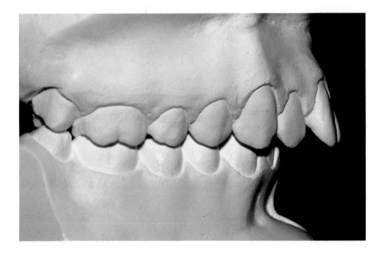

(C)

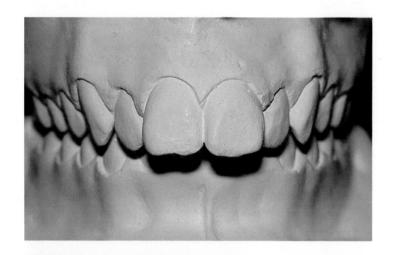

(D)

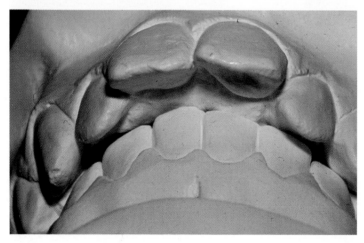

(E)

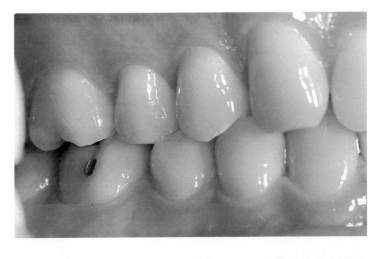

(F)

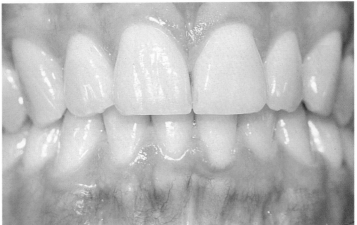

(G)

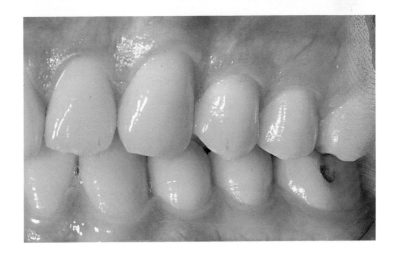

(H)

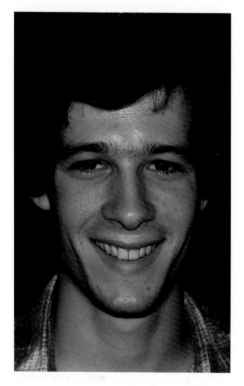

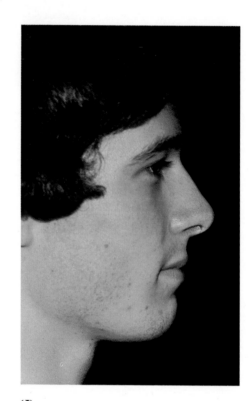

(I)

(J)

vical viscera to move forward due to the increased intraoral space, thereby allowing for improved respiration. These appliances also work very successfully in eliminating the "sucking habit" in children who complicate their malocclusion by habitually sucking various combinations of fingers and thumbs. They also calm the bruxing habit in some deep overbite cases. They normalize function in the patient with abnormal functioning maxillofacial complexes and lead to harmony, stability, and beauty. They accomplish all this in an elegant and humane treatment modality that is easy on the patient's mouth as well as the doctor's back.

"Man is a pliable animal,
a being who gets accustomed
to everything. . . ."

Feodor Dostoievsky
1821–1881

HISTORY AND DEVELOPMENT

Conceived and refined by Dr Balters of Germany in the late 1950s and early 1960s, the Bionator did not just spring forth from his mind new and fully formed like Pallas Athena from the head of Zeus, but rather was the end product of a painfully long and slow series of evolutionary steps wrought with trial and error that go back as far as 1879!

That year was a time of crude beginnings in not only the health sciences but in the more general areas of technology as well. For example, the famous physician and surgeon W. J. Mayo of Rochester, Minnesota, performed abdominal surgery using clamps he designed himself and had to have forged by local blacksmiths. Professional men in the healing arts still travelled about by train or horse and buggy as that year saw the first patent applied for a carriage propelled by an internal combustion engine. When doctors and dentists performed operative procedures on patients, they did so by the light of gas or coal oil lamps, as Thomas Edison had only just invented the incandescent light bulb at his makeshift laboratory in Menlo Park, New Jersey. Orthodontics was taking its first few feeble steps forward too, for it was in that year that Dr N. W. Kingsley wrote, in his treatise on oral deformity,[5] that he had developed a maxillary plate with an inclined plane for the purpose of "jumping the bite" forward in cases of extreme mandibular retrusion. Imagine! Over 100 years ago the idea was conceived of moving the mandible forward as a whole. It wasn't much of a technique at the time, but it represented the important genesis of a concept. The idea was further evolved by a French dentist, Dr Pierre Robin, who published a paper in 1902 describing his "monobloc" appliance to be used for bimaxillary expansion. Incidentally, he also advocated the use of this appliance for the treatment of "glossoptosis," an imaginary condition he believed existed that would result in the destruction of a major portion of the French population! (His orthodontic ideas were all-right, but his theories on holistic medicine were slightly off base!) It's surprising how far the influence of his ideas extended into the twentieth century as some of the major authors of the 1920s and 1930s still referred to some of these original concepts in their texts.[6] But his concept of moving the mandible and the tongue forward to correct mandibular retrusion and free up the esophageal and tracheal passages survives down to this day.

Employing the functional aspects of the muscles in the treatment of malocclusions, an important cornerstone of Bionator treatment philosophy, was an idea first basically conceived by Dr Alfred P. Rogers in 1918. His theories were essentially that exercising the oral-facial muscles in certain ways would aid or correct certain orthodontic conditions.[7-11] The whole world surprisingly followed into line as orthodontists everywhere readily accepted his ideas without the benefit of any true scientific backing. Though the exercises developed by Rogers were believed in and for a while used by almost everyone, no one ever reported a successful treatment using the exercises alone without the concomitant use of appliance therapy. Even the prestigious authors Häupl, Grossman, and Clarkson in their *Textbook of Functional Jaw Orthopaedics* list these exercises as an adjunct to therapy.[12] One of their illustrations relative to this subject shows a child demonstrating one of Rogers' muscle exercises advocated for the treatment of a distoclusion. It portrays the child standing with its head and neck hyperextended and its arms extended and rotated backward. The appearance of the child in this position can't help but remind one of the hood ornament of a Rolls Royce! All these exercises are obsolete now, but Rogers' concept of the functional importance of oral-facial musculature in orthodontic treatment is one of the most important theories we build on today. Oral myofunctional therapy is an important adjunct to modern orthodontics and is a direct descendent of the principles first conceived and defined by Rogers.[13]

The period just prior to World War I saw a plethora of appliance designs developed for both functional appliances and active plates of one sort or another throughout Europe. But the spotlight was stolen from this area of endeavors by a talented and influential orthodontist from across the Atlantic,

Figure 2-4 (A) Note excessive curl to lower lip and exaggeration of mentonian groove resultant to excessive overjet and deep overbites which also may result in **(B)** lower incisor damage of lingual gingival crest area adjacent to cingula of maxillary anteriors.

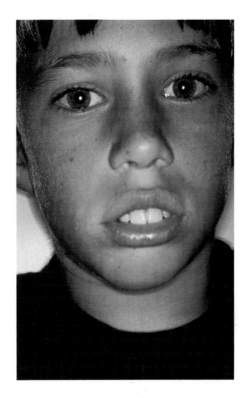

(A)

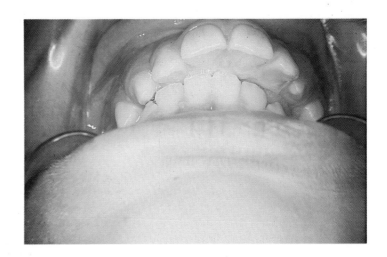

(B)

Edward H. Angle. For 30 years his concept of fixed appliances and nonextraction expansion of the dental arches using heavy forces dominated the orthodontic world. These ideas were at first for a short time very unpopular in Europe because few of the doctors understood the multibanded techniques; and if they did, the cost was so prohibitive that few of the patients of that era in Europe could afford them. Thus removable appliance techniques struggled on. It was hoped that somehow the latter could serve to replace the former as a means of delivering economic orthodontic care to the masses.

But then an individual arrived on the scene who took all the various ideas and theories about using the functional appliances to treat dental malocclusions, and making order out of chaos, coordinated the appropriate information, and after some initial trial and error and homespun experimentation, devised an appliance that reflected the true genius that he was. His name was Viggo Andresen, and his appliance was the Activator.[14]

Andresen was originally a Dane, but he eventually became director of the orthodontic department in the Dental School at Oslo, Norway. He believed in the theories, expounded by Roux and Wolfe in the 1890s, that changes in biomechanical function bring about corresponding changes in both internal structure of bone as well as the actual external shape. He believed that in the case of a Class II malocclusion, the most common variety, an appliance could be constructed so as to hold the mandible down and forward and force the jaw to close in a more normal orthopedically balanced relationship; the stimulation of the appliance on the teeth during this action would cause not only the muscles to reposition themselves but also thereby cause the bone to actually reshape itself in order to accommodate the teeth in the new position, and therefore a more correct relationship between the maxilla and the mandible would result. Over a period of treatment time, he felt the entire maxillofacial complex would adapt to the new jaw relationship dictated by the shape and fit of the appliance worn in the mouth. He also believed these changes would be permanent and would not require any form of retention once treatment was complete, as the muscles and teeth would have repositioned themselves and the bone would have reshaped itself into a new, more correct, and more functional form that was

---

Figure 2-5   (A) Forces of muscles on denture bases. In both adaptive and endogenous tongue thrust situations, anterior component of force during swallowing is greater than opposing counterbalancing forces of lips and perioral musculature. Tip of tongue improperly thrusts and seals horizontally forward in nasopalatine area (probe) instead of sealing vertically against palate, resulting in pointed or "gothic" arch form of maxillary denture base **(B). (C)** After correction with proper FJO techniques, note improved arch form.

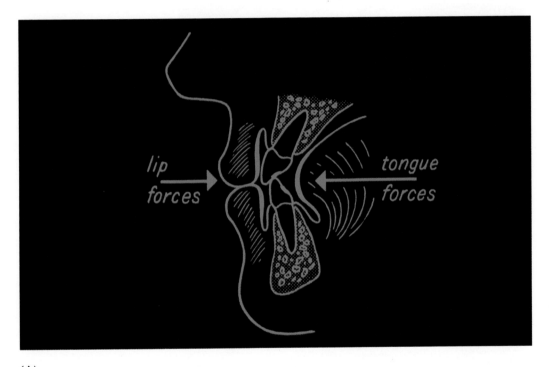

(A)

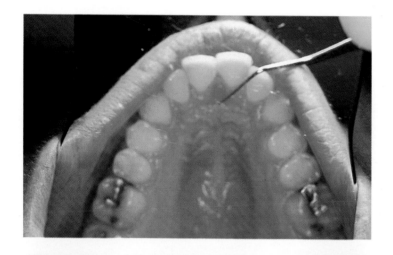

(B)

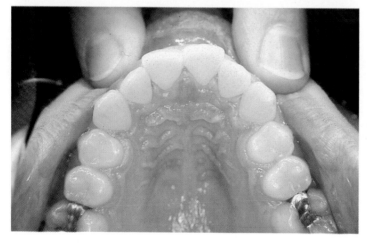

(C)

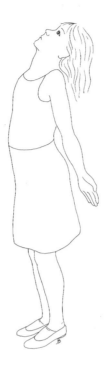

Figure 2-6 Exercise described by Rogers to aid in correction of a distoclusion.

both naturally and biomechanically stable. The appliance he designed, in order to fulfill the theoretical requirements of the time, was to fit loosely in the mouth and was made in such a way that it allowed the jaws to close in only one way, the new corrected advanced and opened position. The appliance design would actually force the jaws to simulate, and thereby activate, this new functional relationship, hence the name "Activator."

Andresen believed that many malocclusions were functional in origin and that if "form followed function," it followed that correct function would eventually lead to correct form. This of course means correct muscle function. One may now at once see how the theories of Kingsley, Roux and Wolfe, and Rogers unite in the metamorphosis of Andresen's functional appliance theory of action. The Activator he constructed did in fact transmit the tissue-forming functional stimuli of the perioral and masticatory muscles, tongue, and teeth to the periodontal tissues, alveolar bone, and temporomandibular joint bringing about the eventual resolution of the structural Class II deformity. Its use was confined to Class II, Division 1; Class II, Division 2; and pseudo-Class III malocclusions. The appliance consisted of an upper maxillary plate with an anterior flange extending into the lingual area of the mandibular arch that on closing held the lower jaw in a forward position

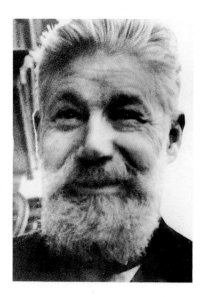

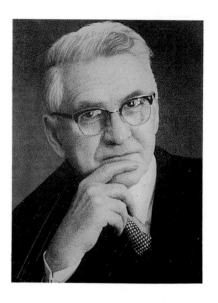

Figure 2-7   Viggo Andresen   **Figure 2-8**   Karl Häupl

relative to the maxilla with a bite opening of approximately 5 mm between the posterior teeth. The appliance also had a labial bow or labial archwire across the maxillary anterior teeth for the purposes of stabilizing the appliance and retracting overly protruded maxillary anterior teeth. The appliance was meant to be worn by the patient only at night, and its projected treatment time consisted of 18 to 24 months. The life of each appliance was about 9 months. They were initially made of vulcanite. Therefore, several appliances were required to be fabricated in order to complete a case. Usually once the appliance was inserted, there were no adjustments needed after therapy had begun.

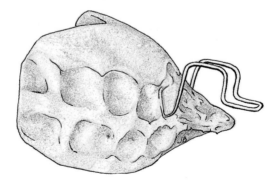

Figure 2-9   Andresen-Häupl Activator; original vulcanite model.

Andresen built his concepts on a firm basis of experience and observation. Though the appliance he designed was bulky and caused considerable difficulties in speech for the patient, it had all the crude elements of the Bionator that was eventually to evolve from it. But the appliance itself was by no means crude in either its treatment regimen, or results. Some initial enthusiasts even referred to it as the "miracle appliance." It was truly a milestone in the development of removable orthodontic appliances. But it may have been lost forever in the shuffle of the times had not fate intervened and a very important circumstance taken place. After having been appointed a professor at the dental school at Oslo, Andresen (and as it turns out, the rest of the orthodontic profession) had the good fortune to strike up an alliance with a fellow staff member at the same institution, the Austrian-born periodontist and pathologist Karl Häupl.

A physician by training, Häupl was a superb scientist of considerable international reputation. He had not been involved with orthodontics until he had met Andresen and therefore bore none of the then prevalent prejudice against Andresen's new ideas. When Andresen showed him the results obtained with his Activator, Häupl was extremely excited, for Andresen's findings coincided exactly with results he had already seen independently relative to tooth migration and tissue and bone reaction. Together they further developed the appliance-induced mandibular advancement technique, refined it, and unlike previous individuals, were able to support their clinical observations with sound research data. Then came the best stroke of luck. Häupl was offered the prestigious position of director of the dental clinic at the University of Prague. From such an eminent position, he had great leverage in convincing other European orthodontists that Andresen's method of "functional jaw orthopedics," a term they coined together, was not only an effective therapeutic method but that it was "biologically superior" to all previous existing techniques! This along with other important and timely supportive data from men like A. M. Schwarz, whose active plates could move individual teeth [15] and whose methods complimented and enhanced Activator therapy, coupled with the proof of men like A. H. Ketcham [16,17] from America, that heavy forces of fixed appliances caused pathologic root resorption, brought the European orthodontic community to its feet in applause for the new biologically superior method of removable appliance therapy. Incidentally, it was Ketcham's observations that also caused the change in philosophy on the American side of the Atlantic with respect to fixed appliance therapy that led to the development of more precise, light-wire forces for tooth movement such as the Angle edgewise appliance. [18] It was the time back in America that marked the beginning of the modern-day multibanded techniques. But it was too late. It was the mid-1930s and a certain portion of clinicians in Europe had already gone enthusiastically down the path of functional appliances and active plates. Unfortunately, Germany had already gone down the path of National Socialism, and an entire world girded for war.

But even this miracle appliance was plagued with difficulties in the early stages of its development, and not everyone in Europe agreed as to its effectiveness. There were dissenters. One of the controversies raised centered around the inability of some clinicians to obtain permanent mandibular repositioning. [19-26] This was probably due to the incorrect nature of some of the construction bites used at the time and the lack of understanding of this important step in the beginning. The bites were generally, at first, not taken with the mandible in an inferior or protruded enough position. By not gaining enough interocclusal space between the posterior teeth or without enough tension on the muscles of the jaws from proper protrusion of the mandible, the Activator's action and efficiency is greatly diminished. The construction bites were initially taken with the mandible opened just beyond the physiologic rest position. Generally, this was not enough. Gradually, as more clinicians experimented with the technique, they realized that the construction bite had to be taken with the mandible in a more open and protruded position. [27-29] But despite these initial difficulties, the Activator was used in many thousands of cases throughout Europe with outstanding results. [30-45]

Moreover, one of the problems with wearing the Activator was its size. It was a bulky appliance at best; and by virtue of the full palatal covering, it made speech very difficult. This was not considered an important drawback as the Activator was to be worn only at night. Another difficulty with this appliance, and with all appliances of that time, was that they had to be made out of vulcanite. When minor tooth movements were desired, gutta-percha melted with chloroform was used and "layered on" in order to make the appliance a little thicker behind the tooth that was to be moved. Another method of individual tooth movement advocated the drilling of holes in various places in the vulcanite and gluing in small wooden pegs that would put pressure upon the teeth to be moved when the appliance was inserted. Gutta-percha and hickory sticks! Not the most convenient of techniques; nevertheless, the early orthodontists of these times still managed effective therapy. If only they would have lived in the age of acrylic. Modern dentists are lucky.

Figure 2-10 **(A)** Modern streamlined Bionator as compared to old-style Andresen-Häupl Activators which were much bulkier and worn only at night. **(B) (C)** Original vulcanite Activator from over a half century ago. **(D)** Shiny spots (blue) appear where teeth rub against acrylic in an attempt to erupt. As with old Activator technique, when such shiny spots appear on flanges of Bionators, they should be reduced with acrylic burs to allow posterior teeth to erupt uninhibited by acrylic. **(E)** Not only should acrylic over teeth be ground away to eliminate anything inhibitory to eruption, but also acrylic eruption of gingival crest should be relieved.

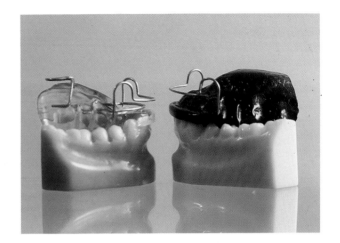

(A)

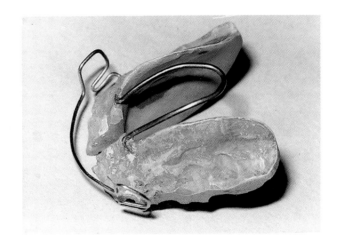

(B)

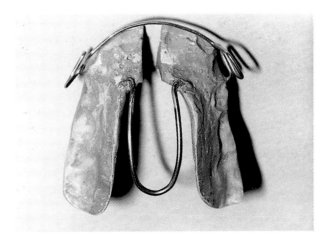

(C)

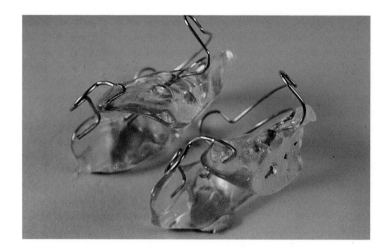

(D)

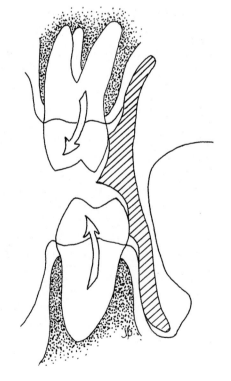

(E)

With the advent of modern acrylic, a new world of feasibility was created for the orthodontist using functional appliances. Its light weight, strength, low porosity, and ease of manipulation made this "wonder" material ideal for creating intraoral orthodontic devices. The late-model Activators were made out of acrylic, rather than vulcanite, once this material became available. But they were still made in the traditional black color as were the original models in order to facilitate grinding high spots and various other adjustments. The black acrylic made the spot that needed reduction easier to see because the appliance was finished in a dull or satin surface. Thus, any excessive contact by the teeth on the appliance would cause a shiny spot to appear denoting the place where an adjustment was needed and where acrylic should be reduced. The new acrylic materials were important in facilitating a number of new designs that appeared after World War II which all traced their theoretical origins to the original Andresen-Häupl Activator prototype.

The evolution of the entire spectrum of removable functional orthodontic appliances in Europe had an interesting and human chapter written one auspicious evening in 1939. A European Orthodontic Society (EOS) meeting was held in Wiesbaden, a German city just west of Frankfurt, at which the aging and white-bearded Andresen was the guest of honor. All had come to pay tribute to the great man who founded the basic tenets of FJO therapeutics. Held at the Kurhaus on Wilhelmstrasse, the list of those in attendance that historic evening ran like an orthodontic who's who of the great European orthodontic practitioners of the time. With Korkhaus presiding, some of the attendants at the meeting that night besides Andresen were none other than Häupl, Petrik, Nord, and Schwarz, to name a few. As the evening waned and the festivities began to subside, a few stragglers hovered around Andresen at the president's table on into the late hours of the night. And then an event took place that might have gone unnoticed and may have been lost to history for its seemingly trite insignificance; yet when considered from the advantageous perspective of hindsight, it turns out to be an occurrence that was at once both incisively retrospective and at the same time strikingly prophetic. Andresen, in a form of German heavy with his Norwegian accent, suddenly looked at an attentive, young man standing next to him and "out of the clear blue" slapped him on the shoulder and said softly to him, *Junger Mann, da haben Sie ein Kind in die Welt gesetzt, und dann kommen die anderen und sagen wie es heisst.* ("Young man, you bring a child into the world, and then the others come and tell you what to name it.") History will never know how much of an insight Andresen had when he spoke those words, nor whether he could foresee the full impact of its prophetic truth. After observing the course of orthodontic history we now see how important this statement has become. For the young man he so addressed was to eventually become himself one of the founding fathers of more modern European removable appliance technique and a man whose preliminary appliance designs served as advanced prototypes for the evolution of a long list of subsequent "named" appliances (not including the Bionator, ironically!) that sprang up throughout Europe in the postwar era. But this was to come years after the 1939 EOS meeting at the Kurhaus in Wiesbaden, where the aforementioned Silesian-born, 18-year-old senior medical student, and son of a prominent German dentist, first met Viggo Andresen and was so advised. That young man was none other than the eminent Hans Peter Bimler![46]

A brief survey of the "Bimler museum" of functional appliance designs reveals the core material from which many, if not all, of the modern European functional appliances derived their lineage. Ideas and principles of therapeutics were borrowed from and reincorporated back and forth throughout the several postwar decades of functional appliance evolution in Europe. These ideas and appliance types often complimented or paralleled the basic tenets of the design that was eventually to evolve into the final form of the Bionator. Each of the major appliance types had its own particular contribution to make in the development of removable functional appliance philosophy. Of course, many of the German ones owe a debt to their most immediate conceptual source, H. P. Bimler, but all of them may be fundamentally traced back to the original theories of Andresen!

Bimler Series of Appliances

Bimler, gradually over a period of years, developed a series of three major types of appliances[47-50]: the Bimler A, B, and C types with six variations for each type. They are designed to address every major type of skeletodental malocclusion. In his never-ending quest for efficiency, Bimler uses his vast experience and enormous technical skills to design appliances that incorporate the action of two or three other more basic appliance designs into one somewhat complicated device that can serve to treat the entire case, start to finish. Obviously this requires consummate skill and a level of experience beyond the basic appliance level of operation. Yet these concepts are not without their price in that the complexity of the appliance designs make for frequent breakage and difficulty in chairside adjustment for those clinicians less gifted with adroit tactile skills at wire bending. Other named appliances that were in vogue during the decades of the postwar era also owe their conceptual heritage to the Bimler appliance.

Figure 2-11 **(A)** Early functional orthodontists sometimes resorted to adding small wooden pegs or modules of gutta-percha to move individual teeth with their prototype vulcanite appliances before the advent of acrylic. **(B)** Early model Activator with wooden pegs for labial movement of upper centrals.

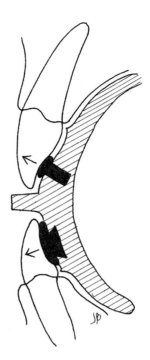

(A)

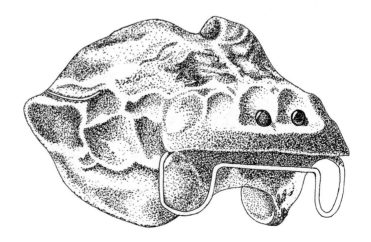

(B)

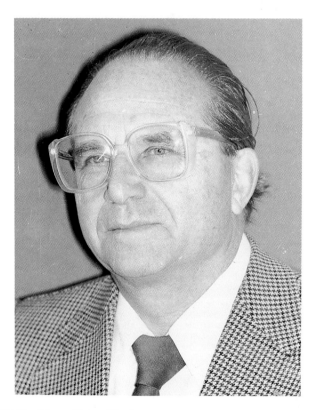

Figure 2-12(A)   Hans Peter Bimler

Herren Activator

One of the first modifications to appear was the Herren Activator developed by Dr Paul Herren in 1953. The Herren Activator is based on principles which are completely opposed to the kinetic philosophies of Andresen. Herren, in conjunction with Gerber, performed experiments showing that

Figure 2-12   Bimler appliances. **(B)** Type A. **(C)** Type B. **(D)** Type C.

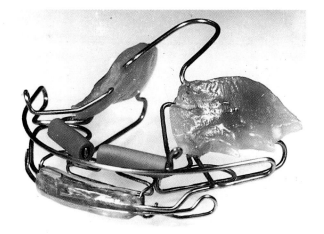

(B)

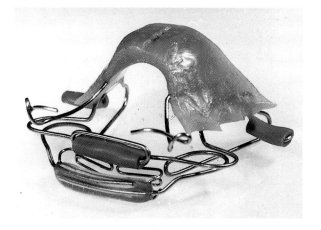

(C)

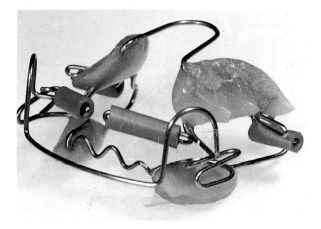

(D)

muscle activity is diminished during sleep and therefore there would be very little appliance activity at this time. The Herren Activator is held in place firmly against the maxilla with arrowhead clips; and the construction bite is taken such as to propulse the mandible in a quite forward position, almost at the limits of tolerance of the patients in some instances. It is still a nighttime-only appliance, to be worn for a minimum of nine hours each night.

Bow Activator of A. M. Schwarz

Another appliance developed soon afterward was the Bow Activator of A. M. Schwarz in 1956.[51] Schwarz was influenced and fascinated by the elastic properties of the Bimler Appliance; and with contributions from Wunderer, he designed the Bow Activator. It consisted of an Activator split in half horizontally, the two halves of which were connected by an elastic metal bow with a safety-pin curve in it to provide a springing action that would absorb the shock of the jaws closing on it, thereby activating and stimulating the muscles and alveolar processes. Sometimes this connecting bow would be given a helical loop. The construction bite was taken with a minimal amount of forward repositioning of the mandible, but the appliance could be adjusted at this connecting bow over a gradual period of time to advance the mandible further forward and to gradually increase the vertical. The results obtained from this appliance were marginal due to the lack of durability inherent in its design and the ease with which it could become distorted. Again, it was a nighttime-only appliance.

Karwetzky Appliance

A close relative of the above appliance was the Karwetzky Appliance which was a U-Bow Activator developed in 1964. It was more effective because it was made with thicker wire in the bow and was therefore stronger. It was also a nighttime appliance but required three hours of daytime wear in addition.

Cutout or Palate-Free Activator of Metzelder

There was also the Cutout or Palate-Free Activator of Metzelder.[52] This appliance was almost the same as a Bionator but still reflected its Ac-

Figure 2-13 Bow Activator of Schwarz. **(A)** Class II appliance. **(B)** Class III appliance. **(C)** Cutout or palate-free Activator of Metzelder. **(D)** Elastic open Activator of Klammt. **(E)** Kinetor of Hugo Stockfish.

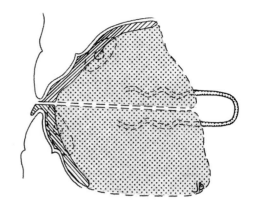

(A)

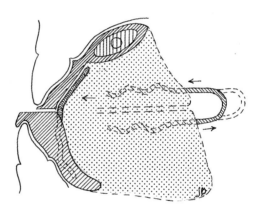

(B)

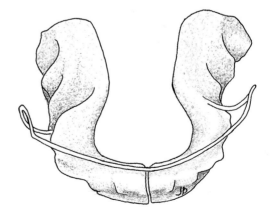

(C)

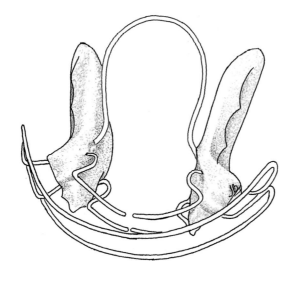

(D)

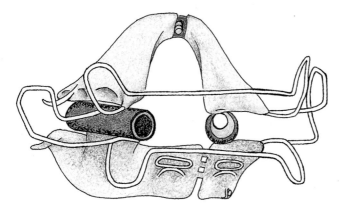

(E)

tivator lineage. It had no palatal covering and no Coffin spring to lend strength and stability to the appliance. It could therefore not be used to facilitate retraining the tongue as well as appliances that possessed the Coffin spring. Because of its shape and lack of stability in the mouth, some authors and clinicians felt the patients would be less likely to wear it; but it did have the advantage of being both a night and a day appliance.

Klamnt Open Elastic Activator

Yet another device was the Klamnt Open Elastic Activator.[53] This Activator's reduced size made it easier and more comfortable for the patient to wear, especially during the daytime. It was created independently and yet parallel to the Bionator. However, it possesses a more complicated design and several more wires in it, which brings about the problem again of breakage and difficulty of adjustment. It definitely shows its Bimler influences in this regard.

The Kinetor

Another appliance was the Kinetor developed by Dr Hugo Stockfish[54,55] in 1951. It was a nighttime-only appliance and required a treatment time of 2 to 4 years. Daytime wear of two to three hours per day was advised for the first year and a half. It was a combination of functional principles with the active operation of various screws and springs added to the appliance. Again, it is a complicated system and subject to breakage, difficulty of construction, and adjustments. It does have the capabilities of expanding the arches in all three directions, sagittally, vertically, and horizontally with jackscrews; but it does violate the principle of simplicity. It is almost as complicated as the Bimler.

Emergence of the Bionator

At last we reach the Bionator of Balters. It was developed in 1968, but surprisingly this is not the end goal of our process of appliance evolution. This appliance was a great advancement over the Andresen Activator as it was less bulky and possessed an open palate with a Coffin spring but no anterior cap. It also possessed buccinator loops to help retract invaginating buccal tissues. Balters was an enthusiastic proponent of balancing the forces of the lips, cheeks, and tongue. He believed that any disturbance in the balance of these anatomical components would result in a malocclusion. He believed the tongue to be the center of reflex activity for the oral cavity. His appliance was the direct forefather of the appliance that we now know today

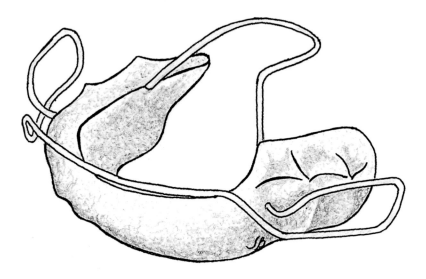

Figure 2-14 Balters Bionator of early 1960s.

as the Bionator. But what we in America refer to as a Bionator is actually a modified Bionator that technically should be referred to as the reduced Activator of Schmuth, after the man who developed it in 1973. Dr G. P. F. Schmuth of Bonn modified the original Balters appliance, keeping the acrylic part similar but retaining the old labial bow of the original Andresen-Häupl Activator. He also added a midline jackscrew to the lower lingual plate. This solved two problems: (1) The original Bionator had a high incidence of fracture in this area, so this allowed for simple strengthening of the appliance. (2) It also allowed for the lateral expansion of the dental arches to a certain degree. He also eliminated the buccinator retraction loops and added a labial cap of acrylic to the lower lingual portion of the appliance to prevent the supraeruption of the lower anteriors. This anterior cap also provided a surface against which the upper anteriors could articulate. The lip of the cap also prevented the lower anteriors from being "dumped" forward. So what we now have is a Bionator that is not actually a Bionator, and a functional appliance that is not purely functional. The jackscrew in the lower anterior area makes this appliance part active plate. But as fair Juliet once mused from her balcony, "What's in a name?"

The appliance we use here in America is incorrectly referred to as a Bionator. But it is a name that has become so ingrained in the general orthodontic community that to change it now would be not only academic but unnecessary. We have what we need, the best appliance available today to meet our goals. It is the end product of a long series of evolutionary "appliance mutations," but stands squarely and firmly on the broad and brawny shoulders of its Neanderthal predecessor, the somewhat distant and more primitive Andresen-Häupl Activator, to which it owes its lineage. But this meandering trail of appliance evolution is not yet quite complete, as there is still one more step to traverse. That final step is to the level of what may be termed as the "super-Bionator" of the present day which we will discuss shortly: the Orthopedic Corrector I.

"Simplify, simplify"

Henry David Thoreau
1817–1862

APPLIANCE DESIGN

Along with the attributes of efficiency and ease of manipulation by both the clinician and the patient, simplicity of design is one of the most important hallmarks of a great functional appliance. Considering all that it does, when it comes to this particular trait, the Bionator is all-time champion. It is truly the essence of conservative use of materials. Nothing is wasted. All that exists on the appliance has a specific purpose, usually several coinciding at once. Therefore before attempting to change or adjust any of the component parts of this appliance, it would be in the clinician's best interest to understand their respective purposes fully, for some are truly not what they appear at first sight.

The Labial Guide Bow

This is the first text that refers to the labial bow as a "guide" bow. Actually that's what it is. When the appliance is inserted in the mouth, the only way a patient can close on it is in a protruded mandibular position. The side plates of the appliance have interproximal projections of acrylic on them which nestle into the interproximal spaces of all bicuspid and molar teeth. But when the patient speaks, or for any other reason moves the jaw up and down, the proprioceptive sensory nerves of the maxillofacial complex sense the smooth coordinated action of the labial bow as it slides up and down over the six upper anterior teeth and gingivae. These receptors help activate the orofacial muscles to keep the mandible in the protruded position as it closes to keep the appliance moving vertically in a smooth and coordinated motion. Patients learn to do this surprisingly quickly and have no trouble preventing the "crash" of the bow against the incisal edges of the upper teeth during closing by the mistake of not having the jaw protruded enough. The labial guide bow also acts to hold the inner surface of the upper lip away from the premaxilla and anterior teeth. The space or clearance of about 1 mm or less between the wire and the labial surfaces of the teeth is sufficient to break the directness of the force vector of the weight and strain of the upper lip in this area. This is very important because it must be remembered that when the patient is wearing the appliance, the increased vertical dimension of the occlusion of the rest position puts a myotonic tension on the perioral musculature. This tension is also increased when the lips attempt to seal during swallowing. This increased upper lip pressure can rotate a premaxilla, teeth and all, right down in a distal direction without something to stop it. Hence the labial bow. Anchored against the acrylic base of the appliance, and by means of this through force vectors to the mesial of the upper first molars, the labial guide bow holds the upper lip out away from the teeth and bone just enough that little or no movement of this type will occur. This is also why the bow needs periodic adjustment to be kept from contacting these teeth. Adjustments are performed of this nature every 4 to 5 weeks. The myotonic stretch placed on the orofacial muscles by the appliance with the mandible in a protruded position causes a *distal drive*[35,40,41] to be exerted on the maxillary teeth through the interproximal evaginations of acrylic. As the musculature gently, yet steadily attempts to pull the mandible back to the original pretreatment Class II position, it exerts a force on the maxillary posterior teeth to drive them distally. In so doing, the appliance ends up in a more distal position cephalometrically relative to its starting place at the beginning of treatment. Since the premaxilla and upper anterior teeth are not bound by either the labial bow or any appliance acrylic, they feel none of this distal drive. As a result they stay in the same relative cephalometric position while the posterior segments of teeth and the entire appliance itself drifts distally. (Special note: this is especially so in cases where second molars have been removed. However, in cases of skeletal Class II mandibular advancement with Bionator-type treatment in which there is a complete absence of any form of crowding, Dr Witzig prefers to leave the second molars in place until the completion of treatment. At that time the option exists of removing either the second or third molars as per the dictates of patient age, other needs of the case, and/or the treating clinician's own preference. The labial guide bow trails along behind it until it holds up against something, namely the maxillary anteriors. Unless the labial guide bow is adjusted at this point to be kept away from the anterior teeth, this distalizing process will not be able to continue as the appliance will "hang up" on the premaxilla. The force of appliance movement in the distalizing direction caused by the stretched musculature is not strong enough to push both the posterior segments and the anterior premaxilla in a distal direction at the same time. But on the other hand, this may be desirable in some cases. For instance, in many Class II Division 1, cases, it is for this specific reason that the appliance is able to correct the protrusion of the premaxilla and the flaring out of the upper anterior teeth. If the labial guide bow is adjusted so as to make light contact with these teeth, the combination of lip weight and a slight distal drive is enough to pull the premaxilla with the protruding teeth into a more correct, less protruded arch form. This is what is known as pulling the premaxilla "down." If, when this type of movement is needed, the labial wire is adjusted to contact the gingival one third of the crowns of the upper anterior teeth, it will produce predominantly a downward force. However, by adjusting the labial guide bow to contact the anterior teeth closer to the incisal edges, both a downward and lingual pressure will be applied. But these pressures are not great.

Since the greatest amount of myotonic tension exists during the first 3 months the appliance is worn, before the muscles and mandible have repositioned themselves, the labial bow is usually kept off of the front teeth at this time to take full advantage of the distalizing forces made available to push the maxillary posterior segments distally and aid in the correction of Class II to Class I. During the fourth month of treatment this vector of tension is less; so the labial guide bow is then adjusted down onto contact with the maxillary anteriors. The increased vertical dimension of the mandible relative to the maxilla at this time produces a force vector of stretch on the orbicularis oris against the premaxilla to assist in the rotation of the teeth and bone to a more conventional arch form. In cases where there is severe maxillary protrusion, the labial guide bow must be adjusted at quite regular intervals, sometimes as often as every 2 weeks. However, the amount of correction of premaxillary protrusion, or upper anterior flaring, possible by the above method is limited. If protrusion of the upper anteriors is formidable, arch preparation with appliances specifically designed for such purposes prior to Bionator insertion is indicated.

The early activators used the labial bow for the active movement, rotation, and tipping of maxillary anterior teeth. But these earlier appliances had palatal acrylic (or if they were really early, vulcanite) in their designs that butted up against the lingual surfaces of these teeth and acted as a fulcrum point against which the bow could be activated to gain mechanical advantage and exert active forces on the teeth. Bionators, of course, are open in the anterior palatal area. So this type of rotational active movement is difficult at best. Ironically this labial bow, so often associated with active movement or retention of teeth in so many other appliances and retainers, is one of the most passive and truly functional components of the Bionator.

The Coffin Spring

Another piece of hardware on this appliance is the famous Coffin spring. Shaped like the Greek letter "omega," it is nothing new in orthodontics, for it too goes back to the 1880s as part of an active plate made of vulcanite and piano wire! Today it serves three main functions to the Bionator.

First, many feel it acts as a tongue trainer. It helps correct the deviant swallowing pattern and tongue thrust by causing the base of the tongue to seal itself against the soft palate during swallowing and thus prevents the tip of the tongue from slamming up against the lingual surfaces of the anterior teeth and the premaxillary rugae area.

Secondly, the Coffin spring can be used as an active component in moving the buccal posterior segments laterally. In unison with opening the midline labial expansion screw, it may be adjusted with a three-pronged pliers to expand gradually along with the rest of the appliance when moderate amounts of arch widening are desired.

Thirdly, but not least importantly, for entirely practical reasons the Coffin spring is great for giving the appliance strength, durability, and stability in the mouth.

Acrylic Side Plates

The acrylic side plates, or wings, perform two important functions. First, the surfaces facing the teeth have interproximal projections of acrylic on them that hold the jaws in a super-Class I position. The mandible has to be in this position in order to close properly so that each acrylic projection intermeshes with its appropriate interdental space. Secondly, the surfaces of the wings facing the tongue, which are smooth, act as a screen holding the tongue out of the way of the posteriors preventing the tongue from widening out over the occlusal surfaces of these teeth. This eliminates the tongue as an obstacle to the desired alveolar bone growth needed to correct insufficient vertical.[56] But the acrylic wings can have a slight "active plate" component to them also. For as the midline screw and Coffin spring

---

Figure 2-15 (A) (B) Labial Guide Bow. Note on this transluminated set of clear plastic models how the wire exits at distal cuspid area, loops up over cuspid eminence, then courses across upper anteriors at their gingival third, about 1 mm from the labial surfaces of the crowns of the teeth.

Figure 2-16 Coffin Spring. Clear plastic models divulge position of Coffin spring relative to palatal vault and roots of maxillary teeth.

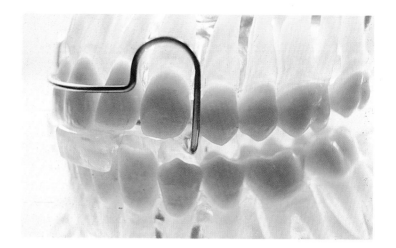

(A)

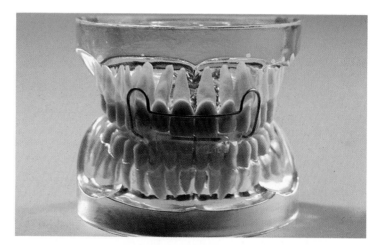

(B)

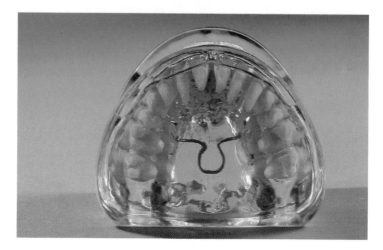

Figure 2-16

are expanded gradually, the side plates gently push against the lingual surfaces of the upper and lower posterior teeth and gingivae simultaneously to moderately widen the dental arches. The greatest amount of active plate effect is produced in the lower anterior area where the combination of acrylic and expansion screw have their most direct effect. A certain amount of lower anterior crowding may be relieved by means of opening the midline screw and adjusting the acrylic properly as it expands bilaterally. The interproximal projections of acrylic also act as interdental wedges to "crack everything loose" tooth movement–wise in the beginning stages of treatment. This is accomplished by simply having the patient open the midline screw a small amount to cause the acrylic to "wedge" into the interproximal spaces, thus breaking the contacts. It is these same projections which are ground off later to speed up the increase in vertical dimension. This will be discussed in more detail in the section on adjustments. The guiding surfaces between these interproximal projections serve to direct the supraerupting posterior teeth in the desired occlusal-facial direction.

Figure 2-17 **(A)** Interproximal projections of acrylic (IPAs) wedge interproximally between posterior teeth. **(B)** Critical IPA mesial to upper first molar. This particular IPA is never reduced as it acts as the anchoring portion of appliance against maxillary dental arch. **(C) (D)** One of the purposes of the appliance's acrylic wings is to prevent "lateral thrusting" of the tongue during swallowing out over posterior teeth impeding their natural eruption, and contributing to deep bite problems. Note seemingly bilateral posterior open bite in this case in both right (C) and left (D) posterior quadrants. **(E) (F)** When the patient swallows note how tongue occludes open space thus perpetuating inhibited eruption of these teeth. Chronic tongue posture over posterior teeth during non-swallowing functions is also thought by some to contribute to poor vertical development. Acrylic wings of Bionator keep tongue out of these areas.

Figure 2-18 **(A)** Anterior Bite Plane or Cap. **(B)** As anterior cap area is expanded laterally (a) by activation of mid-line expansion screw, the effect on the four lower anteriors is dependent on interproximal acrylic (at points marked x). Slight cuspid rotation may also be possible under certain circumstances. Dumping lower anteriors forward is also a possibility provided the lip of the cap is removed (c) to allow anteriors to tip forward, as mandible tends to draw back during early months of treatment due to muscle tension. (*Courtesy of Schwarz, AM, Gratzinger, M:* Removable Orthodontic Appliances, *Philadelphia, WB Saunders Co. 1966.*)

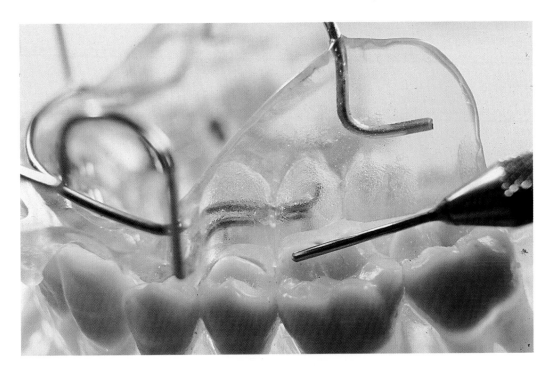

(A)

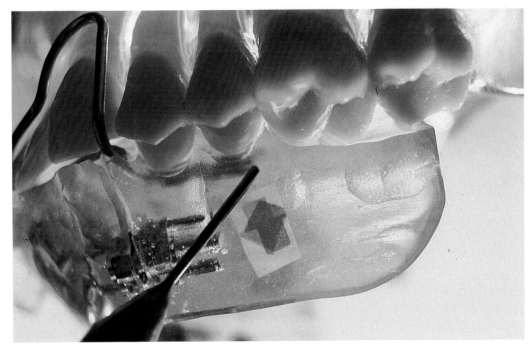

(B)

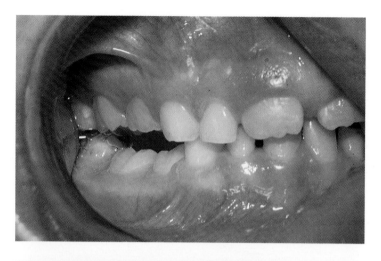

(C)

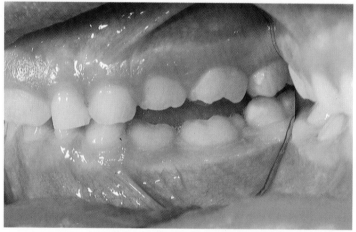

(D)

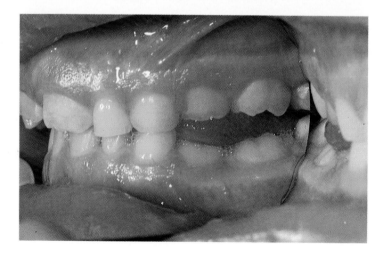

(E)

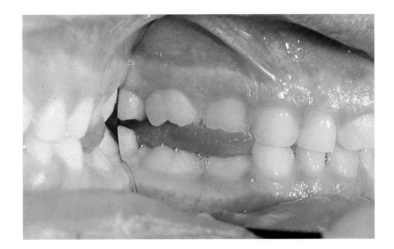

(F)

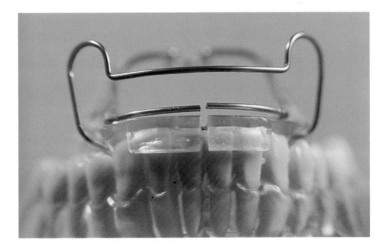

Figure 2-18A

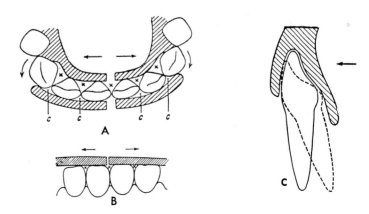

Figure 2-18B

The Anterior Cap

The anterior cap serves first of all as a bite plane against which the anterior incisors articulate. It can be easily seen that the thickness of this plate is what is responsible for the interincisal distance, hence the amount of myotonic stretch felt by the jaws while the appliance is in the mouth. The anterior acrylic cap lips over the edge of the lower incisor teeth just enough to formally catch them and prevent them from being flared forward. It must be remembered that during appliance wear all the facial musculature is stretched and is straining to pull the mandible back to its more retruded original position. With the appliance braced against the maxilla, this delivers a distal drive to the maxillary posterior segments. But it also correspondingly delivers an anterior drive via the lower lingual plate area to the lower incisors. Sometimes this anterior movement is desirable and the cap can be adjusted so as to permit labial crown torque.[57] The inner surface of the cap area should be smooth and free of any interdental projections of acrylic and should not impinge too tightly on the lingual gingivae.

Expansion Screws

At one time there were more than 250 different brands of orthodontic expansion screws on the market. Several have survived to this day and have proved themselves worthy over the years with an excellent performance record. Screws of inferior quality will have a tendency to "back-turn" on themselves and close under the intense pressures of the oral environment.

The midline screw, added to the Bionator by Schmuth, surrenders the purity of the appliance as a functional apparatus, and places it partly in the realm of the active plate. It is so common an addition that here in America, if a laboratory receives an order for a Bionator, it automatically places this screw in the appliance whether specified or not. One quarter of a complete revolution of the central cylinder expands the screw by 0.25 mm. One complete 360-degree revolution is equal to one full millimeter. As stated previously, this midline screw also lends strength to the appliance at its naturally weakest point.

Orthopedic Corrector Side Screws

At this point we should delve into just what the Orthopedic Corrector I is. It is the brain child of Dr John Witzig, and represents the next step up

Figure 2-19 **(A)** Mid-line Expansion Screw. **(B)** Screw opened. **(C)** Position of mid-line expansion screw relative to lower anterior teeth. (*Courtesy of Ohlendorf Co., St. Louis, MO.*)

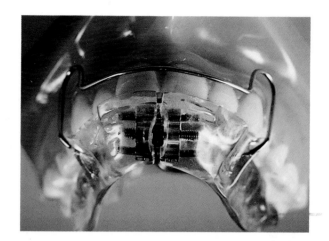

(A)

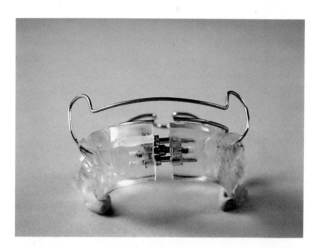

(B)

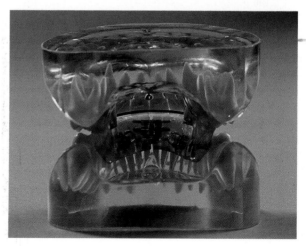

(C)

from the level of the Bionator to that of what might be termed a super-Bionator. It is an appliance that is identical to the original Bionator except for one important addition. Dr Witzig knew that some cases required so much mandibular advancement that the construction bite for the appliance could not be taken in a far enough forward position to accomplish the complete change from Class II to Class I. This was usually due to the patient's inability to tolerate having their jaw comfortable in such a protruded state. Originally, the simple solution at that time was the "two-Bionator" treatment plan. The first appliance was made from a construction bite that was taken as far forward as the patient could comfortably tolerate. After a period of treatment with this first Bionator, the jaw would be repositioned about half of the desired distance from Class II to Class I, at which time new models were taken and a new construction bite was made in a more protruded position still. Since the mandible had already been repositioned part of the way forward in the previous months by the first Bionator, the new construction bite could now be taken in the fully corrected position without undue stress to the patient. It was the second Bionator that allowed the doctor to treat the case to completion.

The Orthopedic Corrector I is nothing more than a Bionator with a set of side screws mounted on either side of the lower lingual area that when opened allow the lower anterior cap to advance more protrusively than the rest of the main body of the appliance. As the side screws are gradually opened, the cap moves more labially; and in order to close the lower anterior teeth into the undersurface of the cap correctly, the mandible must be steadily protruded by the corresponding amount. Of course, when this process has begun, the interproximal acrylic projections between the lower posterior teeth must be ground down so that the teeth do not collide with them as the mandible slides forward in the newer, more protrusive position. It must be remembered that the main bulk of the body of the appliance anchored against the maxilla stays in the same relative position. Therefore, these additional side screws prevent the need for making a whole second appliance in severe skeletal Class II cases where the first appliance would only be capable of taking the mandible half the distance or less to the desired treatment end. It must also be remembered that the mandible must always be protruded beyond the true end position desired at completion of treatment. If the mandible is protruded only to the ideal position and not beyond, the true final position will never be realized by the mandible as there is a certain minimal amount of "stretch" that must be effected by the insertion of

Figure 2-20 **(A)** Orthopedic Corrector Side Screws. **(B)** OCI mid-line screw. Forestadent 01-150-1522 flanked by two 01-134-1315 expansion screws in the Orthopedic Corrector configuration. (*Courtesy of European Orthodontic Products, St. Paul, MN.*)

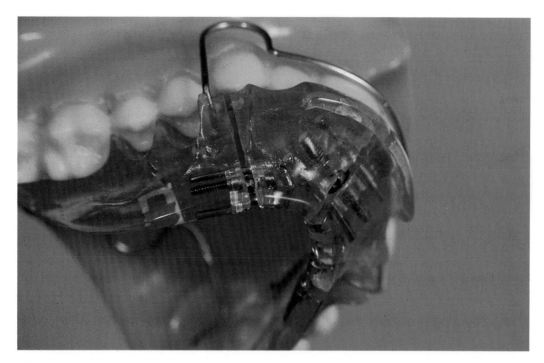

(A)

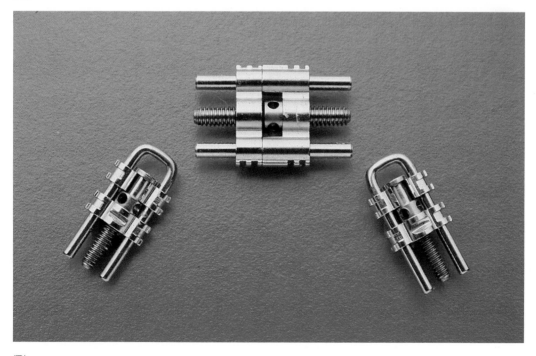

(B)

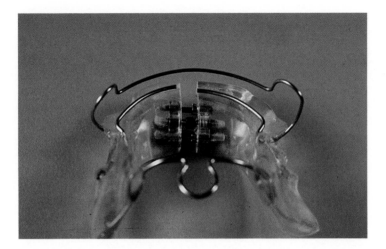

Figure 2-21 Lingual Retention Wire. In this instance the wire is shown after being cut to accommodate mid-line expansion screw activation.

the appliance before any changes will appear in the mandible's permanent position. Merely protruding the mandible 1 to 2 mm past its pretreatment physiologic rest position (albeit retruded) will not be enough to stimulate growth or permanent advancement. Therefore the appliance-induced protrusion should always be at least several millimeters past the ideal end-of-treatment position. Careful government of appliance wear prevents any possible (though highly improbable) development of posttreatment Class III mandibular positioning.

Lingual Retention Wire

The lingual retention wire is a component of the Bionator that has a considerable degree of confusion and discord associated with it. Sometimes it is used, sometimes not. But when it *is* used, it must be used properly.

The original purpose of the wire, usually of a 0.040 gauge, is to act as a buttress against the lingual surfaces of the four upper anterior teeth to prevent their migration lingually. This is very important in cases where the upper anteriors are in an original pretreatment, Division 2, retruded-type angulation. Before the Bionator may be inserted, the excessive vertical inclination of the upper anteriors must be corrected with techniques designed to impart labial crown torque to the offending upper incisors. Once these upper anteriors are torqued labially, they must be retained there. Since the Bionator has a natural built-in tendency to pull the upper premaxilla down and in (mostly in), this would be contraindicated in a case that has just had the upper four anteriors pushed out labially prior to Bionator insertion. Hence the value of the lingual retention wire. It is always used on Bionators that follow Division 2 arch form correction techniques, being fitted snugly against the cingula of the advanced incisors to aid in retention.

Conversely, if the case starts out as a Class II, Division 1, the opposite would be true. The upper anteriors start out being torqued too far labially and the retracting aspects of the Bionator on these teeth are highly desirable. But if the lingual wire is processed into an appliance used for such purposes, the snug fit of the wire along the cingula of the upper anteriors would defeat this purpose. Hence in these circumstances, the wire is left *off* the appliance. But the status of the maxillary anterior incisor angulation is not the only factor to consider when determining whether or not to incorporate the lingual retention wire into the Bionator. Another element to consider is the behavior of the tongue.

Tongue thrusts are a major etiologic factor in many anterior open bite problems.[58-61] (This will be discussed further in subsequent chapters.) One of the handy aspects of the lingual wire is that it may be commandeered from its original design purposes to act as an aid in retraining a forward thrusting tongue in both the conventional Bionator and the specialized Bionators designed to close down anterior open bites (also discussed in subsequent chapters). It may not normally be a standard component of such appliances, but if it's felt that tongue thrust is of major concern in the makeup of a particular case, its use may prove quite valuable and should be specified on the laboratory prescription.

Thus, it may be seen that this particular little wire should be given special attention when specific appliance designs for Bionators are considered.

"If the hive is disturbed by
rash or stupid hands,
instead of honey,
it will yield us bees."

Ralph Waldo Emerson
Essay VII "Prudence"

ADJUSTMENTS

Though stories exist of patients being given Bionators and having "disappeared" from the office for 6 months at a time only to return having everything lining up perfectly, it is not the general rule nor the advised method of approach for treatment but rather the exception. It has been stated that the less you do to these appliances, the better. This also is a gross simplification. It is true that the major amount of orthopedic and orthodontic treatment is actually done by the appliance itself, but this assumes the careful guidance and supervision of the patient by the treating doctor. The adjustments performed on these appliances are what govern and guide the direction and flow of the treatment. It is by means of various adjustments to the appliance that the doctor keeps control over the case and brings about the desired treatment results for his patient. The adjustments are a very important part of functional appliance therapy. They can be easily facilitated and understood by the treating doctor, yet it is the adjustment of these appliances that brings the most amount of concern, apprehension, and confusion to the neophyte when first beginning treatment with these methods. After careful analysis, it can be seen that there is no magic to the methods of the Bionator nor the way it accomplishes what it does. The adjustments of the appliance are logical steps taken for specific purposes in order to obtain very clear-cut results. It is by means of these adjustments that treatment is facilitated and expedited in the attainment of goals set about by the treatment plan. By correctly administering the adjustments at the proper time, treatment time is reduced and better results can be obtained. It must be remembered that the idea behind a functional appliance like the Bionator is to cause the mouth to readapt around the appliance and to reshape itself around the object that resides intraorally in a growing, functioning matrix. As the mouth, jaws, muscles, and teeth reshape and readapt themselves around the guiding slopes of this object, the adjustments to the appliance do nothing more than help stimulate these adaptions to take place more quickly and easily. Adjusting these appliances during treatment is very similar to placing ropes on a small tree in order to hold it straight until its growth is well along the way. Adjustments are nothing more than applied common sense. It can mean the difference between a case where the doctor has to struggle over a protracted period of time to obtain mediocre results, and a case where the doctor is gratified by an expedient, complete, and beautiful conclusion.

As stated earlier in this chapter, the Bionator is an *arch-aligning* appliance. It is assumed that the maxillary and mandibular arches are of a reasonably traditional Roman arch shape when the appliance is inserted. However, it is realized that in all practicality very few cases will be seen where the upper and lower arches are already of desirable Roman arch shape merely needing realignment from Class II to Class I. Most cases will be initially compromised in maxillary and/or mandibular arch form to some degree. In many instances the arches will be suffering from some form of arch deformity, the most common of which is a tendency toward a more pointed or "Gothic arch" shape. Generally cases requiring mandibular advancement also require slight to moderate amounts of lateral development. The adjustments of the Bionator and Orthopedic Corrector are therefore divided into four basic categories.

The first is that group of adjustments concerned with lateral "expansion," or more correctly, "development." The second is concerned with that of increasing vertical. To be technically correct, there should be a third category for the Orthopedic Corrector I, and that is for those adjustments concerned with secondary mandibular advancements. Not all adjustments fall under these categories of course. The fourth is that concerned with patient comfort, individual tooth movements, or other specific problems that arise. But again, this miscellaneous group of mavericks is governed by the same principles that governed the other adjustments, and that is: the common sense steps taken to provide a specified result. What does the doctor want, and what does the patient need, and what must be done to the appliance in order to respond to these needs?

Insertion Adjustments

At the initial insertion appointment, sometimes certain adjustments are made to seat the appliance correctly in the patient's mouth or simply to allow the appliance to be inserted without patient discomfort. One of the first things the doctor might observe upon inserting the appliance into the patient's mouth is that the loops of the labial bow might impinge on the gingival tissues around the cuspids causing discomfort. Either by using the fingers or, preferably, a three-pronged pliers, the labial bow can be adjusted so that it clears the gingival tissue around the maxillary anterior teeth by approximately a millimeter. It should not contact either the teeth or the gingivae anywhere along its course from one side of the maxillary arch to the other. The top of the loop of the labial bow, as it courses over the gingivae of the cuspid area, is the most common site for this offense. Simple and easy adjustment of the wire with appropriate pliers relieves this situation.

Another problem often encountered when appliances are first inserted is that the acrylic wings might impinge too tightly upon the gingival tissue in the submandibular areas. The acrylic of the submandibular area extends down below the gingival crest of the posterior teeth in a fashion somewhat similar to a mandibular denture. These flanges should not extend into the sublingual area but merely extend as far as 2 or 3 mm below the lowest depression of the gingivae along the lingual surface of the mandibular molars. Should these wings impinge on the gingivae, a sore spot identical to that of an improperly fitting denture will appear. Usually the patients can detect the pressure of the acrylic on the gum tissue immediately and can point out the specific area at fault. Simple reduction with acrylic burs is all that is necessary followed by slight polishing to obtain a satin finish. Occasionally a small bubblelike projection of acrylic will be left after processing the appliance. Again the patient will detect this immediately. Simple visual inspection and reduction with acrylic burs alleviates the problem.

Occasionally a Coffin spring will press against the palatal tissues excessively causing a slight indentation on the palatal gingivae. This again is easily adjusted with a three-pronged pliers. The posterior margin of the palatal wings in the Coffin spring area should also be inspected so as not to impinge on the palatal tissues too firmly. This would also result in a denturelike ulceration.

Most of these problems are infrequent and insertion of the appliance goes smoothly. The chief concern of the patient is always the odd feeling of having a "mouthful" of acrylic, but a positive and encouraging attitude should always be displayed by the doctor as initial impressions are important for the patient. The patient should always be complimented and encouraged on how well they managed to insert the appliance and fit it to their mouth. At this time it is important to instruct the patient that their mouth will "water" for a day or so until they become accustomed to the appliance and that their speech will be inhibited slightly. But at this time it is also good to remind them of the story of Demosthenes. He was the Greek orator who lived over 2000 years ago and was burdened in his young manhood with a speech impediment. In an effort to overcome this handicap, he went down to the seashore every day, put small pebbles in his mouth and practiced talking, enunciating, and articulating every syllable he spoke to the point where, even with a mouthful of rocks, he could be clearly and distinctly heard over the sound of the waves. He grew up to become the greatest Athenian orator that ever lived. Sometimes it's the patient and not the appliance that needs the adjustment.

*"Science is organized
knowledge."*

*Herbert Spencer
English Philosopher
1820–1903*

Figure 2-22 **(A)** To open cuspid loop of labial guide bow, flat portion of flat-on-round pliers is placed on inside of loop bend. When using small 3-pronged pliers, single prong is placed outside loop bend. To close cuspid loop, plier actions are reversed. **(B)** Compensatory bends are placed at bend in wire where it courses across labial surface of teeth to keep it at proper horizontal level with respect to crowns.

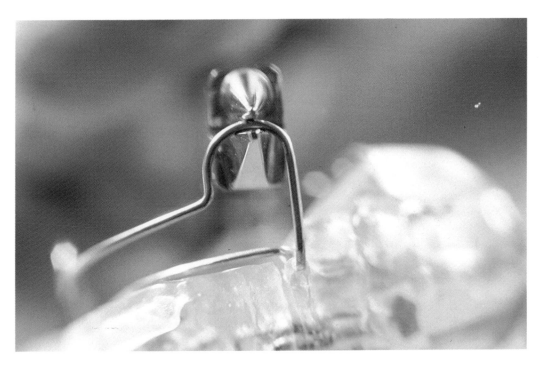

(A)

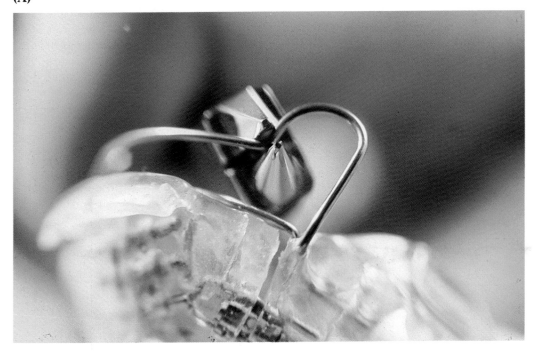

(B)

Adjustments to Widen the Arches

Arch widening was not the primary purpose for which the Bionator (Orthopedic Corrector I) was designed, but it can accomplish moderate amounts of this type of movement by virtue of opening the midline screw in the lower anterior cap area and expanding the Coffin spring.[62] It must be remembered that the appliance expands both the maxillary and mandibular arches simultaneously. So if a discrepancy exists in arch size between the upper and lower, the smaller arch, usually the upper, should be expanded to the appropriate corresponding size independently before the Bionator is inserted. If the Bionator is used to expand a lower anterior arch laterally, the upper arch will not be expanded by the same amount. Relief of moderate crowding in the lower anterior area is the Bionator's main forte as far as lateral development is concerned. Slight lateral development posteriorly may be realized by concomitant Coffin spring expansion.

Lateral development in the lower anterior area is usually the first adjustment made in the treatment time-line after initial insertion appointment adjustments and after "priming" the appliance with several once-a-week turns. After the first month of wear, which allows for the appliance to "settle in" and the patient to accomodate to it, lateral mandibular anterior arch development may be initiated if desired. Expansion screws are commonly used for this purpose. The patient is instructed to turn the midline screw one 90-degree increment once every Sunday. They operate on a principle that one 360-degree revolution of the central cylinder expands the wings of the jackscrew apart by 1.0 mm. Therefore, one 90-degree quarter turn expands by 0.25 mm. This minute amount of expansion is easily tolerated by the patient as it merely "snuggles" the appliance firmly against the inner walls of the upper and lower jaws. After 1 week the expansion has taken place and the appliance once again fits loosely in the mouth, ready for the next turn of the screw. The patient feels no discomfort during this time whatsoever.

Upon initiating lateral development after the first month of wear, it is very important to remember to cut the lingual retaining wire, if present, that runs lingual to the upper anteriors at the midline to allow the appliance to expand. Once this lingual wire is cut, the two halves of the appliance are held together by only three metal objects: (1) the labial bow, (2) the midline jackscrew, and (3) the Coffin spring. As the appliance screw gradually expands, the labial guide bow and the Coffin spring require periodic ad-

---

Figure 2-23 **(A)** Lingual retention wire should be cut prior to screw expansion. It also may be cut and bent to apply pressure in a labial direction to a tooth, although this is not its primary function. **(B)** Expansion screw opened.

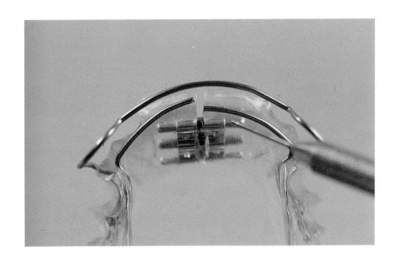

(A)

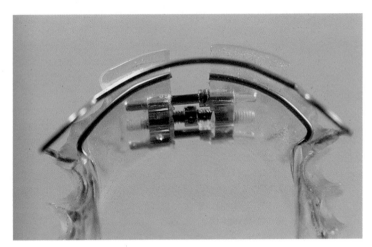

(B)

justment to allow undistorted expansion of the appliance to continue smoothly.

Since the appliance expands laterally by 1 mm per month as a result of one-quarter revolution or one 90-degree turn every week, and since the patient is seen at approximately 4- to 6-week intervals, the normal monthly check appointment is the appropriate time to adjust the Coffin spring and labial guide bow.

To expand the Coffin spring, simply place a three-prong pliers in the apex of the loop with the two prongs on the concave surface and the single middle prong on the convex surface of the loop and flatten out the curve by squeezing the pliers just enough to feel the wire give or "kink" slightly. This expands the loop and pushes the posterior sections of the acrylic wings of the appliance laterally to keep up with the lateral expansion of the appliance in the anterior cap region provided by the midline expansion screw. Using a flat-on- flat or similar pliers, place slight compensatory bends at the corners of the omega bends to relieve the stress in the wire at these two areas that occurs after the initial expansion of the loop of the Coffin wire. Only slight pressure is needed so as to just be able to observe a small change in the wire. Excessive pressure would overexpand the appliance posteriorly resulting in poor fit. But with a little practice and judicious use of the pliers, the technique can easily be mastered. The "feel" is similar to that used when adjusting wrought wire clasps on temporary acrylic partial dentures. Coffin spring adjustment, however, is much more forgiving. After expanding, the appliance can be inserted into the mouth and the patient will usually be able to detect the extra snugness of fit in the posterior areas.

This process may be continued until the appliance has been expanded 4, 5, or even 6 mm. As always with any form of expansion, *overcorrect* a little to allow for a slight amount of relapse. However, if this much expansion, or development, is needed, it is usually obtained with appliances designed expressly for that purpose prior to Bionator treatment.

Adjusting the labial guide bow for the first 3 months consists of merely keeping the wire off of the anterior maxillary teeth and gingivae. This is not as easy as it sounds, for every time the patient presents himself to the office for routine monthly checking appointments during the first 3 or 4 months, it seems as if the labial bow is always riding right down on the facial surfaces of the maxillary centrals or laterals or riding on the gingivae over the cuspids. Adjustments are then made with various wire-bending pliers to keep the wire 1 mm away from the teeth and gingivae. The patient is dismissed only to return next month with the wire right down on the gums and enamel again!

Figure 2-24 **(A)** Expansion bend of Coffin Spring to widen appliance posteriorly. **(B)** Compensatory bends to relieve tension in wire caused by expansion bend of loop portion of spring.

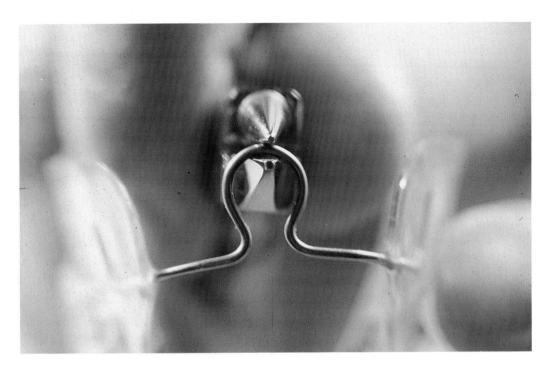

(A)

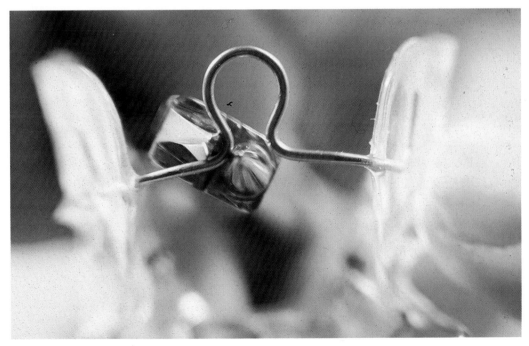

(B)

Adjustment procedures for the labial guide bow are similar to that of the Coffin spring with respect to compensatory bends. Expand the canine loops with a three-prong pliers, first one side, then the other. Then the bow will be out and away from the anterior area, but the bow will cross over the anterior teeth at a raised level compared to its position prior to the adjustment. So with a small flat-on-flat or curved-on-flat pliers, place compensatory bends at the angles where the bow makes a 90-degree turn at the end of the canine loop to cross over the anterior teeth. Open the angle slightly to a more obtuse degree until the bow travels across at the desired level relative to the clinical crowns of the teeth. But with time the bow drifts toward the teeth again.

This is due to two reasons. The first is a result of the lateral expansion of the appliance which we have just discussed. As the appliance expands slowly, the distance between the flanges where the guide-bow wire is inserted on each side of the appliance increases as they separate, and the arc of the bow must necessarily shorten and flatten out slightly. This brings the wire closer to the labial surfaces of the teeth. But this is not the major reason for the drift of the bow toward the teeth. In fact, it's not even a very important component of the cause. The major reason the bow "drifts inward" is that there is a distal drive applied to the maxilla by the tension of the facial muscles that are stretched as the mandible is held forward in a protruded position. This occurs for about the first 3 or 4 months until the muscles reposition themselves to accommodate to the new jaw position. The distal drive on the maxilla moves the posterior maxillary teeth distally slightly,[62] *especially* if second molars are removed; and in so doing the entire appliance, which anchors against these teeth, drifts distally with them. This in turn brings the labial guide bow, which is trailing behind, into contact with the premaxilla. Hence the need for adjusting the wire.

During the course of lateral development in the lower anterior area, some separation may occur between the lower incisors. This is entirely nor-

Figure 2-25   Over an extended period, Bionator treatment is capable of moderate amounts of arch widening in growing child. **(A) (B)** Pretreatment narrowness of maxillary arch in mixed dentition. **(C) (D)** Correction of arch form by means of moderate amount of lateral development effected by use of mid-line expansion screw anteriorly and activation of Coffin spring posteriorly. No other lateral development or expansion appliances were used on this case. Treatment was initiated at 9 years of age. Three separate Bionators were used over course of treatment and case development.

Figure 2-26   **(A) (B)** Commonly observed examples of eruptive forces naturally occurring in teeth. Supra-erupted right mandibular first molar due to missing opposing maxillary first molar and second bicuspid (also note distal drift of maxillary first bicuspid).

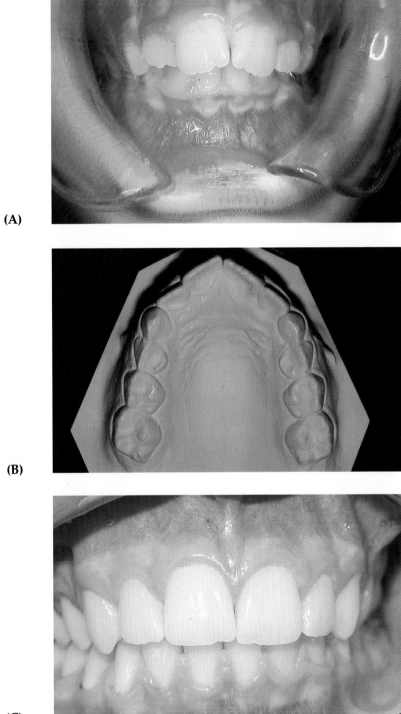

(A)

(B)

(C)

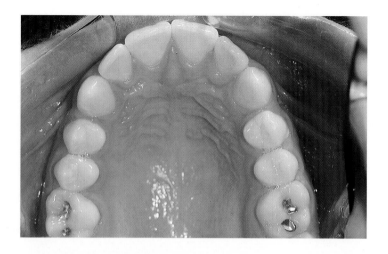

(D)

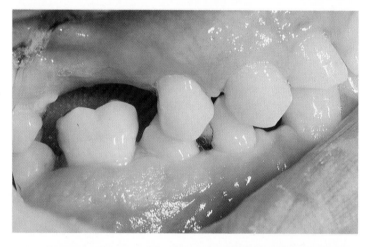

Figure 2-26A

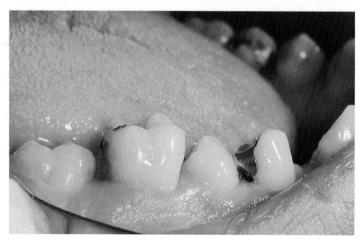

Figure 2-26B

mal and it must be remembered that it is always easier to close spaces than to open them. Teeth always drift forward. As always, overexpand slightly to compensate for slight relapse.

At the completion of this phase of treatment, the space between the flanges at the site of the midline screw may be filled in with quick-cure acrylic and polished to both facilitate appliance strength, stability, and patient tongue comfort.

"Our remedies oft in ourselves do lie,
Which we ascribe to heaven, the fated sky."

All's Well That Ends Well
William Shakespeare

Adjustments to Increase the Vertical

The increase in the vertical dimension of occlusion during Bionator therapy is not so much the result of what the appliance does as what the appliance allows. What it allows is for the inherent natural forces that exist in the alveolar processes to bring about the continued eruption of the posterior teeth, thus opening the bite by bringing the teeth into contact sooner during the arc of mandibular closure.[63-79]

Every dentist has observed patients at one time or another who have had a lower third molar or lower third and second molar removed years previously and as a reult have come to have the upper third molar supra-erupted down into the empty space so that its occlusal surface is well below the plane of occlusion of the remaining maxillary teeth. The phenomenon of mesial drift of posterior teeth into an extraction site anterior to these teeth is also common knowledge. These forces that cause teeth to constantly attempt to erupt occlusally and drift mesially were placed there by Nature to help compensate for occlusal and interproximal wear, keeping the contacts tight and the vertical stable. It is the principle of this force that the Bionator so ingeniously takes advantage of to facilitate the correction of lost or insufficient vertical. These forces are brought into action by the functional stimuli produced by wearing the appliance. Nature does the work; the doctor takes the fee!

The very first adjustments the doctor will make on the appliance to aid in the increase of vertical will be those previously mentioned concerned with the initial insertion of the appliance into the mouth. Soon after the appliance is inserted, there will be a minute increase in vertical as it forces a slight but rapid uprighting of the posterior teeth. Usually the lower molars that are inclined lingually upright slightly as the appliance settles in and snugly nudges into place as it seats itself during the first week of wear. In this action, it is acting more like an active plate, forcing the movement of teeth due to pressure. This effect can also be enhanced in those cases where lingual tipping of posteriors exists by opening the midline expansion screw a little during the first few weeks of treatment. This opening of the screw acts to drive the interproximal projections of acrylic into their respective interproximal spaces and breaks the contacts just enough to aid in getting things moving. One 90-degree turn of the midline expansion screw every Sunday usually does the job. As previously discussed, this process may be continued past the second or third week if moderate lateral lower anterior arch development is required.

After the patient has successfully worn the appliance for a month or so, it should be checked for wear facets on the surfaces of acrylic that cover the lingual cusps of the posterior teeth. These facets are often small and difficult to see. They appear as shiny spots against the satin finish of the acrylic surface. If detected, reduction with a common acrylic bur is recom-

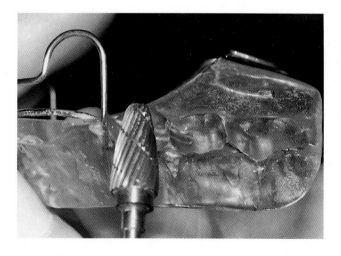

(A)

Figure 2-27 **(A)** Acrylic burs are used to grind away interproximal projections of acrylic (IPAs) from appliance at about three month stage of treatment to allow for vertical eruption of posterior segments. **(B)** As acrylic is reduced, note that care is taken not to touch IPA mesial to maxillary first molar. This portion of appliance must always remain intact as it serves to anchor entire appliance against maxillary dental arch. **(C)** After reduction of anything that might serve to hinder path of vertical eruption of posterior teeth, only acrylic mesial to upper first molar remains. **(D)** Left side of appliance has IPAs reduced properly to allow eruption. Right side remains unadjusted for comparison.

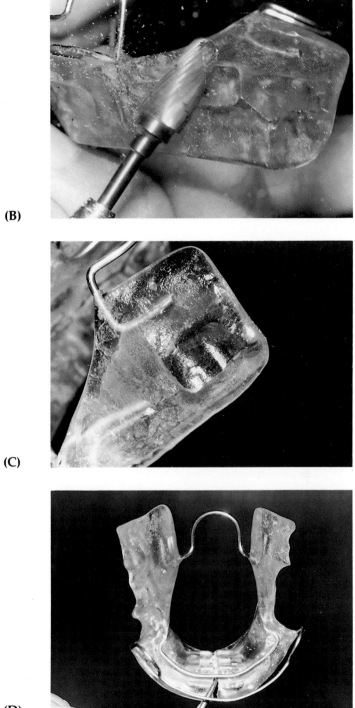

(B)

(C)

(D)

mended, however, some feel their elimination is not that critical of a concern at this time. Later on in treatment their removal *is* critical.

After approximately 3 months of wear, another "fine tuning" type of adjustment can be made. Since the appliance has a distal drive to maxillary posterior teeth, some clinicians feel it aids in the increasing of vertical to reduce the acrylic on the *distal* sides of *maxillary* interproximal projections slightly as this will allow more room for the teeth to be tipped into as they are nudged distally. The acrylic that butts up against the mesial surfaces of the maxillary posteriors is *not* to be touched with the bur; only the acrylic that butts up against the *distal* surfaces of these teeth is to be reduced. Be especially careful not to touch the acrylic that butts against the mesial of the maxillary first molar as that anchors the entire appliance. Some clinicians, however, do not feel that this slight mechanical advantage is significant enough to bother with, and they simply don't do it. It was an adjustment technique far more utilized in conjunction with the older-style Activator therapy.

As the teeth move into their new-found space, slight as it may be as a result of the distal drive of the appliance on the maxilla, the upper posterior teeth are tipped distally, uprighting them slightly which in turn increases the vertical. The first really major adjustments that occur are during the fourth month of wearing the appliance. At that time the acrylic that protrudes into the interproximal spaces between the lower posterior teeth may be reduced by simply grinding them away with acrylic burs. This removes the interferences to eruption that these little projections represent to the individual teeth. Their original purpose was to hold the mandible in the protruded position by interlocking with the teeth. After 3 to 4 months, though the condylar growth is not yet fully complete, the muscles have repositioned themselves enough to hold the mandible in the newer, more advanced and corrected position so that they are no longer needed. With a pencil, mark the crest of acrylic that abuts against the lingual surface of the teeth where they meet with the gingivae. Reduce this ridge of acrylic to allow room for the gingivae to grow and accompany the erupting teeth. *Anything* that contacts the teeth or marginal gingivae will impede eruption and must

---

Figure 2-28 Closing of temporary posterior open bite during Bionator treatment. **(A)** Posterior open bite commonly observed at about half-way point during Bionator therapy when mandible is advanced and actually repositioned with a concomitant increase in muscle length. This always occurs more rapidly than alveolar development vertically, hence posterior open bite. **(B) (C)** This is only temporary, however, and the occlusion eventually comes into full contact and full vertical development during remaining half of Bionator treatment. This process may be speeded up by increasing thickness of acrylic on bite cap.

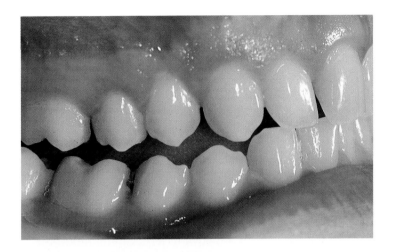

(A)

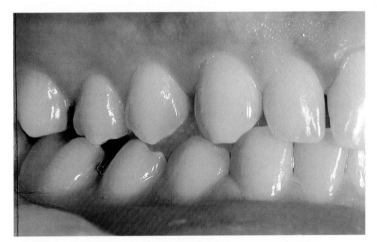

(B)

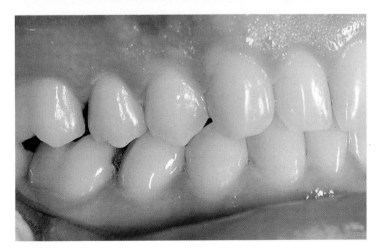

(C)

be removed with acrylic burs. The mandible at this point in time of treatment should be stable enough not to want to draw back. The anterior cap still remains, and that in combination with the muscles is enough to keep the mandible forward. Condylar growth gradually "catches up" to make up the difference, seeking its own level. Therefore, at this time these projections may be removed so the eruption of the lower teeth may proceed at an unhindered, accelerated rate.

It is usually customary to wait until the fifth month to remove the interproximal projections from between the maxillary teeth to take advantage of any remaining distal drive to the maxilla before muscle repositioning causes that force to become diminished. It must be noted that it is of the utmost importance that the acrylic bracing up against the mesial of the maxillary 6-year molars remain *intact* and *not be touched* with the acrylic bur! The reasons for this are obvious after careful reflection. If this is removed, there will be nothing left to brace the appliance against the maxilla, and the first time it is inserted after the acrylic in this critical area is ground away, the appliance will slide distally due to muscle tension and stretch from the lower jaw, and the only thing to stop its distal movement would be the labial bow which would immediately impinge on the maxillary anterior teeth and gingivae.

After 3 to 4 months of wearing the appliance, the tendency toward a posterior open bite develops. This is disconcerting to the doctor unfamiliar with Bionator treatment when he first notices it, but it is a good sign that things are going well and that the patient is wearing the appliance for an adequate amount of time each day. What is happening? The jaw repositions itself faster than the teeth can erupt, a common phenomenon. The patient closes with the anterior teeth in the new corrected position with improved overbite and overjet relations and is unable to "retrude" the mandible to the older pretreatment skeletal Class II retruded position. But at the 4- to 5-month point as the doctor observes the occlusal plane, he sees that a gap appears between the upper and lower posterior occlusal surfaces. This gap is greatest usually at the first bicuspids, diminishes slightly at the second bicuspids, and maybe disappears altogether at the area of the first molars which may or may not be in occlusion. But this situation corrects itself as treatment progresses and the spaces start to close up vertically. The space between the upper and lower first bicuspids closes up *last* as they have the greatest vertical distance to travel. They sometimes close themselves up after all treatment is complete and the appliance has been removed. Grinding away the interproximal acrylic merely gives this process a head start so that it is as close to being occluded as possible at the end of the Bionator treat-

---

Figure 2-29 **(A)** Normal cap thickness. **(B)** Acrylic added to cap to speed posterior eruption.

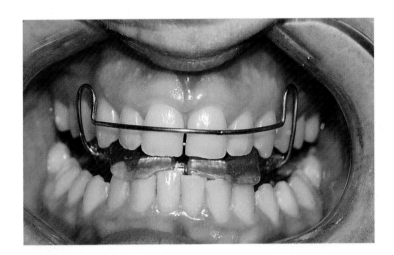

(A)

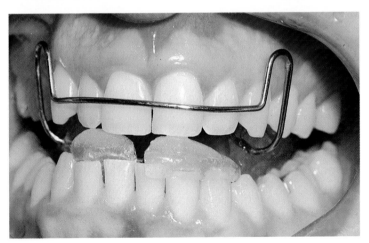

(B)

ment when the appliance is taken away. Both man and Nature appreciate efficiency of time.

Another technique for helping the eruption of the posterior teeth is adding quick-cure acrylic to the superior surface of the anterior cap. If the bite needs to be opened on the appliance to help speed up the increase of vertical, acrylic can be added to the area of the cap where the maxillary incisal edges articulate on the cap's flat surface of acrylic. After applying the quick-cure acrylic in a semipaste form to prevent it from running, the appliance can be inserted into the mouth and the patient instructed to close and hold in the newer, more open bite, usually a 1- to 2-mm increase. When the acrylic becomes fairly firm but not completely set, it may be removed and placed in a bowl of hot water to quicken the setting. It is then trimmed and polished so the new surface of the cap is reasonably flat again. The indentations of the teeth will act as a guide to the level to which it should be polished. Since the incisors are now separated by a greater distance due to the increased thickness of the cap, the posterior teeth will also be separated by an increased amount. This stimulates the posteriors even more to seek out their opposing neighbors, thus speeding up the eruption slightly.

"Where nothing is, a little doth ease."

Fifteenth Century Proverb

Acrylic Projections and the Orthopedic Corrector I (Adjustments to Advance the Mandible)

At this point it would be appropriate to discuss the adjustments concerned with that variant of the Bionator, the Orthopedic Corrector I. It's the addition of the side screws to the Bionator that creates the Orthopedic Corrector. This permits forward repositioning of the front half of the appliance. After about the third or fourth month of wear when the patient's muscles have readjusted themselves enough that the strecth on them is greatly reduced, the side screws of the Orthopedic Corrector I may be activated. This moves the anterior cap and front lower half of the appliance away from the

---

Figure 2-30   (A) As side screws of the Orthopedic Corrector I are activated to advance mandible, lower acrylic projections enveloping lower posterior teeth must be removed **(B)** and **(C)** from both sides of appliance to allow unhindered advancement of mandibular arch.

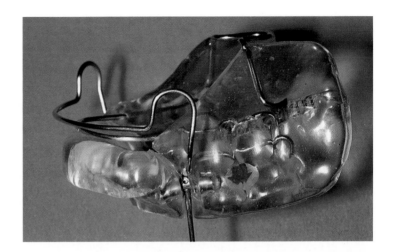

(A)

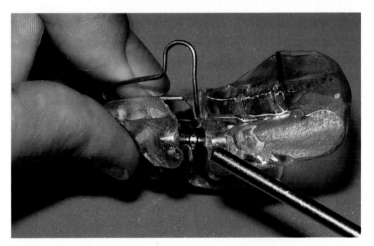

(B)

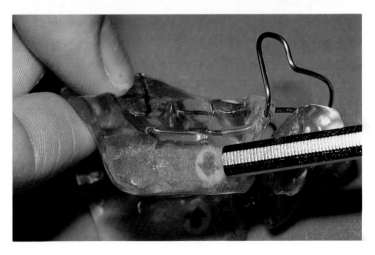

(C)

ORTHOPEDIC CORRECTOR I
Patent Pending

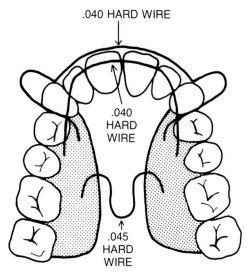

.040 HARD WIRE

.040
HARD
WIRE

.045
HARD
WIRE

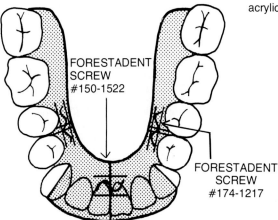

FORESTADENT
SCREW
#150-1522

FORESTADENT
SCREW
#174-1217

(D)

INDICATIONS:
1) Class II to Class I
2) Increase vertical in deep overbite cases
3) Excellent results in skeletal Class II treatment
4) Mixed dentition or permanent dentition treatment

Note 1:
   To this appliance can be added several modifications for specific tooth movement, rotations, tongue training, space closure, etc., depending on the case. These are taught in the advanced technique seminars.

Note 2:
   This appliance will treat the above indications to the finest, most stable results, in the shortest period of time, of all orthopedic or functional appliances in use today.

Construction Note:
   The upper incisors contact the lower incisor acrylic capping.

maxilla, labial bow, lingual wire, and lateral wings, which remain anchored against the maxillary first molars and stay in the same relative cephalometric position. But to correctly enable this process to happen, it is imperative that the acrylic projections between the lower posterior teeth be removed flush with the base of acrylic. For as this portion of the appliance advances as a result of the opening of the lateral expansion screws, the mandible has to protrude farther and farther forward to close into the underside of the cap correctly. With the acrylic wings remaining behind, braced against the maxilla the advancing lower posteriors would crash into the stationary acrylic projections of the lower part of the appliance if they weren't removed. It would be impossible to open the side screws and lengthen the appliance in this manner without making these reductions. This appliance is designed to prevent the need for the construction of a whole second appliance in severely retruded skeletal Class II or TMJ involvement–type cases. One problem occasionally encountered in the Orthopedic Corrector I is the development of ulcers or stripping in the lingual gingival area just below the lower anterior crowns. Careful monitoring of this area during side-screw activation and advancement of the lower cap component of the appliance guards against this event. The acrylic in the lower lingual cap area might have to be relieved in such a way that just the crowns of the lower incisors contact the interior of the cap. This would leave the lower lingual gingival tissue free of contact with cap acrylic.

"It is far more difficult to be simple than to be complicated."

John Ruskin
1819–1900

Miscellaneous Adjustments

For many, whenever their eye first falls on the word "miscellaneous," they automatically think this term to mean "go on to the next part as this is nondescript and unimportant." But the two adjustments listed here are of the *utmost importance* in understanding how to get the most out of a Bionator or Orthopedic Corrector I.

First is the adjustment of the labial bow. As stated previously, it is kept off the teeth and gingivae for the first 3 months of wear. Then at the beginning of the third or fourth month it is adjusted using various favorite wire-bending pliers so that it contacts the maxillary teeth as much as possible to provide, in conjunction with the forces of the upper lip, lingual crown torque to bring these teeth inward when desired. If the wire is adjusted so that it rides across the gingival third of the maxillary anteriors, the resultant force vector of the pressure of the lip and pull of the appliance through the wire will bring about predominantly a *downward* force to this area. However, if the wire is adjusted such that it rides across these teeth at the incisal one third close to the edges, the resultant vector will be in both a *downward and lingual direction*. The area for wire contact selected is a function of the shape of the premaxilla and position of the teeth. The doctor simply chooses the site for wire contact by virtue of the result he desires.

But again, it must be remembered that major orthodontic changes of this type should be taken care of with more efficient appliances and techniques designed for this purpose prior to Bionator therapy. Another thing to remember is that as the crowns of the maxillary anteriors are regressed or torqued lingually by the above process, the *lingual* wire must be cut (if present) at its midpoint and bent back out of the way so as not to interfere with this movement.

Now we shall consider an adjustment procedure that accomplishes the exact opposite of the above. Instead of initiating lingually directed crown torque on the upper anteriors, we shall look at how to flare the lower anterior incisors labially.

The acrylic cap over the lower anterior teeth serves to stabilize the appliance in the mouth and acts as a bite plate to hold the anterior incisors apart. As a result, the entire upper and lower arches are held apart at a prescribed distance which is a product of the thickness of the construction bite. The anterior cap not only comes up to the incisal edges of the lower front teeth but actually lips over the edge and down the facial surfaces of them for 2 or 3 mm. This is because the stretch applied to the facial muscles by the action of the appliance holding the jaw forward causes not only a distal drive to the maxilla but an equal and opposite anterior drive to be expressed in the lower incisor area. If the acrylic cap did not lip over the incisal edges of these teeth, they would be pushed and flared out labially. If this is in fact what is desired, all the doctor has to do is take a fine-pointed acrylic bur and grind the acrylic away that just lips over these incisal edges, but not off the incisal edges themselves, so that the force vector will flare them labially yet not allow supraeruption to occur. This is a simple yet effective method of correcting a higher interincisal angle down to the clinical norm of 130 degrees plus or minus 6 degrees. Many deep bite cases suffer from too high an interincisal angle, ie, the lower anteriors are too straight up and down. They should have a graceful labial flare to them to obtain the desired 130-degree angle relative to the long axis of maxillary incisors.

If during this process of acrylic "lip removal" off the cap an individual tooth requires more movement than the others, it can be moved individually by the acrylic drop method. After some flaring has taken place so that some space starts to develop, a small drop of quick-cure acrylic may be carefully

Figure 2-31   (A) Right side of appliance cap as it appears normally, acting to hold lower anteriors stationary. Left side of appliance has cap removed to "dump" lower anteriors forward during first three months of treatment. **(B)** Intraoral view of Bionator with labial lip of cap removed to tip lower anteriors forward—thereby increasing interincisal angle, and thickened incisal portion to help speed up eruption posteriorly— thereby increasing the vertical.

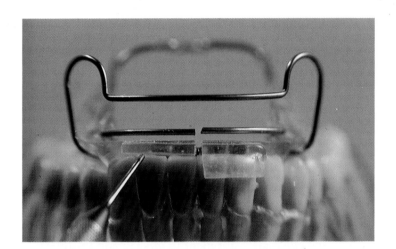

(A)

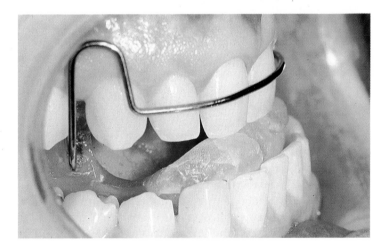

(B)

placed on the inside surface of the cap that butts up against the lingual surface of the tooth in question. This will place more active pressure on the tooth concerned than the others as the appliance seats in the mouth resulting in more rapid labial movement bringing it into line with the others. Care must be taken that not too much acrylic is added as this would result in an unseatable appliance and a sore tooth. A thickness of about 1 mm, or as close as possible, is ideal. It is best to add a sufficient amount, let it harden, and grind it back to the desired thickness. Alternately try the appliance in and out until the patient notices only firm, yet gentle pressure on the given tooth. This step can be repeated every week until the tooth is moved to the desired position. But this technique is adequate for moving these incisors only relatively short distances individually. Grinding the lip off the cap can flare a group of incisors together quite a ways. However, to move one or two teeth 3 or 4 mm, treatment with fixed bands or bonded brackets is easier and quicker. This will be discussed in subsequent chapters.

Once the desired angulation of the lower anteriors is achieved, if the appliance is still required to be worn awhile (2 to 4 months or more), the lip should be added back on to the cap once again to keep the incisors in place and prevent further labial tipping. The best way to do this is simply to "snap" a set of upper and lower alginate impressions, pour them up, and send them to the laboratory along with the appliance where technicians have the adequate equipment to quickly and neatly restore the lip to its proper shape and texture. This can be done in a day if such laboratories are nearby or in five to seven days if done through the mail. (Still not enough time for any significant relapse to take place.) This can be done in the doctor's laboratory, but the procedure must be done by experienced hands and with the aid of a pressure cooker of some sort, for if not done properly, the addition will quickly snap off as it is in an extremely high-stress area. It may also be done directly in the mouth. Add a piece of rope wax to the dried and isolated lower anterior area in the mouth and form it into the interproximal spaces and place the appliance in the mouth. The rope wax across the lower anteriors should leave the top 3 to 4 mm of the crowns exposed at the incisal portion. With the wax as an inferior and lateral border, and the top of the cap as a superior border, you now have an area isolated into which quick-cure acrylic may be added or "flowed in." After initial set, remove carefully and harden in hot water. Trim and polish and the lip is restored.

Another adjustment that might be employed on certain occasions that could be put in this miscellaneous category is the utilization of the lingual wire that runs behind the upper anteriors. Sometimes this can be bent with a three-pronged pliers, either when the wire is still intact or after it has been cut at the midline, such as to place the peak of the kink right behind the lingual surface of a particular tooth to be moved labially. The conditions have to be right to employ this technique, however, since it is difficult at best to achieve. There must be a perfect fit of the wire around the back side of the upper anteriors; and the wire must not be bent into the surface of the tooth too far, as it will not allow the arc of the upper six teeth to be cradled in the sling of the two wires correctly, ie, the labial guide bow and the lingual retention wire. If there is any crowding whatsoever to complicate the movement of the malaligned tooth in question or if the distance it is to be moved labially is too great (2 to 3 mm or more), it is better to level, align, and rotate the teeth to a correct arch form with brackets or other techniques prior to insertion of the Bionator. Never use a device for a purpose other than that for which it was designed in the first place. Saws make poor hammers.

"I agree with no man's opinions.
I have some of my own."

Ivan Turgenev
1818–1883

THE CONSTRUCTION BITE

After obtaining a good set of working models of the upper and lower arches, a construction bite must be taken to send to the laboratory so that the models may be related to one another correctly and the appliance can be constructed. This wax bite is the blueprint for the appliance and determines just how the power of the appliance will be delivered to the tissues, bones, and teeth. It is the most important part of functional appliance therapy aside from the doctor's skills and the patient's cooperation. The ease of treatment, length of duration, and ultimate outcome of the entire case can be determined by this simple little piece of wax.

The development of the technique for taking the wax bite has quite a long and colorful history and it has, as you have probably already guessed, been fraught with controversy.

The debate goes all the way back to the days when Andresen developed the first Activators. He believed the appliance he developed along with Karl Häupl worked on a principle of changing the functional patterns of the muscles by means of stimulating the protractors and elevators and stretching the retractors by means of an appliance that was oversized and yet still passive in the mouth. It did not, however, displace the mandible beyond the physiologic rest position relative to the vertical and was 3 mm short of the limit of the patient's tolerance relative to the protrusive aspect. He believed the appliance delivered intermittent forces to the teeth and bones as the muscles functioned around it, and that the appliance needed to be worn only at night.

The first to oppose this view was Selmer-Olsen[80] who said muscles couldn't be stimulated at night, for this was the time Nature used to give them complete rest. He said it was the stretching of the muscles that was the source of the stimulation, and the corresponding reflexive contraction or possibly even natural tension caused a force to be delivered to the teeth through the direct transmission of force vectors from the intervening appliance. He believed the tooth-moving forces delivered to the teeth by the appliance were a form of potential energy (stretch) and not a representation of kinetic energy (function). He said Andresen's opinion that a vertical opening of more than 2 mm (Andresen recommended a 2- to 4-mm opening between molars relative to vertical bite opening) was *beyond* the physiologic rest position. Selmer-Olsen believed the usual rest position of the mandible during sleep was at an interocclusal distance of 2 mm between the posteriors on the average and any appliance that forces the mandible to a greater distance than that was actually forcing the mandible to reside beyond the rest position vertically. This would therefore induce stretch to the muscles. He believed it was this stretch that caused the eventual orthodontic repositioning. He said Andresen was wrong if he thought he could hold a jaw at a greater distance than 2 mm beyond the rest position and still have only a passive, truly functional appliance.

Grude,[81] a colleague of Andresen, tried to smooth things over by saying if an appliance was constructed within the physiologic rest position, it worked according to Andresen's theories; but if it happened to be constructed at a vertical beyond the limits of the rest position, an entirely different mechanism took over and worked according to Selmer-Olsen's views. Little did he, or the entire orthodontic community for that matter, know how right he was!

Well, all that wasn't good enough for Herren[82] whose opinion was that the Activator didn't work according to Andresen's theories at all, even if it was constructed within the physiologic limits of rest position. He believed that an equilibrium existed about the whole stomatognathic system between the biologic structures on the one hand and air and gravity, etc, on the other.

Figure 2-32 (A) Materials needed for proper wax construction bite registration include thermostatically-controlled water bath capable of warming wax to 138° to 140°F and special pink base plate wax. Once sheet of wax is heated properly in water bath, it is folded to provide adequate thickness to register bite. **(B)** Desired protrusion of lower arch and jaw past upper in common Bionator Class II deep bite treatment. This is necessary to stimulate mandibular repositioning forward, but it must be remembered that amount of forward repositioning always stops 2–4 mm back of position the jaw is held in by the appliances. (*Courtesy of European Orthodontic Products, St. Paul, MN.*)

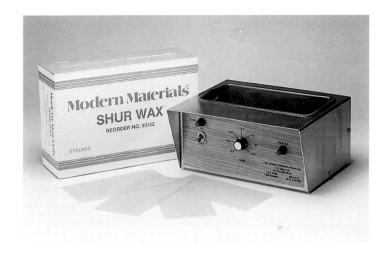

(A)

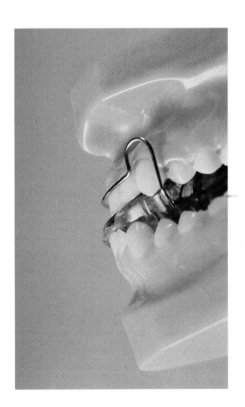

(B)

This equilibrium is disturbed by the use of an appliance. He said there were *many* rest positions while sleeping, all dependent on the patient's posture, effects of air, gravity, etc, and the appliance allowed only one of these rest positions to be assumed regardless of the sleeping posture of the patient. Therefore the pressures caused by the disturbances of this equilibrium, actually an effort of the mouth to return to an equilibrium, brought about the orthodontic and orthopedic changes dictated by the shape of the appliance. He believed also in active forces as did Andresen but thought that mandibular movements only played a minor role.

Harvold[83] said to never mind sleeping, you've got to go *active*! Stretch the muscles, that's what does the job. The more stretch, the better. Like Andresen, he took the construction bite with the jaw 3 mm short of the patient's limit of tolerance relative to the protrusive position but with a whopping 8- to 10-mm vertical opening beyond the rest position! Later on, Woodside was to go even further, to 12 to 15 mm beyond rest! Graber and Neumann[84] said you could figure it out mathematically. Use a combination of bite opening and protrusion to equal 10 mm! In other words, if you open the bite 4 mm between the occlusals posteriorly, then advance the mandible by 6 mm.

For many years in the United States the bites were taken in an incisal end-to-end position, as recommended by Balters of Germany, with an interincisal opening of 2 to 3 mm. If the centrals are in orthodontically poor position to make estimation of such a bite untenable, alignment of the laterals is used.

When taking bites for Class II Bionators, Witzig[85] recommends using a bite with 2- to 3-mm interincisal clearance at the centrals or laterals and a mandibular advancement such that the lower centrals are 2 to 3 mm protruded beyond the upper centrals or laterals. Schmuth, on the other hand, reverts back to the original construction bite of Andresen, a concept well over a half century old!

Thus we have come full cycle. But as a result of this journey, certain truths do rise to the surface. The mandible with its musculature must be held in an advanced and open position in order to effect a change. For the Bionator, Orthopedic Corrector I, one way to register a construction bite is as follows:

First have a set of study models handy to help coordinate the checking of the bite for correct positioning of the mandible. What is desired is that the jaw be positioned such that there is approximately a 2- to 3-mm space between the incisal edges of the upper and lower anterior teeth. It must be remembered that the arches are expected to be within reasonable limits of what is commonly accepted as "arch form." Some variance can be tolerated, but if it is too difficult to align the incisors, use the molars as a guide and have the patient advance his or her mandible so there is a definite "super-Class I" situation or mild Class III relationship effected. But if the incisors are in reasonably normal position, they may act as the best guide. The lower jaw should be positioned forward just enough so that the lower

CONSTRUCTION BITE

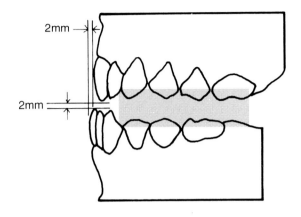

2mm

2mm

Wax construction bite for the mixed dentition and early permanent dentition, when the appliance is worn all the time, except while eating and during active sports.

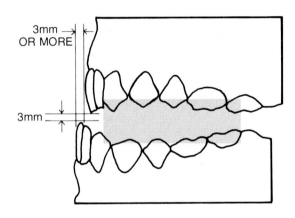

3mm OR MORE

3mm

Wax construction bite for high school students, college students, and adults, when the appliance will be worn 12 or more hours out of every 24 hours, but not during classes.
Reposition the mandible more forward during the construction bite.

Note 1: The pink base plate wax should be warmed in water at 139°F.

Note 2: The folded wax sheet is placed on the lower posterior teeth, away from the anterior teeth.

Figure 2-33

incisal edges are protruded about 2 to 3 mm beyond the upper incisal edges. So, you have a 2- to 3-mm open bite in the anteriors and a protrusion of 2 to 3 mm of the lowers past the uppers, a simple average position. You may protrude the mandible farther if the patient can tolerate it and will cooperate by wearing the appliance with so much protrusion. The same holds true for the vertical registration. The more open the bite, the faster the teeth will erupt. Harvold was right. The more stretch, the faster the vertical increases. But again, the patient's comfort and cooperation must be considered. Seldom is excessive opening or advancement needed. (Note: Construction bites may be varied according to the dictates of certain facial types and growth patterns. This will be discussed in subsequent sections.)

When the bite is opened 2 to 3 mm at the incisal edges, this automatically gives a 4- to 6-mm opening at the posteriors, usually more, which is correct. A protrusion of 2 to 3 mm of the lower anteriors past the uppers also sets up the correct amount of stretch to the facial muscles to stimulate them to change their position and to the condyles to stimulate them to form new osseous tissue to lengthen the mandible in the young patient.

Variations will occur and the judgment of these comes with clinical experience. For instance, in a severe Class II, Division 1, with excessively protruded maxillary anteriors, it might be impossible to get the lowers past the uppers in the anterior region, especially if there is any lingual inclination to the lowers. Then using the molars as a guide will help aid in registration of the degree of protrusion.

With the study models handy, have the patient practice closing to the desired construction-bite position. Guide the patient's jaw to this position with your hands while standing behind him and having him watch himself in a hand mirror. Demonstrate using the model's or your own teeth as a guide. The patient usually has no trouble understanding what you want. Always encourage and compliment him on his efforts. He will be eager to please.

Preparing the wax is another procedure that is subject to the clinician's preference. One kind of wax proven suitable because of its softness, texture, and dimensionable stability is Shur-Wax, pink base plate wax from Modern Materials Mfg Co, St Louis. Most major dental suppliers carry it as a standard item. Other brands of base plate waxes are generally too brittle for best results. Bite rims have a tendency to be too difficult to heat and cool evenly due to the bulk of their thickness.

A means of obtaining water at approximately 138°F is desirable for warming the wax. It is well worth the investment to get a thermostatically controlled water heater for this purpose.

Several methods prove effective for preparing the wax into a bite block. First it can be heated for five to eight seconds in the 138°F water bath and folded into thirds, the resultant oblong again folded in half and roughly hand-shaped to fit the study casts which should still be handy. Reheat the wax again and trim it so it is not contacted by the anterior teeth when the bite is taken. They act as guides and should not be covered by wax as the jaw closes. Another method is to fold the wax sheet into thirds and then curl in the edges so the wax block just fits lengthwise across the mandibular arch. A third method advocates rolling the wax into a tube the size of your little finger and bending it into the shape of the arch, but again take care to bend it so you can clearly see the incisal edges of the teeth in the anterior region to be your guide.

Once the bite block is prepared and properly heated, place it on the lower posterior teeth and have the patient, with the aid of a hand mirror and the doctor's hands, close into the desired position and hold still for ten seconds. This will allow the wax to cool in the mouth just enough that it might be carefully removed without distortion. As the patient opens, a very slight audible "snap" will be heard as the teeth break loose from the suction of the indentations they made with the wax. Remove the bite either by taking hold of it manually or having the patient push it out into your hand with their tongue. Chill in cool water for one minute. It is wise to take several bites. Send the best one to the laboratory along with the models. Experience will give you the confidence of your judgments in this matter. It is not difficult.

Once the bite is taken, the patient is thanked and complimented for being so helpful, and dismissed. You are ready to send the models and wax construction bite to the laboratory for appliance construction. Two sets of models at the beginning of Bionator treatment are advisable, since one should be kept as a permanent record of the condition of the mouth prior to treatment while the other is sent to the laboratory for appliance construction. These models are usually destroyed during processing and cannot be returned for record-keeping purposes or posttreatment conferences.

When constructing a Bionator for the purposes of increasing the vertical dimension only, a slightly different type of bite is taken. In cases such as these, the molars are already in Class I occlusion, but the patient is merely suffering from an excessively deep overbite. Taking the construction bite in the conventional manner would result in the mandible being protruded too far and the final case could end up in a super-Class I or even a Class III situation. To prevent this, the bite is registered in an open position without the mandible being protruded quite as far. When the mandible is merely rotated downward, it retrudes itself, only dentally, by opening on an arc. This causes the lower dental arch to travel distally slightly relative to the vertical plane and therefore distally to the stationary upper dental arch. If allowed to erupt from this slightly retruded point, the mandibular posterior segments could possibly come upward into a slight dental Class II situation. To compensate for this, slight mandibular protrusion is employed in taking the construction bite. The end-to-end position of anterior incisors should be the foremost limit of protrusion necessary for this type of bite. This will correct for the arc rotation displacement distally that is seen when the mandible is rotated on its axis only, and the resultant eruption of the lower first molars will be back to the correct Class I relationship again.

"How poor they are that have not patience!
What wound did ever heal, but by
degrees?"

Shakespeare
Othello

TIME LINE

The key to successful treatment with Bionators and Orthopedic Correctors is the proper application of the knowledge of appliance design, construction bites, adjustments, etc, to a well-coordinated *treatment time line*. This acts as a guide by which the clinician may judge the progress of the case during treatment. Of course, variations will occur, and experience will dictate modifications necessary to each particular case. Generally, however, the treatment follows a fairly generalized pattern that is highly repeatable and therefore predictable. What follows is an idealized time line of Bionator treatment. The progress described is that for the most expedient use of the appliance under the most ideal conditions on the most ideal type of cooperative, growing patient. Usually the total treatment time is longer than the 9 months we describe here and is usually closer to a year. But the first 4 to 6 months are fairly constant and therefore quite predictable for most cases.

The initial visit is a very important appointment from the standpoint of establishing a good rapport with the patient. What is usually needed is very little appliance adjustment but a lot of positive attitude and encouragement on the part of the doctor. The patient's first impression upon having the appliance inserted into his mouth is one of "having a real mouthful!" Offer a simple smile and a reassuring acknowledgment of the fact that this is perfectly normal and to be expected. The patient usually has a look of disbelief on his face when informed that he will get used to wearing the appliance within as little as a week. The patient should be informed that his mouth will water for a day or so because of having a foreign object in it. The mouth interprets the appliance as a particle of food like a piece of hard candy, hence the excess salivation. Inform the patient it is perfectly socially acceptable to slurp in order to gather the saliva in their mouths together to swallow it. They will anyway. Inform them of what the good Prince Albert once said: "When doctors give orders, even kings and princes must obey."

A good way to perform the initial insertion is to place the appliance in the patient's mouth, seating it on the lower teeth; and with the aid of a hand mirror, have the patient watch himself as he closes, having to protrude his lower jaw so the labial guide bow slides easily over the upper anteriors. The first attempts at closing will usually result in biting into the guide bow with the uppers, but this only happens once or twice. Once the patient closes into the appliance correctly for the first time and gets the "feel" of it, this never happens again.

Of course, check the appliance to make sure it does not have any tight spots that rub on the gums or soft tissues which would result in a denture-type sore. Check the Coffin spring to make sure it does not impinge on the palate, and make sure the labial guide bow is at least 0.5 to 1.0 mm away from the maxillary anterior teeth and gum tissues.

Also at this time explain the use of the orthodontic progress diary. These little calendar booklets are usually enclosed with each appliance from the laboratories, or they may be purchased in bulk from various supply houses. Show the patient that you marked the insertion day, and date as a "free day" giving him time to take the appliance in and out as much as he wants the first day to practice getting used to it. But from then on, he is to mark in the book each day the number of hours the appliance is out of his mouth. Accuracy to the nearest minute is not necessary of course, but just a rough approximation of the time that the appliance is not being worn is all that is needed. Parents may help the child with the mathematics involved, but it should be stressed that the *child* should mark the time himself in the book. It should also be stressed that the patient must bring the booklet to each appointment. This keeps the patient's interest up during the long months of treatment and most importantly gives the doctor an idea of the level of patient cooperation and allows the doctor to better predict the length of treatment required relative to the daily amount of time the appliance is being worn.

Before dismissing the patient, remind him of three things. First, that Bionators are essentially "talking" appliances, that is, they work quickest and best when the patient holds them firmly in his teeth and forces the muscles to "talk around them." Remind him of the determination of the great Greek orator Demosthenes. Also remind him that slurping is perfectly OK and will only last a few days. Also make a point to remind the parents not to reprimand a child for doing so; they are self-conscious enough with these new appliances. Extra harassment from well-meaning parents is not needed!

Secondly, remind the patient that he must make every effort to wear the appliances at all times except when eating and during active sports. The patient should mark the number of hours each day in his booklet that the appliance is out. Advise the patient that it is best to get in the habit of marking their ortho progress report diaries at the same time each day. Right before going to bed is a good time. Remind him that he may lose the appliance the first few nights in his sleep only to wake up to find it on his pillow. Assure him that this will not be a problem after some practice and the best way to insure that the appliance will stay in all night is to be well-resolved and disciplined in wearing it all day.

A printed sheet of paper of the above instructions is another handy item to have for this appointment. They can easily be written to your liking and reproduced inexpensively. They should include tips on cleaning the appliance daily with a soft brush and soaking it in mouthwash or a commercial denture cleanser for about ten minutes each day. Remind the patient that when it is out, to be *sure* to put the appliance in its protective case (sent along with the appliance by the laboratories) to prevent its breakage by being sat on, banged by books in school lockers, squashed in pockets, or crunched under any of a various assortment of hard objects. Another tip is that if the child sleeps with a dog in the room, remove the pet from the room until the patient is sure he can sleep all night without spitting out the appliance. When dogs discover appliances lying about, they seem to find the combination of human scent and crunchy consistency irresistible and will happily chew up the little orthodontic devices, Coffin spring and all! Remind the patient with a smile that Fido doesn't really need his teeth straightened with expensive functional appliances. Be firm on this point.

Thirdly, dismiss the patient with a stern admonition that if any time between the present and their next appointment, which should be in about a week or less, the appliance should hurt him in any way, he should go right to the phone and call you—any time, day or night—and mean it! If the appliance is checked over very carefully before the patient is dismissed, and fits properly, there will almost never be a call; and if in the rare event there is a call, it is a very good "practice-builder" to take the emergency. Patients are very important, especially children. They deserve and thrive on attention.

Now, even though you will be seeing the patient in a week or so, it is wise to call him at home after a day or two just to see how he is doing. Talk to the parents and reassure them and remind them of your instructions of the intital insertion appointment. Also be sure to talk directly with the patient. This makes the patient feel special, which he is, and helps deepen the trust betwen patient and doctor. Encourage and compliment the patient on his efforts so far and always pick out the most positive accomplishments that he's made. If progress is exceptionally difficult for one reason or another, never say anything to discourage the patient, but simply remind him that thousands of patients before him have gone through the same thing and that you are very confident he will do just fine. The doctor who makes his patient feel that he is really on his side, through thick or thin, will have very few failures due to lack of patient cooperation.

Once a child develops faith in you, he will come through for you just about every time. Children enjoy being treated as important people. They enjoy being involved and doing things themselves. They enjoy being responsible to you for themselves and learning their own strengths as they go. They seem to possess a totally uncontaminated "malarkey-detector" that allows them to see straight through much of the facade and superficiality adults tend to envelope life in. As a result, only sincerity in developing a true relationship with the child will do. Once this is established between the doctor and his patient, treatment is enormously facilitated.[86-88] Without it, treatment is next to impossible. The appliances can't work sitting on the shelf! This is why the child must be given the impression from the onset that the doctor is dealing directly with him. Parents, though concerned, are on the sideline. You report to them privately as to the child's progress. Thus developing such a relationship with a child patient is a rewarding and gratifying experience, a fringe benefit of functional appliance therapy. Humanity's best and most untainted product, little people are super!

One Week

At this appointment have the patient bring in his orthodontic progress diary booklet and check to see if he is marking it adequately. Compliment him on his efforts. Discuss or treat any problems he is having getting used to the appliance. Check the appliance to make sure the labial guide bow is clearing the teeth and tissues. Encourage the patient and assure him that he is doing fine. Remind him that you always knew he had what it takes to "come through and be a real winner."

At this point some clinicians prefer to "prime" the appliance slightly by having the patient activate the middle screw once a week for a period of a month or so to gain 1 to 2 mm lateral expansion of the appliance in the lower anterior area. The purpose behind this is to drive the projections of acrylic into the interproximal spaces to open up the contacts slightly, and to speed up the eruption of the teeth a little. If contacts are not tight to begin with, this step may be skipped. Of course, if lateral expansion past this point is desired to gain space in a slightly crowded lower anterior arch, the lingual reinforcing wire should be cut at the midline before the appliance is expanded too far, or it will cause torque to be imparted to the appliance and distort its shape or even break it. If you desire to prime the appliance a little, show the patient how to insert the key into the expansion screw and turn it 90° to obtain 0.25-mm expansion. The first time the screw is turned it will be quite firm, so demonstrate for the patient by turning it once for him, then immediately turn it back to the starting position so the patient may try turning it himself. Ask him how it feels upon reinserting it after opening the screw by one-quarter turn, and the usual reply will be that it feels "tighter." Convey approval and tell the patient it will feel that way for a day or so. Inform the patient that now he is to turn the screw once every Sunday until the next appointment which will be in one month. This means the maximum opening of this screw by that time will be 1 mm, not much to worry about. As always, these appointments should be a time for the doctor and the patient to be together alone to take care of these issues. After this is accomplished, the parents may be called into the operatory for a progress report or may be seen in the doctor's private office if necessary to be filled in on what is going on. This makes the patient feel even more special, that he receives the doctor's attention individually and without distraction or interruption of parents and/or siblings in private. Concerned parents are to be given due respect of course, but most of the scheduled appointment time should be just between the doctor and the patient.

Now that the patient is used to the appliance, he may be dismissed with an appointment for a month or so from the present. Remind the patient and the parents to remember to bring the progress diary to the next appointment. If any instructions were given at the present appointment, it is best to jot them down on your own notes for your records and on a piece of note paper for the patient to take home. Patients easily forget or get confused. Written instructions are handy to have and leave no doubts as to what must be done. Again, as always, dismiss the patient with encouraging reassurances that he has done well so far and will do just fine in the months ahead.

First Month

Check the appliance at this time to make sure the Coffin spring and the labial guide bow are still free of the tissues. The labial bow may need some slight adjusting at this point to free it from contact with the maxillary anterior teeth or gingivae. Check for sore spots. Examine the patient's orthodontic progress diary and comment on how well he is maintaining it. If it indicates he has the appliance out more than six hours per day, remind him that this greatly retards the action and effect of the appliance and will lengthen the amount of treatment time needed. Also check to see that the booklet is adequately marked as to number of hours worn, days when the screw was turned, etc. If the records are poor and/or wearing time is down; gently, but firmly, charge the patient to do better and to try harder to comply with your wishes. Be reasonable and allow that there will be some times when it must be out for a while for good reasons, but insist that persistence is the key to rapid and successful treatment. Always pick out something to compliment the patient on, whether it be their record keeping or faithfulness in wearing the appliance. Always try to give the patient some good news as to the progress they are making orthodontically. This can be a little tough at the 1-month stage, but there is usually something in the mouth that is changed. If the patient has been turning the midline screw, the appliance is 1 mm wider, if nothing else! Answer any questions and offer tips on solving any of the minor social problems that may arise as a result of wearing the appliance. Reiterate your instructions on keeping their appliances and their mouths clean. If oral hygiene is a problem, remind the patient that the appliances work faster in clean mouths. Plaque makes teeth slippery, and the acrylic can't grab onto them as well. (As a scientific theory, this one may be on the fringe of an out-and-out fib, but if it helps motivate the patient to brush better, it may be justified!) Offering free samples of denture cleansers of the soaking variety may also help the patient who has trouble keeping his appliance clean to realize the importance of hygiene.

If the case requires that the arches be developed laterally beyond this point, cut the lingual wire at the midline screw. This wire may also be carefully adjusted at this time to move an individual tooth slightly, such as an upper central or lateral neeeding a slight nudge labially. Offer the patient encouragement and support so as to be sure that the overall appointment experience is one of a positive nature. Mark the progress detected in your private notes in the patient's records and the instructions you have given the patient to perform for the next appointment. Also make notes as to what you expect to see (or hope to see) by the next appointment. This is an important step; for on a busy day after seeing several cases, it is hard to remember where you are in a case without adequate notes as to progress and monthly goals carefully written and dated in the patient's records to act as quick reminders. It is also best to record any pertinent statements the patient makes relative to his progress such as: "I forget sometimes" or, "It comes out sometimes at night." Remember, to a child who feels he's on the carpet, "sometimes" loosely translates to "a lot!"

Dismiss the patient on a cheerful, expectant note with an appointment for 4 to 6 weeks. Report progress to the parents and try to compliment the child *in front of the parents* in some way by telling the parent of the good things the child has accomplished. You may choose to call the parents at home that night to discuss things at a more leisurely pace, away from the hectic environment of a busy office.

Second Month

At this time the muscles are at midpoint in the act of repositioning themselves from their original pretreatment status to their new anatomically enhanced locations. The entire muscular repositioning and retraining process takes about 3 or 4 months. The condylar growth in the patient who is still growing has not developed too far yet of course, as that takes more time. Condylar growth can be stimulated until about age 23 to 25 years according to some experts.[89-99] It is this growth that lengthens the mandible, adds height, and aids in the permanent repositioning of the lower jaw from Class II to Class I.

As before, check the appliance for any chipped or rough edges causing sore spots. Check the Coffin spring and labial bow to make sure they clear the tissues. If the patient has been turning the midline screw, the labial bow will probably need adjusting away from the teeth somewhere and the Coffin spring should be expanded just slightly. Check the orthodontic progress diary and comment on the quality, or lack thereof, of the notations. If lateral expansion of the appliance is going on, the lingual wire should have been cut by now. Check it to make sure it is not causing irritations. If it is being used to move individual teeth labially, check for appropriate tension, and adjust if necessary.

Make notes of importance and date them in your own records. Give the patient encouragement and support. Inform the parents of progress noted and dismiss the patient with an appointment to be seen again in 4 to 6 weeks.

Third Month

By now there should be some truly noticeable changes observable by the patient as well as the doctor. The lower jaw should be fully accustomed to its new position by this time, and it quite often is impossible for the patient to retrude the mandible back to the original Class II position. As an interesting sidelight, if the appliance is taken away now, the jaw usually reverts almost completely back to its original position over a period of a couple of months. But if the patient is young enough and has been faithfully wearing the appliance, it is quite often nearly impossible for even the most athletic clinician to manipulate the mandible back to its former retruded position! The muscles simply won't allow it! Of course, each patient is different; neither the doctor nor the patient should be discouraged if this amount of progress is not observed at the 3-month stage of treatment. Occasionally Nature likes to take Her good sweet time. Another month or two and the changes will appear.

Of course, the eruption of the teeth due to alveolar bone growth always lags behind mandibular repositioning.[100] Therefore, if a definite forward position of the mandible is noticed, there will also appear a space opening up between the occlusal surfaces of the opposing bicuspids and sometimes even the molars. The space is greatest between the occlusals of the upper and lower first bicuspids and decreases posteriorly. As the alveolar bone is stimulated by the appliance to increase, the teeth will close up the space by "supererupting" over the next 4 to 5 months.[101] Simply observe the patient's jaw relationship and occlusion as the teeth are closed without the appliance in, and these changes will be noticed. Oddly, the patient notices no problems in chewing even though he is presently suffering from a very short-term posterior open bite! Inform the patient that this is a good sign that progress is excellent. Compliment the patient and offer further encouragement and support.

Make the routine checks of the progress diary and the Coffin spring, labial bow, etc. If the patient is still turning the middle screw, expand the Coffin spring slightly. Again, adjust the labial guide bow so that it is not touching teeth or tissues.

Another area to check is the anterior cap. If the lip of the cap is off for the purposes of flaring the lower anteriors out for the relief of slight crowding, for improper lingual inclination, etc, examine the present state of these teeth. If they have been "dumped forward" enough, send the appliance to the laboratory with a fresh set of models to have it added back on, or add it yourself in the office. This then acts as its own retainer. If individual lower incisor teeth need a little more movement, they can be moved out even with the others in the arch by adding a small drop of acrylic to the area just lingual to the crown of the tooth in question. If the entire group still needs more movement, continue present therapy, *sans acrylic cap lip!*

The appointment after 3 months of wear is *very important,* for the patient is wearing an Orthopedic Corrector I. After 3 months of wear, the patient is ready to start activating the side screws of the appliance to continue the process of advancing the mandible, since by now most of the initial advancement has taken place with the appliance in its present, unopened state.

Either at the 3-month stage if progress is excellent or the 4-month stage of treatment if progress is just fair to normal, these screws may be activated to continue the rest of the mandibular advancement process. But they may only be activated after all the interproximal acrylic projections have been ground off from between the lower posterior teeth. Remember, the main bulk of the appliance stays in relatively the same cephalometric position anchored against the palate by the tension and stretch of the muscles. Only the anterior cap advances as the side screws are turned, requiring the mandible to be advanced further and further to enable the lower incisors to slip up into their normal place inside the cap. If the interproximal projections are not ground off the lower posterior areas once this process begins, the lingual heights of contour of the lower teeth will collide with them as these teeth move further forward away from the main bulk of the appliance with the lower jaw as it seeks out the newly forward-positioned cap.

Instruct patients on proper side-screw activation and demonstrate how to advance the cap by turning *each side* screw *three* turns. Make sure they don't confuse this with the one turn of the midline screw if they are still doing so. Again, have them do this triple turn of the side screws every Sunday night until the appliance has the jaw positioned forward enough to be correct. Write these instructions down or have a small preprinted instruction card to this effect handy to give the patients. Write it in their orthodontic progress booklets also. It's surprising how easily they forget or become confused once they leave the office. Medical terms and instructions are foreign to the mind of the layman. Write it!

Fourth Month

By now there is some condylar growth starting to take place, and the muscle response, which is always ahead of bony changes, should be such that the patient can now habitually close down to the new position, with little or no retrusion of the mandible to pretreatment positions possible at all. The mandible is just about irrevocably repositioned forward. At this stage of treatment, several important things start happening that are brought about by using the correct adjustment procedures.

First, check the labial guide bow. If the teeth are in close proximity to where you want them as far as what is considered proper for upper anteriors, keep the wire off the teeth and gum tissue to prevent possible crowding in this area as a result of the forces delivered to them by the labial bow, appliance, and upper lip. But if the maxillary anteriors are protruded or flared labially, as they commonly are, *now* is the time to adjust the labial bow so that it *contacts* these teeth. Using a favorite wire-bending pliers, usually a three-pronged variety, adjust the bow so that (1) it contacts these teeth at the gingival third, which produces a predominantly downward force to the teeth; or (2) adjust it so it contacts the teeth in the incisal third to produce a downward and lingual pressure. This second type of bow adjustment is the more common.

Second, if the patient is wearing a Bionator, now is a good time to start implementing some of the adjustments to help speed up the increase in vertical. Grind off the interproximal projections of acrylic between, around, and over the upper and lower teeth *except* for the single projection on both sides of the palatal portion of the appliance that butts against the mesial of the upper first molars. This *must not* be touched by the acrylic bur. It is this small portion of acrylic that anchors the entire appliance against the maxilla and provides the stability against which the stretching muscles can stress. Some clinicians mark this area with a pencil or marker of some sort so as to be better able to see it while adjusting and reducing the other areas of acrylic. Some clinicians will also remove the projections from only the lower and wait until the next month to remove them from between and around the uppers. That is a matter of preference and clinical judgment for each case. (Note: If the patient is wearing an Orthopedic Corrector I, these lower projections of acrylic have been removed at the previous appointment to enable the patient to start advancing the cap by turning the side screws. If so, remove the projections from between and around the upper teeth, again being careful *not* to remove them from the area that contacts the mesial of the upper first molars. These two remaining projections are needed to keep the appliance anchored properly against the upper first molars.)

Third, if the cap has been used to flare or "dump" the lower anteriors forward by having its lip removed, check the progress of these teeth; and if they have been moved (or actually tipped) forward enough, send the appliance to the laboratory along with a fresh set of models and have it added back on again; or do it chairside in the manner described previously. If more movement is required, continue "steady as she goes."

By this time in the treatment schedule, there should definitely be some evidence of space opening up between the occlusal surfaces of the upper and lower bicuspids, ie, a posterior open bite. In fact, if the patient has been faithful in wearing his appliance at least 18 hours a day, there may even be some sign of this space starting to close already, as the alveolar bone growth is stimulated by the open bite to effect a supraeruption of these teeth. This is a slow process, however, and there may be some space still remaining in the bicuspid area as late as the 9-month mark, the ideal projected time of completion of treatment. But if this is so, it is of no concern; for with the rest of the teeth and jaws in their proper overbite and overjet relationships and no crowding present to prevent teeth from erupting, these few stragglers will continue to erupt right along the proper path to the correct plane of occlusion even without the benefit of the appliance in the mouth. Let's face it; where else can they go? *Function* will stimulate this final and orderly completion of eruption.

Of course, perform the usual routine tasks of checking the patient's progress diary booklet, commenting on the quality of record keeping, etc.

If it is not up to par, gently, but firmly, remind the patient that this is a very important part of the treatment program and that he is totally responsible for doing his part. But then also, again offer friendly encouragement and support. If the problem is one of not wearing the appliance enough during each day (less than 18 hours), stress the importance of keeping the appliance *in*; and remind the patient, the better he does in this regard, the sooner the treatment will be complete. If you suspect a real problem with this, offer to see the patient more often, like every 2 weeks or so, in a "needs-to-improve" program. A needs-to-improve program is similar to being on "probation"; at least that's what you want them to think. It also sets up the groundwork for withdrawing from the case should you run into the rare patient who simply won't cooperate. Remember, the parents and patient should be informed from the onset that when cooperation stops, the treatment, payments, and responsibility of the doctor for the case *also stops*. Should such a situation arise, always use the utmost care and diplomacy in withdrawing from the case. People are human. They often change their minds; and if they feel the doctor is congenial, sincere, and forgiving, they will be back if they should decide it's time to try again.

The patient should not be indicted as "at fault," but rather as simply "not being ready" for functional appliances. Ours is to treat, not to judge. That is a privilege of higher powers.

Dismiss the patient with a reminder that all his efforts are really going to start paying off now in the next few months to come. They are about halfway through the Bionator treatment program!

Fifth Month

By now things are really in "high gear." The mandible's repositioning forward is usually irrevocable by this stage of treatment. The alveolar bone is also well into the process of increasing its height by this stage of the course of treatment under ideal circumstances in the growing adolescent patient. Thus the temporary posterior open bite is starting to close. The condyles are starting to increase in their thickness at their articular ends, increasing ramus height and therefore ultimately the overall length of the mandible in the process. Vertical- or lingual-inclined incisors on the lower are starting to be pretty well flared forward by the trimmed, lip-free cap; labially protruded upper incisors are starting to be pulled in more vertically by the labial bow. And an attractive young face, and personality too, are starting to develop right along with them. The cygnet is beginning to be replaced by the swan!

Make the usual adjustments and notations. Add the lip of acrylic back to the cap if the lower incisors are where you want them. Adjust the labial guide bow off the upper incisors if *they* are where you want them. But if they were flared forward at the beginning of treatment, they will still most likely have a ways to go inward yet. Check the progress diary and praise the patient. Encourage the patient and remind him that he is on the home-stretch. How quickly and quietly falls the foot of time!

Sixth Month

Again, make the routine adjustments as needed. Check the patient's progress diary and comment on its notation. Observe the progress and note it in your records as to changes observed, etc, as well as what is looked for by the next appointment. Changes in the vertical should be noticeable by now. But remember, the deeper the overbite, the longer it will take to at-tain proper vertical. The alveolar bone grows faster in the molar area than in the bicuspid areas. So as a result, the open bite space will be greater in the bicuspid area for a longer period of time than in the posterior region, where the interocclusal space closes faster. Also, the growth of alveolar bone usually takes place faster and is more noticeable in the mandible than the maxilla, ie, the lower teeth seem to supraerupt faster than the uppers.

Again, adjust the labial bow, the Coffin spring, etc, as needed. (Note: A word of caution here relative to the labial bow. Some clinicians advocate bending the labial bow with their fingers when gross movements are needed. But this should be avoided, as after 4 to 6 months of adjusting, the bow wire can start suffering from metal fatigue. This fatigue is greatest at the right angle bend where the wire comes out of the acrylic of the appliance just distal to the maxillary cuspid. Grabbing the bow with the fingers and bending it for adjustment purposes causes an enormous stress vector to travel right through this area. Where the stress is greatest, the fatigue will be greatest; 99% of all labial bows that break will break right at this bend, leaving a short stub sticking out of the acrylic of the appliance which is dif-ficult at best for laboratories to repair by soldering. To avoid this problem, use a pliers for adjusting the bow. Make the adjustments sequentially. That is, adjust the cuspid loop on one side of the bow, and then the other. Then place the compensatory bends at one corner angle, where the wire turns 90° from the cuspid loop to cross over the labial surfaces of the anterior teeth, then the opposite corner angle. This will prevent excessive stresses from occurring at the point where the bow leaves the acrylic as opposed to mak-ing all the adjustments, both active and compensatory, on just one side at a time. Even so, they still sometimes break at this juncture.) Rough treat-ment by the patient, usually teenage boys, is also a common factor in caus-ing some appliances to break. Again, stress putting the appliance in the protective case any time it is not being worn. If appliances break from func-tion, the laboratory pays the repair fee. If they break from abuse, the pa-tient pays the repair fee. Being crunched under a dictionary in a school locker is not function!

Also at this point in the treatment time line, the patient starts becoming *im*patient for the end. Enthusiasm starts to ebb and cooperation as to wearing the appliance at all practical times starts to diminish. Now is *no time* to "pull up lame." More than ever, encourage and support the patient. Stress that so much can be lost and all the previous months' good efforts, determination, and sacrifices will yield mediocre or even poor dividends if faithfulness to the treatment regimen is not kept up to par. Implore them to "give it all they've got" these last few months on the homestretch. The patient may begin exhibiting faint signs of "burnout"; but remind them that long programs of orthodontic treatment are like a long trip in a car, an academic school year, a marathon, a great symphony, or even like life itself; it usually becomes most difficult at the end. Now is the time to "pour on the coals." Happy results are just around the corner! It's a great life for those who don't weaken!

Seventh and Eighth Months

Routine appointments with routine adjustments and procedures. Some of the simpler cases might even finish up during this time, especially if the child is in a peak growing period and has been faithful in wearing the appliance all the time! If the case is more severe, the patient may have some time to go yet.

If the patient has been opening the midline screws for the purposes of expanding the arches laterally and has stopped now or in the past month or so, it is a nice gesture to fill in the area with quick-cure acrylic. This keeps the opened gap in the appliance smooth and comfortable for the tip of the tongue and helps with the hygiene, keeping plaque from building up in the exposed threads of the screw.

Offer encouragement and understanding to those who are growing weary of treatment or whose record keeping and time of wear seem to be dropping off. Yet at the same time, the doctor must be firm and insist the patient realize the amount of time and money invested so far in this project is formidable. Success is only a few months away. The shortness of time to completion is the best incentive.

In all fairness, patient motivation problems are infrequent. The patients adapt so well to the appliances, are so enthusiastic when they see the results coming along, and are so grateful for not having to wear "regular braces," headgear, etc, that they almost always bubble with enthusiasm and greet you with charming and happy smiles when you see them for their routine appointments. When they realize all these benefits of removable appliance therapy depend on their compliance with your dictates, cooperation is rarely a problem. Parents are supportive in their enthusiasm also. They are excited to see the dramatic changes in the child's facial development and this feeds the positive cycle of growing satisfaction for the treatment methods. When the parents are pleased and the child is pleased, the doctor is pleased and this makes for a happy day. Life needs more of them.

Often as treatment draws to a close the patient becomes lax in marking his diary. But with good treatment results in a patient who is a proven appliance wearer, strict adherence to the dictum of keeping the diary current is no longer a critical issue. Just before graduation, seniors are expected to take a few privileges.

Final Month

There is a certain easy grace that permeates the atmosphere of these final appointments as both the patient and the doctor realize the end is at hand. For the patient, a good feeling of having completed a job well done, for which he was solely responsible; for the doctor, a feeling of a weight of responsibility lifted from his shoulders and a deep sense of satisfaction as he observes a beautiful, broad smile and a well-balanced, happy face— the results of his handiwork. There is a *lot* of smiling that goes on during these appointments, by everybody! Whether the case takes 9, 10, 12 months, or even longer, is obviously a function of patient age, cooperation, severity of the case, doctor skill, etc. Worrying about the strict and exact compliance with a predicted time of completion must be tempered by a wide range of tolerance. Many clinical judgments go into the decision as to when a case is finally complete. The doctor's standards and philosophies mitigated by the patient's desires and level of satisfaction usually are the major factors in determining the completion point. It will always vary from case to case. There is no set rule. The ultimate governing factor might just well be the doctor's own conscience. It might best be simply summed up in the words of that famous philosopher, scholar, and former Major League catcher for the New York Yankees, Yogi Berra, "It ain't over 'til it's over!"

RETENTION

Retainers are rarely used after the completion of Bionator treatment. If the teeth in the arches have been moved a considerable amount prior to insertion of this appliance, or actually in preparation for insertion of this appliance, the Bionator acts as its own retainer during treatment and helps generate its own stability by giving the case its own orthopedic and orthodontic balance.

If the doctor is concerned about relapse, all he has to do is consider the question, "Where are the teeth and mandible going to relapse to?" Are the teeth going to intrude back down into their sockets? Are the condyles going to resorb at their articular surfaces? Are the muscles going to reposition themselves back to their old pretreatment positions again so that they may better attempt to pull the lower jaw and its condyles back to the superior posterior displaced position of the pretreatment state? Hardly.

The worst that can happen is that teeth once moved or tipped will individually relapse back. In these cases the old standard rules for retention apply. Generally, the farther you move a tooth, the longer you should hold it there to allow it to stabilize; 3 to 6 months is usually minimum. If the teeth have been moved by the correct techniques prior to insertion of the appliance, the 9-month treatment time line of the Bionator, which is acting also as its own retainer for these teeth during its own therapy, falls well within this minimum time span.

Rarely, a "tongue thrust" will return to push upper centrals labially again; but simple reinsertion and proper adjustment of the appliance (making it like a Bionator II, discussed later) can correct the problem, and myofunctional therapy may be instituted. Again, this is rare, but the earlier these types of problems are diagnosed and treated, the better.

If the doctor is concerned about some form of relapse for one reason or another, or if the case has been brought a very long way from a very severe deep overbite and/or large overjet situation prior to treatment, the patient may be weaned off the appliance gradually, ie, wearing it only at night for several months, then every other night for several more for a period of time until the case appears to be quite stable. Stability is a result of Nature having Her way. The teeth and jaws are in the orthodontically and orthopedically correct and balanced positions she designed them for in the first place. The clinician merely helped in seeing to it that She got them there without something getting "stuck" along the way. The doctor is merely a facilitator. It was his hands, but Her wisdom.

> *"He wishes not to seem,*
> *but to be the best."*
>
> *Aeschylus*
> Seven Against Thebes
> *525–456 B.C.*

SUMMARY

There are many patients who suffer from deficient mandibles. There are many patients who suffer from lower jaws that are too small and too retruded: jaws that are tucked back and under the overhanging shelf of the maxilla in a Class II situation. The Bionator and Orthopedic Corrector I are the best appliances available today to treat and correct this situation. They help to develop the lower face and relieve possibly strained temporomandibular joints. Many Class II, Division 1, and Class II, Division 2, patients especially, are in danger of suffering from muscular imbalances and temporomandibular joint malarthroses later on in adult life if these deficient mandibles are not brought down and forward into their proper orthopedically correct position with proper overbite and overjet relationships.

The concept of what these appliances are designed to achieve is almost a century old even though the actual specific details of their particular design are relatively new. These appliances are mostly functional in design but are also part active plate.

By properly applying the correct series of adjustments on a well-calculated time line, these appliances will bring a beautiful and stable result. Most of the other ancillary techniques in orthodontics consist of procedures preparing the individual arches to receive this final step, *arch alignment.*

Table 2-1
The Bionator, Orthopedic Corrector

A. Purpose
    1. Class II to Class I
    2. Advance mandible by stimulating condylar growth
    3. Increase vertical by stimulating alveolar bone growth
    4. Increase lower face height
    5. Relieve SPDC and strained TMJs
    6. Mixed or permanent dentitions

B. Construction bite
    Standard Bionator/Orthopedic Corrector I
    1. 2–4 mm interincisal distance
    2. 2–4 mm protrusion past end-to-end incisally

    Bionator to increase vertical dimension only
    1. 2–4 mm interincisal distance
    2. Slight advancement from Class I to super-Class I

SPDC = superior, posterior displacement of the condyle

Case Study Pretreatment and Posttreatment Illustrations— Following Pages

Figure 2-34 Study of classic Bionator case. Skeletal Class II, large overjet, deep overbite condition is obvious from **(A)** frontal views of the face, **(B)** pretreatment study models, **(C)** lateral view of face with its retrognathic facial profile and lip incompetency, and **(D)** lateral view of pretreatment models which exhibit characteristic vertical and horizontal discrepancies. Severity of mandibular retrusion (verified cephalometrically) is clearly shown. **(E)** The construction bite is taken with mandible down and forward and in this case with incisors about end to end since upper incisors are already flared quite far labially. **(F)** Once constructed, appliance forces mandible to reside in same location as per dictates of construction bite. After only four months of Bionator wear, the slight "over advancement" of mandible is evident. This is only temporary and mandible easily settles back to its more correct position. This over-corrected position is due merely to muscle habit. Also appearing at 4 to 5 month stage in this case is characteristic posterior open bite. **(G) (H)** This also is temporary and proper adjustment of acrylic wings of appliance will allow proper vertical eruption of both upper and lower posterior quadrants. **(I) (J)** At completion of treatment, posterior open bite has closed and case is in full dental Class I. **(K)** Final posttreatment models show full correction of original malocclusion. **(L)** Overlapping cephalometric tracings divulge true skeletal correction effected by the Bionator during 12-month treatment time. **(M) (N)** Posttreatment facial views showing fully developed lower facial complex 1 1/2 years after treatment, no retention. **(O–T)** Serialized computer pretreatment and posttreatment cephalometric analyses of a case of mandibular advancement by means of Bionator treatment. **(O)** Pretreatment Modified Steiner analysis (with data), **(P)** Pretreatment Functional Orthopedic analysis (with data), and **(Q)** Pretreatment Modified Bimler analysis (with data) depict classic signs of typical Class II malocclusion with its deep overbite, severe overjet, mandibular retrusive condition. Posttreatment cephalometric analyses of **(R)** Modified Steiner, **(S)** Functional Orthopedic, and **(T)** Modified Bimler depict complete correction of these problems in full advancement of mandible from skeletal Class II to full Class I.

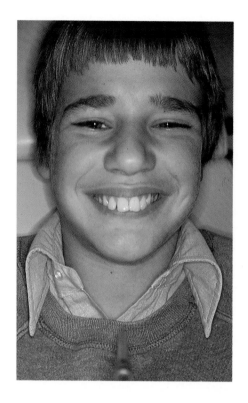

(A)

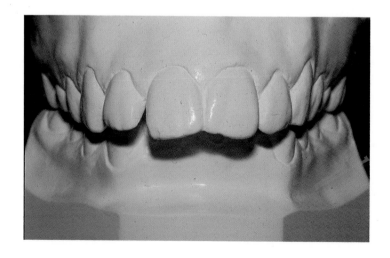

(B)

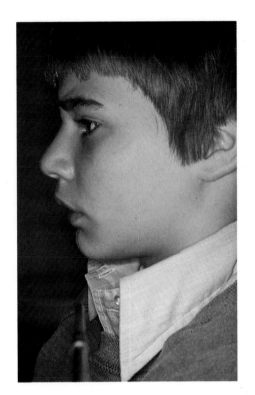

(C)

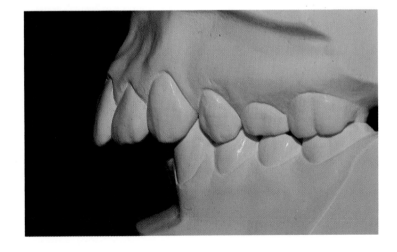

(D)

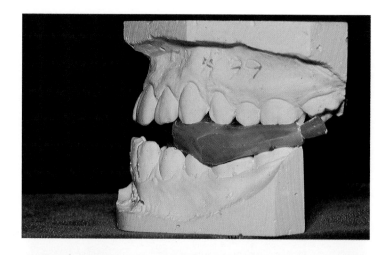

(E)

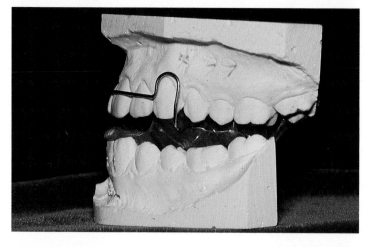

(F)

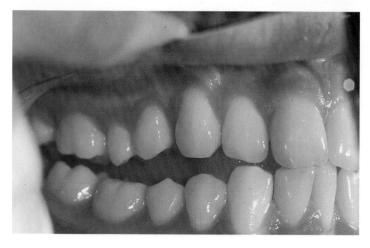

(G)

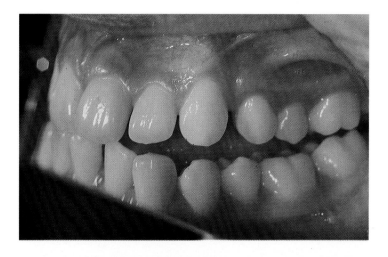

(H)

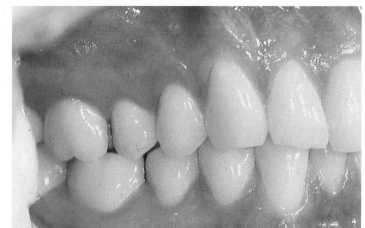

(I)

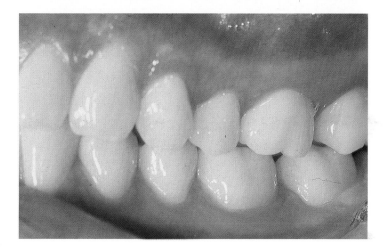

(J)

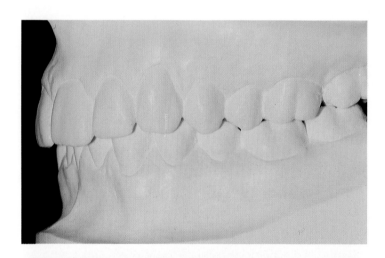

(K)

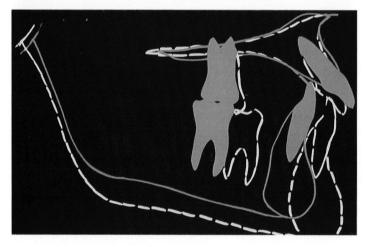

(L)

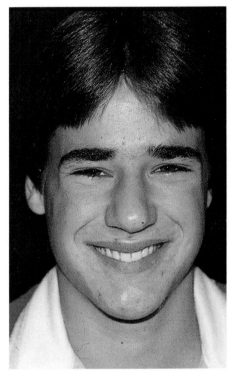

(M)

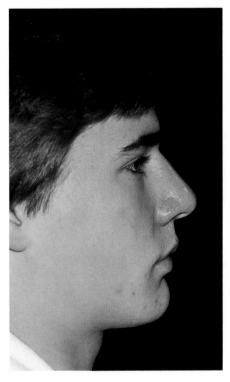

(N)

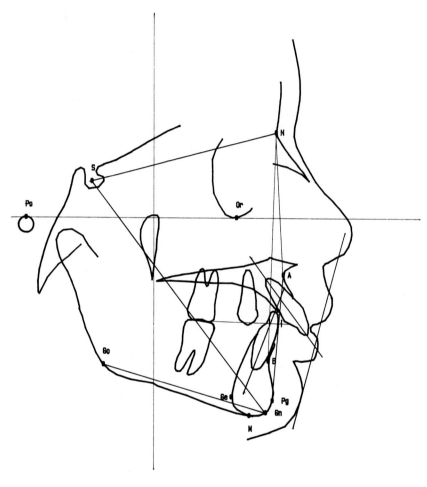

(O)

MODIFIED STEINER ANALYSIS

SKELETAL

MEASUREMENT	NORM	ACTUAL	COMMENT
SNA	80.0° to 84.0°	78.7°	RETROGNATHIC MAXILLA
SNB	78.0° to 82.0°	73.7°	RETROGNATHIC MANDIBLE
ANB	0.0° to 5.0°	5.1°	SKELETAL CLASS II
WITS	-3.0mm to 1.0mm	4.9mm	SKELETAL CLASS II
UPPER FACIAL HEIGHT	50.0%	45.4%	
LOWER FACIAL HEIGHT	50.0%	54.6%	
Go-Gn to SN	28.0° to 36.0°	30.2°	
Y-Axis to SN	63.0° to 69.0°	66.2°	
			Normal skeletal bite.
OCCL to SN	14.0° to 15.0°	16.1°	ANY CHANGE IN POSTERIOR VERTICAL SUPPORT WILL HAVE A THREE-FOLD PROPORTIONAL CHANGE IN ANTERIOR VERTICAL
Pg to NB	1.5mm to 3.5mm	2.2mm	

DENTAL

MEASUREMENT	NORM	ACTUAL	COMMENT
UP1 to NA DIST	4.0mm	9.2mm	
UP1 to NA ANG	20.0° to 24.0°	34.2°	BUCCOVERSION
LOW1 to NB DIST	4.0mm	3.4mm	
LOW1 to NB ANG	23.0° to 27.0°	19.7°	LINGUOVERSION
LOW1 TO UP1	120.0° to 140.0°	121.1°	
A-Pg to LOW1	-2.0mm to 3.0mm	-0.4mm	
6+6 to PTV	15.0mm	13.3mm	BE SURE ENOUGH TUBEROSITY EXISTS TO DISTALLIZE MOLARS IF NECESSARY

SOFT TISSUE

MEASUREMENT	NORM	ACTUAL	COMMENT
UPPER LIP	0.0mm to 2.0mm	2.6mm	
LOWER LIP	0.0mm to 2.0mm	1.3mm	

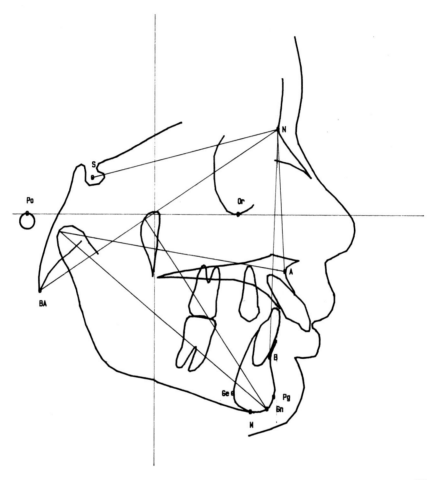

(P)

FUNCTIONAL ORTHOPEDIC ANALYSIS

MEASUREMENT	NORM	ACTUAL	COMMENT
A. RELATING THE MAXILLA TO THE CRANIAL BASE			
A Pt to N Perp	-1.0mm to 3.0mm	2.9mm	
B. RELATING THE MANDIBLE TO THE MAXILLA			
Eff. MAXILLA Lgth	***	91.0mm	EFFECTIVE MAXILLA LENGTH AFTER ADJUSTMENT FOR 'A' PT. LOCATION: 88.1
Eff. MANDIBLE Lgth	109.2mm to114.2mm	107.1mm	SHORT MANDIBLE
Diff=MAX-MAND Lgth	***	19.1mm	
Lower Facial Ht[Vert Dim]	61.8mm to 65.8mm	61.3mm	SHORT VERTICAL DIMENSION
C. RELATING THE UPPER INCISOR TO THE MAXILLA			
Up1 to A Perp	4.0mm to 6.0mm	10.2mm	
D. RELATING THE LOWER INCISOR TO THE MANDIBLE			
Low1 to A-Pg Line	1.0mm to 3.0mm	-0.4mm	
E. MANDIBULAR POSITION			
Pg to N Perp	-6.0mm to -2.0mm	-1.4mm	PROGNATHIC MANDIBLE
F. OTHER USEFUL CEPHALOMETRIC MEASUREMENTS			
SNA	80.0° to 84.0°	78.7°	RETROGNATHIC MAXILLA
SNB	78.0° to 82.0°	73.7°	RETROGNATHIC MANDIBLE
ANB	0.0° to 5.0°	5.1°	
Interincisal Angle	120.0° to140.0°	121.1°	
Mandibular Flane Angle	20.0° to 30.0°	15.9°	
Facial Axis (Ricketts)	86.5° to 93.5°	89.5°	

REFERENCE I.D. GRID

ANTERIOR PROFILE ANGLE	BASIC ANGULAR RELATION	SUBORBITAL FACIAL INDEX	
Class I 0-10° Class II >15° Class III <0°	Upper Basic Angle DLM DLM Lower Basic Angle	Dolico —— Meso —— Prosopic Lepto	FACIAL FORMULA
BONY OVERJET A-B Distance (Projected) Class III (−) Mean -4 to 8 mm * Class II (+)	Factor Ⓐ (+)(±)(−) Factor Ⓑ (+)(±)(−)	**TEMPORAL POSITION** T-TM Distance Short 20-24 Class III Med. 28-32 Normal Long 36-40 Class II	GNATHIC INDEX
INTERINCISOR ANGLE BIPRO <120 DIV 1 120-140 DIV 2 >140	Upper Bicuspid Inclination P.O.R. P.O.R. Lower Bicuspid Inclination	**STRESS AXIS** / **ANGLE CLASS** Per I Post II Pre III	DENTAL FORMULA

* − 0 to 8mm is The American interpretation
− 4 to 8mm is The True Bimler interpretation

PATIENT'S I.D. GRID

10.3	D/M	DOLICHO	FACIAL FORMULA
	-7.1/		
6	16.3	33.6	GNATHIC INDEX
121.1	0/R	POST/II	DENTAL FORMULA

(Q)

MODIFIED BIMLER ANALYSIS

MEASUREMENT	NORM	ACTUAL	COMMENT

FACTOR 1:
| UPPER PROFILE ANGLE N TO A | -1.0° to 1.0° | -3.0° | RETROGNATHIC |

FACTOR 2:
| LOWER PROFILE ANGLE AB TO VERT | | 10.3° | |
| ANTERIOR PROFILE ANGLE (F1+F2) | 0.0° to 10.0° | 7.3° | SKELETAL CLASS I |

FACTOR 3:
| MANDIBULAR INCLINATION | | 17.5° | |

FACTOR 4:
MAXILLARY INCLINATION ANS-PNS	-3.0° to 3.0°	-7.1°	NASAL FLOOR CONTRIBUTES TO OPEN BITE
LOWER BASIC ANGLE (F3-F4)	15.0° to 30.0°	24.6°	BALANCED GROWTH (MESO)
ALVEOLAR HEIGHT		-1.6mm	

FACTOR 5:
CLIVUS INCLINATION	60.0° to 70.0°	67.0°	MEDIUM POSTERIOR CRANIAL BASE
UPPER BASIC ANGLE (F5+F4)	60.0° to 70.0°	59.9°	DOLICHO PROSOPIC
FACIAL HARMONY		D/M	OPEN VERTICAL: D/L
SUBORBITAL FACIAL INDEX (A1M/AC)	1.00 to 1.05	0.91	DEEP FACE

FACTOR 6:
| STRESS AXIS | | 119.1mm | CLASS II (POST) |

FACTOR 7:
| N-S INCLINATION | | 14.3° | |

FACTOR 8:
| MANDIBULAR FLEXION | -5.0° to 5.0° | 16.3° | HYPERFLEXION - UNDER-DEVELOPMENT OF MIDDLE FACE; FAVORABLE IN CLASS III CASES; IT WILL BE REDUCED IN BITE OPENING IN TREATMENT |

LINEAR MEASUREMENTS
MAXILLA LENGTH (AT)		51.7mm	
TEMPORAL POSITION (T-TM)	23.0mm to 32.0mm	33.6mm	LONG T-TM WILL LEAD TO SKELETAL CLASS II
OVERJET OF BONY BASES (A1-B1)		6.0mm	
MANDIBULAR LENGTH (B1-TM)		79.3mm	
MANDIBULAR DIAGONAL		106.9mm	
MANDIBULAR HEIGHT		76.0mm	
HORIZONTAL TOTAL		85.3mm	

ANGLES
UPPER INCISAL ANGLE		127.2°	
LOWER INCISAL ANGLE		111.7°	
INTERINCISAL ANGLE	120.0° to 140.0°	121.1°	
GONIAL ANGLE	105.0° to 120.0°	123.8°	LEPTOGNATHIC
IMPA		94.2°	

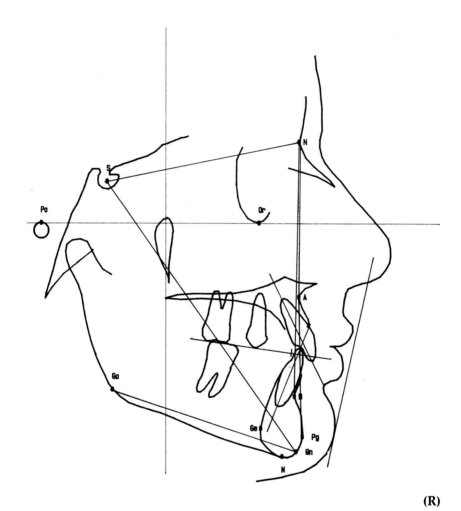

(R)

MODIFIED STEINER ANALYSIS

SKELETAL

MEASUREMENT	NORM	ACTUAL	COMMENT
SNA	80.0° to 84.0°	78.6°	RETROGNATHIC MAXILLA
SNB	78.0° to 82.0°	77.7°	RETROGNATHIC MANDIBLE
ANB	0.0° to 5.0°	1.0°	SKELETAL CLASS I
WITS	-3.0mm to 1.0mm	3.4mm	SKELETAL CLASS II
UPPER FACIAL HEIGHT	45.0%	44.6%	
LOWER FACIAL HEIGHT	55.0%	55.4%	
Go-Gn to SN	28.0° to 36.0°	29.4°	
Y-Axis to SN	63.0° to 69.0°	65.4°	
			Normal skeletal bite.
OCCL to SN	14.0° to 15.0°	19.0°	ANY CHANGE IN POSTERIOR VERTICAL SUPPORT WILL HAVE A THREE-FOLD PROPORTIONAL CHANGE IN ANTERIOR VERTICAL
Pg to NB	1.5mm to 3.5mm	3.5mm	

DENTAL

MEASUREMENT	NORM	ACTUAL	COMMENT
UP1 to NA DIST	4.0mm	6.7mm	
UP1 to NA ANG	20.0° to 24.0°	26.8°	BUCCOVERSION
LOW1 to NB DIST	4.0mm	3.1mm	
LOW1 to NB ANG	23.0° to 27.0°	21.3°	LINGUOVERSION
LOW1 TO UP1	120.0° to140.0°	131.0°	
A-Pg to LOW1	-2.0mm to 3.0mm	1.0mm	
6+6 to PTV	17.0mm	14.3mm	BE SURE ENOUGH TUBEROSITY EXISTS TO DISTALLIZE MOLARS IF NECESSARY

SOFT TISSUE

MEASUREMENT	NORM	ACTUAL	COMMENT
UPPER LIP	0.0mm to 2.0mm	1.7mm	
LOWER LIP	0.0mm to 2.0mm	2.1mm	

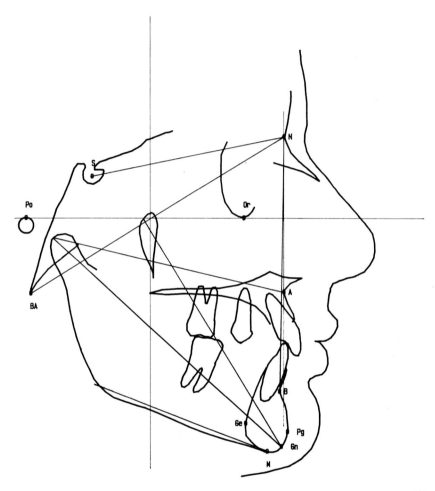

(S)

FUNCTIONAL ORTHOPEDIC ANALYSIS

MEASUREMENT	NORM	ACTUAL	COMMENT
A. RELATING THE MAXILLA TO THE CRANIAL BASE			
A Pt to N Perp	-1.0mm to 3.0mm	-0.1mm	
B. RELATING THE MANDIBLE TO THE MAXILLA			
Eff. MAXILLA Lgth	***	94.2mm	
Eff. MANDIBLE Lgth	119.4mm to124.4mm	121.4mm	
Diff=MAX-MAND Lgth	***	27.1mm	
Lower Facial Ht[Vert Dim]	66.3mm to 71.0mm	68.2mm	
C. RELATING THE UPPER INCISOR TO THE MAXILLA			
Up1 to A Perp	4.0mm to 6.0mm	6.7mm	
D. RELATING THE LOWER INCISOR TO THE MANDIBLE			
Low1 to A-Pg Line	1.0mm to 3.0mm	1.0mm	
E. MANDIBULAR POSITION			
Pg to N Perp	-6.0mm to -2.0mm	1.4mm	PROGNATHIC MANDIBLE
F. OTHER USEFUL CEPHALOMETRIC MEASUREMENTS			
SNA	80.0° to 84.0°	78.6°	RETROGNATHIC MAXILLA
SNB	78.0° to 82.0°	77.7°	RETROGNATHIC MANDIBLE
ANB	0.0° to 5.0°	1.0°	
Interincisal Angle	120.0° to140.0°	131.0°	
Mandibular Plane Angle	20.0° to 30.0°	18.1°	
Facial Axis (Ricketts)	86.5° to 93.5°	88.9°	

REFERENCE I.D. GRID

	ANTERIOR PROFILE ANGLE	BASIC ANGULAR RELATION	SUBORBITAL FACIAL INDEX	FACIAL FORMULA
	Class I 0-10° Class II >15° Class III <0°	Upper Basic Angle DLM DLM Lower Basic Angle	Dolico Meso — Prosopic Lepto	

	BONY OVERJET		TEMPORAL POSITION	GNATHIC INDEX
	A-B Distance (Projected) Class III (−) Mean -4 to 8 mm * Class II (+)	Factor ④ (+) (±) (−) Factor ⑧ (+) (±) (−)	T-TM Distance Short 20-24 Class III Med. 28-32 Normal Long 36-40 Class II	

	INTERINCISOR ANGLE		STRESS AXIS	ANGLE CLASS	DENTAL FORMULA
	BIPRO <120 DIV 1 120-140 DIV 2 >140	Upper Bicuspid Inclination P.O.R. Lower Bicuspid Inclination	Per Post Pre	I II III	

* − 0 to 8mm is The American interpretation
− 4 to 8 mm is The True Bimler interpretation

PATIENT'S I.D. GRID

FACIAL FORMULA	2.5	M/M	MESO
		−5.8/	
GNATHIC INDEX	1.7	14.7	35.2
DENTAL FORMULA	131	0/R	PRE/I

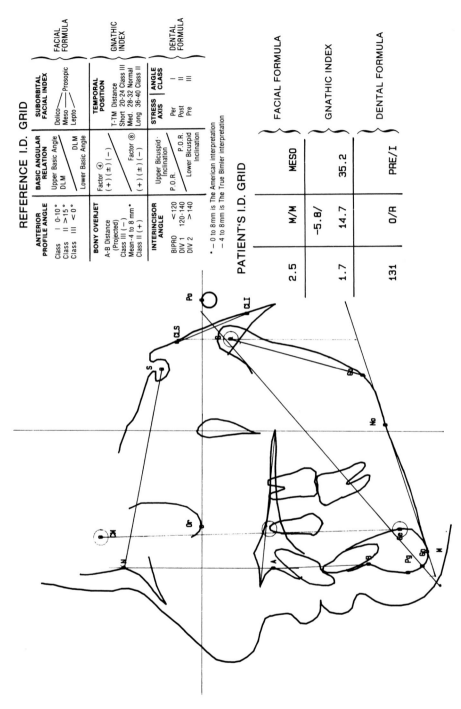

(T)

MODIFIED BIMLER ANALYSIS

MEASUREMENT	NORM	ACTUAL	COMMENT

FACTOR 1:
  UPPER PROFILE ANGLE N TO A   -1.0° to 1.0°   0.1° ORTHOGNATHIC

FACTOR 2:
  LOWER PROFILE ANGLE AB TO VERT   2.5°

  ANTERIOR PROFILE ANGLE (F1+F2)   0.0° to 10.0°   2.6° SKELETAL CLASS I

FACTOR 3:
  MANDIBULAR INCLINATION   18.9°

FACTOR 4:
  MAXILLARY INCLINATION ANS-PNS   -3.0° to 3.0°   -5.8° NASAL FLOOR CONTRIBUTES TO
                                                         OPEN BITE

  LOWER BASIC ANGLE (F3-F4)   15.0° to 30.0°   24.7° BALANCED GROWTH (MESO)

  ALVEOLAR HEIGHT   -0.2mm

FACTOR 5:
  CLIVUS INCLINATION   60.0° to 70.0°   68.3° MEDIUM POSTERIOR CRANIAL
                                                  BASE

  UPPER BASIC ANGLE (F5+F4)   60.0° to 70.0°   62.5° MESO PROSOPIC

  FACIAL HARMONY   M/M   NEUTRAL (L/L, M/M, D/D)

  SUBORBITAL FACIAL INDEX (A1M/AC) 1.00 to 1.05   1.02 MEDIUM

FACTOR 6:
  STRESS AXIS   119.6mm CLASS I (PRE)

FACTOR 7:
  N-S INCLINATION   11.3°

FACTOR 8:
  MANDIBULAR FLEXION   -5.0° to 5.0°   14.7° HYPERFLEXION - UNDER-
                                                 DEVELOPMENT OF MIDDLE FACE;
                                                 FAVORABLE IN CLASS III
                                                 CASES; IT WILL BE REDUCED
                                                 IN BITE OPENING IN TREATMENT

LINEAR MEASUREMENTS
  MAXILLA LENGTH (AT)   52.7mm
  TEMPORAL POSITION (T-TM)   23.0mm to 32.0mm   35.2mm LONG T-TM WILL LEAD TO
                                                       SKELETAL CLASS II
  OVERJET OF BONY BASES (A1-B1)   1.7mm
  MANDIBULAR LENGTH (B1-TM)   86.2mm
  MANDIBULAR DIAGONAL   120.8mm
  MANDIBULAR HEIGHT   89.8mm
  HORIZONTAL TOTAL   87.9mm

ANGLES
  UPPER INCISAL ANGLE   116.7°
  LOWER INCISAL ANGLE   112.4°
  INTERINCISAL ANGLE   120.0° to 140.0°   131.0°
  GONIAL ANGLE   105.0° to 120.0°   123.6° LEPTOGNATHIC
  IMPA   93.5°

REFERENCES

1. Ricketts RM, Roth RH, Chaconas SJ: *Orthodontic Diagnosis and Planning.* Rocky Mountain/Orthodontics, 1982, vol 2, p 380.
2. Moore AW: Orthodontic treatment factors in Class II malocclusion. *Am J Orthod* 1959;45:323–352.
3. Anderson JP: A cephalometric study of the relative position of mandibular condyles before and after treatment of Class II division 1 malocclusions, thesis. University of Washington, Seattle, 1955.
4. Strang RHW: *A Textbook of Orthodontics,* ed 3. Philadelphia, Lea & Febiger, 1950;544.
5. Kingsley NW: *A Treatise on Oral Deformity with Appropriate Preventive and Remedial Treatment.* New York, Appleton & Co, 1880.
6. Häupl K, Grossman WJ, Clarkson P: *Textbook of Functional Jaw Orthopaedics.* London, Henry Kimpton, 1952, p 72.
7. Rogers AP: Exercises for developing the muscles of the face with a view to increasing their functional activity. *Dent Cosmos* 1918;60:857–876.
8. Rogers AP: Muscle training and its relation to orthodontia. *Int J Orthod* 1918;4:555–577.
9. Rogers AP: Making facial muscles our allies in treatment and retention. *Dent Cosmos* 1922;64:711–730.
10. Rogers AP: Living orthodontic appliances. *Int J Orthod* 1929;15:1–14.
11. Rogers AP: The behavior of the temporomandibular joint in response to the myofunctional treatment of distoclusion. *Int J Orthod* 1935;21:426–438.
12. Häupl K, Grossman WJ, Clarkson P: *Textbook of Functional Jaw Orthopaedics.* London, Henry Kimpton, 1952, p 200.
13. Straub WJ: The etiology of the perverted swallowing habit. *Am J Orthod* 1951;37:603–610.
14. Andresen V: The Norwegian system of functional gnatho-orthopedics. *Acta Gnathol* 1936;1:5–36.
15. Schwarz AM, Gratzinger M: *Removable Orthodontic Appliances.* Philadelphia, WB Saunders Co, 1966.
16. Ketcham AH: A preliminary report of an investigation of apical root resorption of vital permanent teeth. *Int J Orthod* 1927;13:97–126.
17. Ketcham AH: A progress report of an investigation of apical root resorption of vital permanent teeth. *Int J Orthod* 1928;15:310–325.
18. Angle EH: The latest and best in orthodontic mechanism. *Dent Cosmos* 1929;71:164–174, 260–270, 409–421.
19. Bjork A: The principles of the Andresen method of orthodontic treatment, a discussion based on cephalometric X-ray analysis of treated cases. *Am J Orthod* 1951;37:437–458.
20. Softley JW: Cephalometric changes in seven "post normal" cases treated by the Andresen method. *Dent Rec* 1953;73:485–494.
21. Jakobsson SO: Cephalometric evaluation of treatment effect on Class II, division 1 malocclusions. *Am J Orthod* 1967;53:446–457.
22. Harvold EP, Vargervik K: Morphogenetic response to activator treatment. *Am J Orthod* 1971;60:478–490.
23. Ahlgren J: Late results of activator treatment. *Br J Orthod* 1976;3:181–187.

24. Moore AW: Observations on facial growth and its clinical significance. *Am J Orthod* 1959;45:399–423.
25. Trayfoot J, Richardson A: Angle Class II, division 1 malocclusion treated by the Andresen method. *Br Dent J* 1968;124:516–519.
26. Weinberger TW: Extra-oral traction and functional appliances—a cephalometric comparison. *Br J Orthod* 1973;1:35–39.
27. Harvold EP, Vagervik K: Morphogenetic response to activator treatment. *Am J Orthod* 1971;60:480.
28. Hotz RP: Application and appliance manipulation of functional forces. *Am J Orthod* 1970;58:459–478.
29. Woodside DG: Some effects of activator treatment on the mandible and the midface. *Trans Eur Orthod Soc* 1973;443–447.
30. Grude R: The Norwegian system of orthodontic treatment. *Dent Rec* 1938;58:529.
31. Engh O: Treatment with the Andresen activator. *Trans Eur Orthod Soc* 1951;200–208.
32. Bjork A: The principles of the Andresen method of orthodontic treatment, a discussion based on cephalometric X-ray analysis of treated cases. *Am J Orthod* 1951;37:457.
33. Korkhaus G: Present orthodontic thought in Germany. *Am J Orthod* 1960;46:270–287.
34. Brown RW: Cephalometric study of mandibular length change during F.J.O. treatment, thesis, University of Michigan, Ann Arbor, 1959.
35. Moss JP: Cephalometric changes during functional appliance therapy. *Trans Eur Orthod Soc* 1962;327–341.
36. Meach CL: A cephalometric comparison of bony profile changes in Class II, division 1 treated with extra-oral force and functional jaw orthopedics. *Am J Orthod* 1966;52:353–370.
37. Marchner JF, Harris JE: Mandibular growth in Class II treatment. *Angle Orthod* 1968;36:89–93.
38. Freunthaller P: Cephalometric observations in Class II, division 1 malocclusions treated with the activator. *Angle Orthod* 1967;37:18–24.
39. Ahlgren J: A longitudinal clinical and cephalometric study of 50 malocclusion cases treated with activator appliance. *Trans Eur Orthod Soc* 1972;48:285–293.
40. Demisch A: Effects of activator therapy on the craniofacial skeleton in Class II, division 1 malocclusion. *Trans Eur Orthod Soc* 1972;48:295–310.
41. Hausser E: Functional orthodontic treatment with the activator. *Trans Eur Orthod Soc* 1973;427–430.
42. Reey RW, Eastwood A: The passive activator: Case selection, treatment response and corrective mechanics. *Am J Orthod* 1978;73:378.
43. Wieslander L, Lagerstrom L: The effect of activator treatment on Class II malocclusions. *Am J Orthod* 1979;75:20–25.
44. Cohen AM: A study of Class II, division 1 malocclusions treated by the Andresen appliance. *Br J Orthodont* 1981;8:159–163.
45. Stoeckli P: Personal communication, Annual Meeting of the European Orthodontic Society, Barcelona, Spain, 1979.
46. Bimler HP: Personal communication, Wiesbaden, West Germany, July 18, 1984.
47. Bimler HP: Dynamic functional therapy. *Trans Eur Orthod Soc* 1973;451–456.
48. Bimler HP: Possibilities and limitations of treatment in Class II cases. *Trans Eur Orthod Soc* 1956;55–67.

49. Bimler HP: *The Bimler Appliance: Construction and Adjustment.* Great Falls, Mont, V Nord, 1966.

50. Bimler HP: Some etiologic factors in Class III malocclusions. *Trans Eur Orthod Soc* 1970;115–129.

51. Schwarz AM, Gratzinger M: *Removable Orthodontic Appliances.* Philadelphia, WB Saunders Co, 1966.

52. Graber T, Neumann B: *Removable Orthodontic Appliances.* Philadelphia, WB Saunders Co, 1977, pp 247–252.

53. Graber T, Neumann B: *Removable Orthodontic Appliances.* Philadelphia, WB Saunders Co, 1977, pp 253–268.

54. Stockfisch H: The Kinetor. *Trans Eur Orthod Soc* 1973;457–461.

55. Stockfisch H: Possibilities and limitations of the Kinetor bimaxillary appliance. *Trans Eur Orthod Soc* 1971;317–328.

56. Kraus F: The vestibular and oral screen. *Trans Eur Orthod Soc* 1956;217.

57. Parkhouse RC: A cephalometric appraisal of cases of Angle's Class II, division 1 malocclusions treated by the Andresen appliance. *Dent Pract* 1969;19;12: 425–433.

58. Harvold EP: The role of function in the etiology and treatment of malocclusion. *Am J Orthod* 1968;54:883–897.

59. Peat JH: A cephalometric study of tongue position. *Am J Orthod* 1968;54:339–351.

60. Brodie AG: Anatomy and physiology of head and neck musculature. *Am J Orthod* 1950;36:831.

61. Hanson ML, Logan BW, Case JL: Tongue thrust in preschool children. Pt II. Dental occlusal patterns. *Am J Orthod* 1970;57:15–22.

62. Grude R: Myofunctional therapy. A review of various cases some years after their treatment by the Norwegian system had been completed. *Nor Tannlaegeforen Tid* 1952;62:1–28.

63. Quinby HC, quoted by Weinberger BW: *Orthodontics, a Historical Review of Its Origin and Evolution.* St Louis, CV Mosby Co, 1926, vol 2.

64. Davenport IB: Correction of undershutting jaw by raising and jumping the bite. *Dent Cosmos* 1905;47:252.

65. Hopkins SC: Bite planes. *Am J Orthod* 1940;26:107–119.

66. Belger I: Cephalometric analysis of growth in subjects using bite plates. *Angle Orthod* 1956;26:42–49.

67. Bahador MA, Higley LB: Bite opening, a cephalometric analysis. *J Am Dent Assoc* 1944;31:343–352.

68. Atherton JD: The effect of removable appliance therapy on facial pattern. *Br Dent J* 1963;114:512–514.

69. Hemley S: Bite plates, their application and action. *Am J Orthod* 1938;24:721–736.

70. Sleichter CG: Effects of maxillary bite plane therapy in orthodontics. *Am J Orthod* 1954;40:850–870.

71. Menezes DM: Changes in the dentofacial complex as a result of bite plane therapy. *Am J Orthod* 1975;67:660–675.

72. Breitner C: Bone changes resulting from experimental orthodontic treatment. *Am J Orthod Oral Surg* 1940;26:521–546.

73. Carlson H: Studies on the rate and amount of eruption of certain human teeth. *Am J Orthod Oral Surg* 1944;30:575–588.

74. Kloehn SJ: Guiding alveolar growth and eruption of teeth to reduce treatment time and produce a more balanced denture and face. *Angle Orthod* 1947;17: 10–33.

75. Salzman JA: *Principles of Orthodontics,* ed 2. Philadelphia, JB Lippincott Co, 1950, p 807.
76. Softley JW: Factors concerned with closed bite. *Br Soc Stud Orthod* 1947;200–209.
77. Dunn R: Vertical overbite or arrested vertical development in the molar and premolar region. *Int J Orthod* 1926;12:8.
78. Broadway RT: Depression of lower incisors. *Trans Br Soc Orthod* 1957;70.
79. Richardson A, Adams CP: An investigation into the short and long term effects of the anterior bite plane on the occlusal relationship and facial form. *Trans Europ Orthod Soc* 1963;375–382.
80. Graber T, Neumann B: *Removable Orthodontic Appliances.* Philadelphia, WB Saunders Co, 1977, p 134.
81. Grude R: The Norwegian system of orthodontic treatment. *Dent Rec* 1938;58:529.
82. Herren P: The activator's mode of action. *Am J Orthod* 1959;45:512–527.
83. Harvold EP: *The Activator in Interceptive Orthodontics.* St Louis, CV Mosby Co, 1974.
84. Graber TM, Neumann B: *Removable Orthodontic Appliances,* ed 2. Philadelphia, WB Saunders Co, 1984, p 189.
85. Witzig JW: *Orthodontic and Orthopedic Principles and Appliances.* Minneapolis, 1979.
86. Lustman SL: Emotional problems of children as they relate to orthodontics. *Am J Orthod* 1960;46:358–362.
87. Feldstein L: Problems of orthodontists in treating adolescents. *Am J Orthod* 1959;45:131–140.
88. Lewis HG, Brown WAB: The attitude of patients to the wearing of a removable orthodontic appliance. *Br Dent J* 1973;134:87–90.
89. Baume LJ, Haupl K, Stellmach R: Growth and transformation of the temporomandibular joint in an orthopedically treated case of Pierre Robin's syndrome. *Am J Orthod* 1959;45:901–916.
90. Gresham H: Mandibular changes in Andresen treatment of Angle Class II malocclusion. *NZ Dent J* 1952;48:10–36.
91. Ozerovic B: Some changes in occlusion and craniofacial pattern obtained during treatment with removable orthodontic appliances. *Trans Eur Orthod Soc* 1972;329–337.
92. Baume LJ: Cephalo-facial growth patterns and the functional adaptation of the temporomandibular joint structures. *Trans Eur Orthod Soc* 1969;79–98.
93. Rushton MA: Growth at the mandibular condyle in relation to some deformities. *Br Dent J* 1944;76:57–68.
94. Enlow DH, Harris DB: A study of postnatal growth of the human mandible. *Am J Orthod* 1964;50:25–50.
95. Enlow DH: *Handbook of Facial Growth.* Philadelphia, WB Saunders Co, 1975, p 102.
96. Koski K: Cranial growth centers: Facts or fallacies? *Am J Orthod* 1968;54:566–583.
97. Moss ML, Rankow RM: The role of the functional matrix in mandibular growth. *Angle Orthod* 1968;38:95–103.
98. Pimenidis MZ, Gianelly AA: The effects of early postnatal condylectomy on the growth of the mandible. *Am J Orthod* 1972;62:42–47.
99. Meikle MC: The role of the condyle in postnatal growth of the mandible. *Am J Orthod* 1973;64:50–62.
100. Hellman M: The face and teeth of man. *J Dent Res* 1929;9:2.
101. Brash JC: The growth of the jaws, normal and abnormal, in health and disease, in *Growth of the Jaws and Palate.* Dental Board of the United Kingdom, 1924, pp 59–61.

CHAPTER 3
The Great Second-Molar Debate

Sometimes as an unforeseen accident of the times, a solution to a problem is derived, such as the bicuspid extraction philosophy, which may at one time solve that singular problem but at the same time create others far more serious in its wake. This is the situation which has come about in the field of orthodontics due to the problem of dental crowding within the arches and how to relieve it. As we have previously stated, the Bionator is an arch-aligning appliance, and is predicated by its very definition on proper arch form, ie, arches free of dental crowding. Therefore, decrowding of the arches becomes a very important step in orthodontic therapeutics, especially prior to Bionator therapy. Yet just *how* this is accomplished can have both a profound and permanent effect on the face, the stability of the occlusion, and most importantly, the preservation of the functional integrity of the temporomandibular joint!

And therefore, not prematurely, but rather by necessity, we enter the very heart of traditional orthodontic therapeutics: the need for increased arch length and how to get it! This mandates that one address the most significant concept developed to date for solving the problem of excessive crowding: the sacrificial extraction of teeth to provide sorely needed space into which remaining teeth may be realigned. It is a virtual "inner sanctum"

155

of the orthodontic world in which up to the present time the reigning high priest has been the concept of bicuspid extraction which has ruled unchallenged over generations of venerating followers.[1-6] It has been so since the days of the turn of the century when its first proponents such as Calvin Case and Martin Dewey first parted ways with their instructor and contemporary E. H. Angle and his "non-extraction dogmas" of arch expansion. This technique proscribes the bicuspids as the individual teeth arbitrarily deemed expendable, while all other teeth, with the exception of third molars, are revered as inviolate. Third molars are considered even more expendable than bicuspids. It was a technique never designed with the face, the stability of the occlusion, nor the health of the TMJ in mind, merely the decrowding of arches.

It was a technique that seemed logical and was time-honored. It bore the promise of expediency and excellent results. It is also predicated upon fixed appliance usage, a necessary means of handling the orthodontic problems associated with the technique once spaces have been created by the extraction of the bicuspids.

Over the years, all sorts of paraphernalia have been ingeniously devised to move teeth, usually against their will, into the newly created quarter-inch gap in the arch resulting from the extraction of the condemned bicuspids. Elaborate mechanisms of anchorage and retraction, balance and counterbalance, force and counterforce have been conceived and elaborated upon by dedicated and talented practitioners to facilitate these necessary movements, alignments, and retentions.[7-13] Orthodontic practitioners strived valiantly to overcome the problems inherent in the technique and in so doing became not only proud, but adamant and even on occasion complacent in their ability to move and realign individual teeth. The somewhat isolated concerns of merely straightening teeth drew their paramount attentions. Theirs was a standard for the world!

But as the methodologies became more and more sophisticated, the minute observance of detail became such a preoccupation for some that during their noble attempts to solve the staggering problems of four-bicuspid-extraction-oriented orthodontia, if you will forgive the pun, a little of the total face of the overall treatment goal became mottled behind the quiddities of technique.

Yet for the most part, the American orthodontic community embraced this standard with open arms and became secure in it to the point of dogmatically professing it as the only technique to be used when extractions were indicated. At least the orthodontic procedures seemed well researched and documented. However, the most fundamental issues were never challenged. No one ever questioned the possibility that their standard might be suspect, nor their beliefs called to question. The theory seemed invincible. All seemed well with the world.

But colder eyes quietly watched from a distance and their shrewd preception sensed a need for a new direction in thinking as the problems inherent in the bicuspid extraction system rose to the surface and became apparent. Too many facial profiles became "dished-in," too many occlusions relapsed to improper arch form, too many temporomandibular joints became dislocated with condyles being driven up and back off the posterior end of the disc. It was not a matter of whether or not to extract to aid in the decrowding of arches, but rather of which tooth to extract. An alternative method had to be sought. As far as extractions were concerned, another tooth had to be selected. After careful consideration, another tooth was selected, one with a naturally built-in replacement factor associated with it and one that shocked the highly conservative members of the "four-bicuspid extraction establishment." The "second molar replacement" principle was a concept the general orthodontic community as a whole had never been educated to, nor was it familiar with it in clinical practice. Needless to say, they were not prepared to deal with it once it was thrust upon them. Its implications that their four-bicuspid extraction methods had been ill-conceived and errant from the start was a notion incomprehensible to their heretofore unchallenged positions. With insecurity and apprehension being some of the natural human by-products of such a wholesale and overwhelming assault upon what up until then had been a highly respected status quo, the conservative establishment endeavored to resecure its position. Thus a monumental controversy was ignited; the great second-molar debate!

Historically speaking, debates on extracting one tooth or another are nothing new to orthodontics. These controversies go back to the turn of the century to the very founding father of modern-day orthodontics himself, Edward H. Angle.

A Pennsylvania farm boy, he graduated from the Pennsylvania College of Dentistry in 1878 and immediately entered into the practice of or-

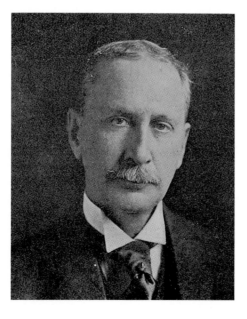

Figure 3-1 Edward Hartley Angle

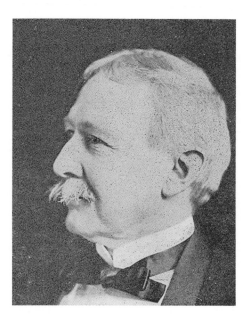

Figure 3-2 Calvin S. Case

thodontics. After a brief stint out West, and some time in private practice in Minneapolis, he became first, Professor of Orthodontics at Northwestern University School of Dentistry, and then eventually settled in a similar job at Washington University in St Louis. He devoted his whole life to the field of orthodontics and was determined to isolate it as a specialty of dentistry. He wrote what has become "the Bible" of orthodontics of the first half of this century[14] and his "Angle classification" system of defining the three main types of malocclusions is used throughout the world to this day.[15] He developed many forms of orthodontic devices and his edgewise appliance[16] has been used by more orthodontists on more cases than any other fixed appliance developed up to the present time.[17]

In 1900 he opened his own private school in St Louis solely for the purpose of teaching orthodontics. It consisted of an 8-week course. The following year he helped form the American Society of Orthodontics still headquartered in that city.

But he was, for all his scientific training and acumen, negatively adamant on one issue: that of the extraction of teeth for the purposes of relieving crowding in the dental arches. He was very much against this procedure and here is where he spawned his greatest criticisms from his colleagues and students, some of whom would contribute greatly to the field of orthodontics in their own right.

One of the most intense opponents of the Angle philosophy was Calvin Case. An instructor in orthodontics at the Chicago College of Dental Surgery, he was a teacher throughout his life. He also wrote a book that was second only to Angle's in popularity, *The Techniques and Principles of Dental Ortho-*

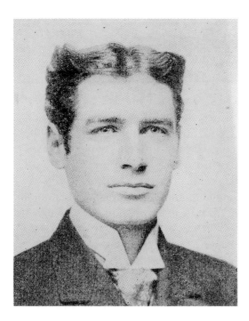

Figure 3-3 Martin Dewey

pedia, published in 1908. He, unlike Angle, did not believe that every tooth had to be present in the mouth to produce a "perfect" correction of a dental malocclusion. He was also one of the first to propose the use of light-wire forces and the use of retainers after treatment to aid in stabililty.

Another arch dissenter to the Angle method was one of Angle's own students, Martin Dewey. A graduate of Keokuk Dental College, Dewey, who was later to earn an MD degree also, joined the Angle School of Orthodontia during its first year and stayed on after graduation to become an instructor. But his opposition to Angle's views on extractions and his refusal to accept Angle's dogmatic claims of the superiority of certain treatment methods over others led to Dewey's resignation.

Since the orthodontic college founding business looked pretty good, he formed one of his own in 1911 in Kansas City. He too wrote a book, *Practical Orthodontics*, published in 1914, and helped found what is now known as the *American Journal of Orthodontics* (then the *International Journal of Orthodontia*).

Other great men of the time too were alienated by the strictly narrow teachings of Edward Angle. Among them was the famous Albert Ketcham. His criticisms of certain Angle techniques[18,19] brought about a severe counterattack from Angle. All sorts of arguments continued back and forth among these founding fathers which engendered bitter feelings that lasted lifetimes. The beginning of orthodontia in America was a rocky road indeed.

But since those early days it has become quite generally accepted that in certain cases of extreme crowding, extraction of teeth for the sake of gaining space for the others is a perfectly acceptable procedure. No qualms are felt whatsoever when third molars are removed to relieve potential or actual crowding in the posterior segments. There are even those who postulate that in this regard, we only aid in what Nature is striving for evolutionarily anyway.[20] That is, anthropologically the australopithecines, early forerunners to man, and even *Homo habilis*, and early *Homo erectus* had protruding mandibles with adequate room for third molars. As the species evolved, the skull and face gained in height and decreased in facial angle to facilitate speech. In so doing, the third set of molars gradually became a redundancy, and rather than become vestigial, were more commonly impacted or on occasion simply lost to the gene pool. Now there is speculation that with modern *Homo sapiens* and his even flatter, more vertical face, these third molars have become a complete redundancy and are on the way out genetically. Several million years should prove the accuracy of this theory one way or another!

But often the crowding or decreased arch length is not solely confined to the posterior segments, but rather also extends forward to the anterior areas. This is usually treated by extraction of one of the two pair of bicuspids, with the first bicuspids usually the ones most often slated for the forceps. It is theorized that bicuspid extractions are indicated when nonextraction correction of arch-crowding would result in overexpansion of teeth past the limits of the apical bases.

The more severe the crowding, the better this system works. Cases of slight crowding present a real dilemma to the orthodontist for he is faced with either (1) extraction with a resultant excess of space requiring excessive tooth movement for closure and concomitant arch length shrinkage, or (2) overexpansion of all the teeth without the benefit of extraction and the possibility that this overexpansion will take teeth beyond the limits of the denture base of bone resulting in a high risk of instability and relapse (Angle's old problem).

Over the years many refinements were made in technique to improve results, but in spite of these noble efforts, problems still persisted. Critics of the results obtained with the four-bicuspid extraction methods pointed out that certain untoward sequelae appeared in a great percentage of finished cases. Vertical dimension was often lost, contact points were not always satisfactory, stability was a problem with demands for excessively long retention periods, and arch size and facial fullness were often compromised. Often a "flat" appearance resulted in the premaxillary area or "smile line."

It is easiest to segregate these problems into two main groups, orthodontic and orthopedic. Often the purely orthodontic dental implications were the chief concern of treating clinicians with complete disregard being given to the overall bone reaction on a gross anatomical level to the bicuspid extraction system. It is important to keep both of these categories in mind when evaluating the merit of a given treatment method, for though the teeth are important, they will always come into the office attached to a human being, and the patient as a whole person is even of greater importance.

"If Cleopatra's nose had been shorter, the whole face of the world would have been changed."

Pascal (1623–1662)
Pensées

ORTHOPEDIC CONSIDERATIONS

When one evaluates the orthopedic considerations of the bicuspid extraction system, the two main areas that come to the forefront are the specific area of the temporomandibular joint and the general area of the entire human face.

The Face

Faces are extremely important. Rightly or wrongly (most probably wrongly), they determine the prejudice the world will have either for or against an individual on his journey through life. Children are quick to malign a fellow playmate who suffers from an insufficiently formed, unattractive face. This is torment to the young recipients of such abuse as children are most often sensitive and insecure to begin with. Adolescents fare little better. The social life, and often future adult life, of a young lady is often predicated upon her ability to present an attractive and pleasing face to the world. The very symbol for the female sex itself, ♀, is an allusion to Aphrodite's mirror, used to make sure the goddess of love and beauty herself is suitably attractive in appearance. And as for the men, in all the classical sculptures of antiquity, not a single example of a statue of a male can be found with a severely retruded mandible! The weak and unassuming chin in males has been considered throughout the ages as being simply unmasculine.

Bicuspid extractions affect the face in several ways. First, they result in a narrower smile line of teeth as the arch is necessarily devoid of one less tooth on each side. As the remaining teeth are moved into the empty space, a smaller overall arch results. This can be compounded by retaining the molars by means of headgear in their initial pretreatment positions and pulling everything else back to contact. If the premaxilla is brought in too far, the support for the upper lip is diminished and the lip appears weak at the cuspid eminence lending an aged and "sunken-in" appearance to the corners of the mouth. Since the lower incisors must fit in behind the uppers, the above condition of overretraction of the upper anteriors does nothing to remedy the retruded chin often associated with skeletal Class II cases.

The loss in vertical, often associated with bicuspid extraction cases,[21] only serves to compound the problem of insufficient lower face height. This too lends a slightly older appearance to the overall face.

Another complication associated with mandibular insufficiency is that if such a case is treated by extracting bicuspids and retracting the premaxilla, the nose appears to be longer and a more pointed, "fishlike" appearance to the face results. The nasal bone, cartilage, and soft tissue remain in the approximately same cephalometric position during treatment and, unless drastic measures are taken, their position is strictly a function of genetic growth. As the premaxilla and lip are retracted, the nose remains behind as if it were marooned "high and dry." Though these changes can be subtle, intensifying their situation with improper orthodontics is not a circumstance usually favorably accepted. This "nose-lengthening" process also lends an aged appearance to the face.

One of the most glaring examples of the above is found in a case reported by Eirew[22] where a pair of identical twins were both treated orthodontically for malocclusions. One was treated the conventional way by means of extraction of four bicuspids and fixed appliances. The other was treated without the benefit of extractions by means of a functional appliance to expand the arches. The results were overwhelming. The first twin, the extraction case, suffered so much from the above-mentioned sequelae that comparison to her sister, treated with the functional appliance, caused her such disappointment and consternation that investigation and comparison of the cases had to be dropped. Eirew reports that this first twin felt as though she had been dealt an "unkind blow and she is now the ugly sister." In fact, her sister treated with FJOs does present a far more youthful and pleasing appearance with her broad full smile, flushed cheeks, and pleasingly balanced lips.

If it had to be boiled down to a word, it would be "fullness." Simple perusal of any magazine will divulge numerous examples of both male and female models with this trait evident in their lower faces. A rugged, full, square jaw has always been a trait considered handsome in a man, but women also do well with a fullness to their lower face. The wide high cheekbones and large full lower jaw line are evident on many a female model. Their smiles and lip lines are full and well supported at the corners of the mouth. No gaps appear between the line of sight of the bicuspids and the corners of the mouth upon broad smiling. And, as anyone the least bit observant will tell you, a smile improves any woman's looks by 100%.

Figure 3-4   (A) Initially the teeth of a 16-year-old girl after four bicuspids were extracted appear in beautiful occlusion; but when compared with results the treatment brought about on profile of **(B)**, it at once becomes obvious that extraction of bicuspids and overretraction of anterior parts of both upper and lower dentures left orthopedic aspects of the case wanting.

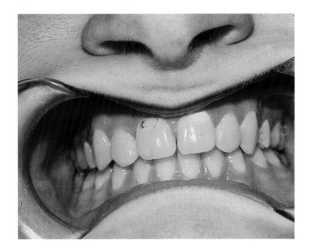

(A)

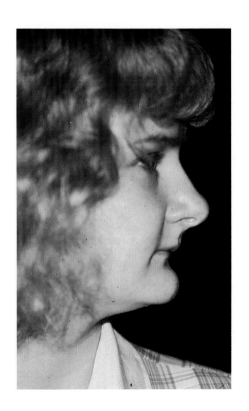

(B)

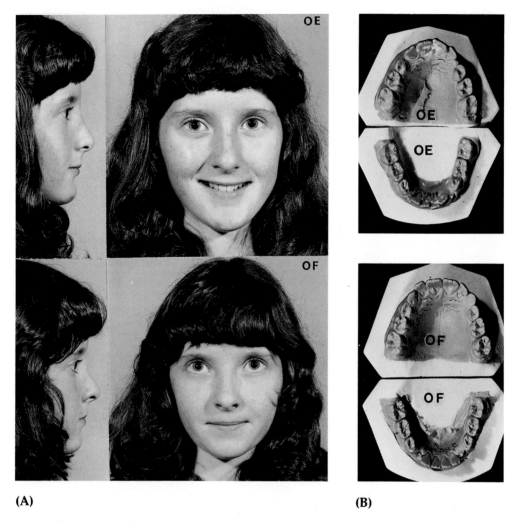

(A)   **(B)**

Figure 3-5 **(A)** Original appearance of identical twins prior to treatment, OE was girl to receive four bicuspid extraction, fixed appliance treatment, while OF was girl to receive treatment leaving all bicuspids intact and a functional appliance. **(B)** Original models of twins showing pretreatment arch form. (*Courtesy of Dr Hans Eirew, Manchester, England.*)

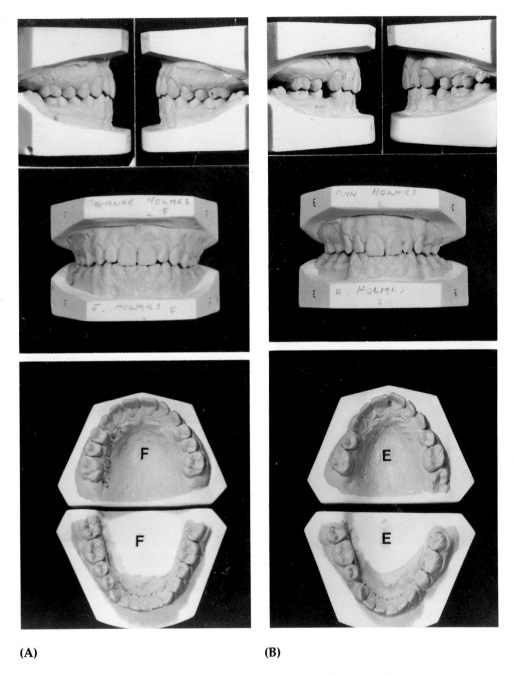

(A)   **(B)**

Figure 3-6 **(A)** Final models of twin treated by functional appliance.
(B) Final models of twin treated by extractions and fixed appliances.

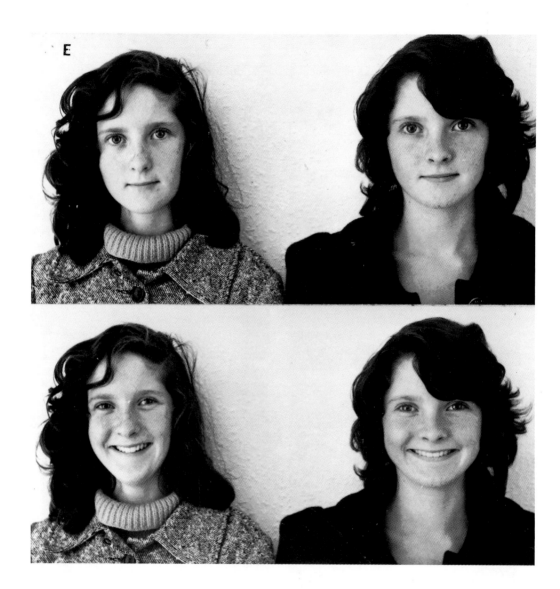

Figure 3-7 Posttreatment comparison of faces. "Res ipsa loquitur."

Bicuspid extraction, by virtue of taking place on a curve, shrinks the radius of that curve and takes away from the fullness of the line of sight to the eye of the remaining teeth. The dental arch shrinks but the oral opening doesn't; and when a patient smiles broadly enough, it can sometimes appear as if there is not sufficient size to the denture to fill the space of the opening and as a result part of the buccal mucosa of the innner cheeks fills in the gap between the bicuspids and the corners of the mouth. This can be detected by the eye in some patients who have had bicuspids extracted and is not as complimentary as a larger, fuller dental arch.

The Temporomandibular Joint.

Another very important area to consider orthopedically is the aforementioned temporomandibular joint. It is an area that has, until recently, received very little attention from the orthodontic community.

Although at present, the concern over bicuspid extraction technique and its untoward effects on the function of the temporomandibular joint seems to be a high priority interest of our modern times, its origins go back almost half a century to the first clinician to ever call attention to it on a major scale, Dr H. E. Wilson of London, England. The extensive pioneering work[23-29] of this shrewd and acutely observant clinician might easily qualify him for the title of "the father of second-molar extraction concepts." And ironically, the evolution of this concept was not the product of an effort to solve problems of an orthodontic nature but was in a roundabout way devised to address problems of an orthopedic nature, ie, the treatment of patients suffering from temporomandibular joint pain and dysfunction.

As an orthodontist, Wilson had been involved in treating patients with temporomandibular joint (TMJ) disturbances orthodontically. He observed that many of these patients had previously had four-bicuspid extraction-type orthodontics and many of these in turn exhibited, in addition to their TMJ problems, a whole host of additional orthodontic problems such as: mesially tilted posterior teeth, distally tilted canines and lower anteriors, persistent deep overbites and, of course, the old standby, relapse! What Wilson discovered to his amazement was that for many of the cases, successful treatment involved the reverse tooth movement to what was performed in the original orthodontic treatment! As Wilson states, "'In an effort to avoid producing conditions that could later be a factor in temporomandibular joint disturbances, an alternative to the four bicuspid extraction method was sought." This eventually led to the second-molar extraction principle of allowing the thirds to erupt in place of the extracted seconds. This obviated the necessity for retracting anterior teeth as there was no bicuspid space to close. Posterior teeth could be distalized to relieve crowding anteriorly while at the same time allowing the face and jaws to continue to be developed down and forward, the natural way, protecting the TMJ in the process. Putting his theory into practice, Wilson studied 500 cases where second molars had been removed allowing third molars to erupt. An extremely high percentage (87%) of those followed exhibited third molars erupting acceptably to place. The very few that did not "can usually be treated simply." (With 500 cases, I wonder if he was trying to outdo Pasteur?!)

Since the position of the teeth in the jaws has a direct bearing on the functioning of the TMJ during their occlusion and the musculature is a vehicle to bring about this occlusion, a thorough knowledge of this anatomical structure is imperative.

It is not the purpose of this chapter to discuss TMJ malarthrosis in detail. However, a brief review of anatomy and a simplified organization of thoughts on the TMJ would be most handy in helping put functional jaw orthopedic methodology into its proper perspective relative to this important anatomical structure.

Defined as a "compression movement articulation," the temporomandibular joint is a ball-and-socket arrangement with an intervening collagenous disc between the ball, the head of the condyle, and the socket, a depression in the base of the temporal bone called the glenoid fossa. Both the head of the condyle and the major portion, the articular surface of the bone, of the glenoid fossa are composed mostly of collagen, unlike most other joints in the body which are hyaline in nature. The disc is quite pliable and elastic and acts as a stabilizer for the head of the condyle as it translates during opening down the slope of the articular eminence, or to be more specific, the posterior surface of the eminentia, or tuberculum. It is attached anteriorly to the superior head of the lateral pterygoid muscle and posteriorly to a very rubber bandlike ligament that is very important. This posterior attachment is known as the bilaminar zone because it contains two layers of fibers with soft loose areolar tissue in between. The area is also highly enervated with nerves and blood vessels. It does not have much shock-absorbing effect and was not designed by Nature to be impinged upon by the head of the condyle. Between the superior surface of the disc and the dome of the fossa, and the inferior surface of the disc and the capitular head of the condyle are two synovial spaces. These upper and lower compartments, as they are referred to, are separate from each other and nonconfluent in the normal healthy joint. They contain synovial fluid. This fluid acts as an ideal lubricant to facilitate movement of the disc and condyle during rotational and translatory movements of the joint.

Figure 3-8 **(A)** A duplicate set of edentulous upper models were waxed up with identical sized teeth (identical mold numbers) for comparison of arch sizes between "extracted arch" and "nonextracted arch." The first molars are set at identical distances from maxillary Hanular notches on both casts and at identical crossarch widths. The model on right has all bicuspids present whereas model on left has a bicuspid missing on each side. The remaining six anterior teeth were reset in as close to reasonable arch form as possible without moving the molars forward. Although it may at first appear as an optical illusion, the set-up on left appears much shorter and wider. Yet when they were set up, both were carefully measured so both sets of second bicuspids would be at exactly the same crossarch width. If the arch were to have anteriors more protruded to compensate for so much retraction caused by missing bicuspids, the overall arch would, of course, have to be narrower. Either way, an arch grossly smaller all around obviously results. **(B)** For more dramatic comparison, one side of denture was set with both bicuspids, other side set with only one. Note amount of arch shrinkage. **(C)** Placing both dentures against each other so that first and second molars coincide, amount of arch shrinkage is once again evident.

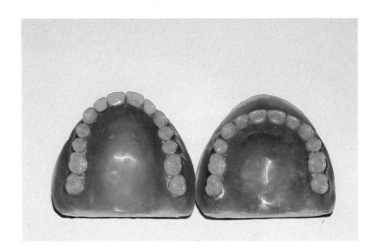

(A)

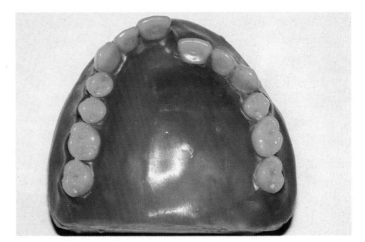

(B)

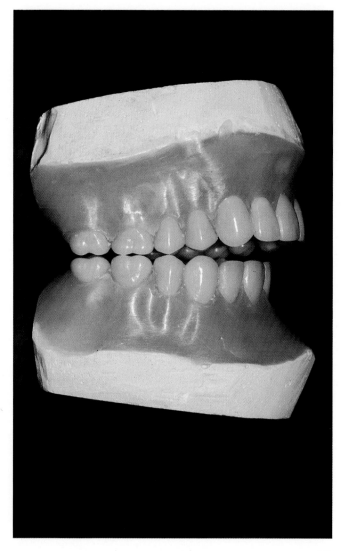

(C)

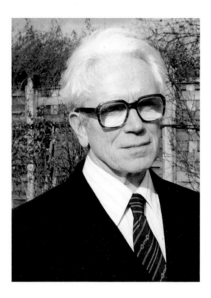

Figure 3-8   (D)   H.E. Wilson

Interestingly, the disc only covers the condyle to about one half to two thirds over the top of the most superior part of the condyle or, more specifically, the capitulum. It lies on the anterior portion of the condylar head in the anterior slope of the glenoid fossa as if poised like a sled on a hill waiting to cradle and guide the condylar head down the slope to the articular eminence, or tuberculum, a convexity of the temporal bone at the "end of the run." In so doing, it provides joint stability and smooth operation all the way. The entire arrangement is sort of like an upside-down ski slope. The disc is always poised on the more anterior aspect of the capitulum or actual articular surface of the condyle at an angle of about 45 degrees to the horizontal. However, sometimes it may not always remain exactly poised between the capitulum and tuberculum in certain cases of TMJ malarthrosis, rather it may be deranged by being displaced anteriorly. But it never makes the mistake of going too far up over the top, ie, retracting too far posteriorly and superiorly up over the head of the condyle. The entire apparatus is enclosed in a sort of collagenous cocoon of ligaments that forms a gristly, tough covering called the capsule. These ligaments serve to help keep everything in place, but they are not elastic like the ligaments of the bilaminar zone. They can be stressed and stretched during improper or imbalanced joint function to the point of permanent distortion.

It is very important to understand what happens to the disc during function and what conditions could bring about dysfunction.

Why is the disc attached to a muscle at one end and a highly elastic ligament at the other? No one knows. But there are some pretty good ideas around as to how this strange arrangement works. When the mouth is opened, the condyle rotates and almost immediately begins its translation down through the anterior portion of the glenoid fossa. Now it must be re-

Figure 3-9 Temporomandibular joint (TMJ) anatomy, function and
pathofunction. **(A–G)** Normal function. **(A)** Sagittal section of left TMJ.
(B) External anatomy of temporomandibular joint (left side). **(C)** Intra-
articular disc and capsule of TMJ in its normal structural relationship.
Intra-articular disc (A) is in normal position between artricular eminence
of the temporal bone and head of the condyle of the mandible with
teeth and jaws in fully-closed occlusally-balanced positions. Disc is
biconcave and made of dense fibrous connective tissue. It is attached to
condylar poles medially and laterally by tough collateral ligaments
(B). Posterior to distal edge or heel of disc and contiguous with it is the
highly vascular and neurally enervated bilaminar zone, or retrodiscal
tissue, containing posterior ligament (E). Anteriorly the front of the disc
(toe) is attached to superior head of the lateral pterygoid muscle (C)
while inferior head of the lateral pterygoid muscle (D) is attached to the
condylar neck on its anterior slope just below condylar head.
(D) Mid-sagittal section through TMJ (A) articular eminence or tuberculum, (B) intra-articular disc displaying classic 2:1:3 proportional ratios
of thickness anteriorly at toe, narrowing at midsection and widening
again to its thickest at posterior end or heel, (C) condylar head (upper
surface which lies adjacent to inferior border of disc is referred to as
capitulum), (D) highly sensitive bilaminar zone and posterior attachment, (E) superior belly of lateral pterygoid muscle, (G) external
auditory meatus. **(E)** TMJ condyle/disc assembly is capable of purely
rotational movements about an axis of hinge rotation (circular arrows
and dot at center). As mandible rotates (dotted line), it is capable of
fullscale translation movements as mandible moves down and forward
in a wide arc of opening. Stereoscopic design of biconcave disc and its
ability to move back and forth with translatory movements of condylar
head (capitulum) allow it to cradle condyle with full shock absorbing effect in all phases of lower jaw movement, especially during closing and
full force loading of the joint as in mastication, deglutition, or bruxism.
(F) Beginning of translation: as condyle moves down and forward as
mandible opens, disc travels with it, stabilizing condyle against articular
eminence and providing an ideal surface against which loading forces
may be absorbed. Tension begins to be expressed in elastic posterior
ligament, or attachment, as disc assembly begins to move down and
forward as result of the anterior pull of the lateral pterygoid muscle.
(A) tuberculum, (B) capitulum, (C) superior head of lateral pterygoid,
(D) inferior head of lateral pterygoid, (E) superior posterior ligament,
(F) inferior posterior ligament, (G) superior synovial compartment,
(H) inferior synovial compartment anterior area, (I) inferior synovial
compartment posterior area.

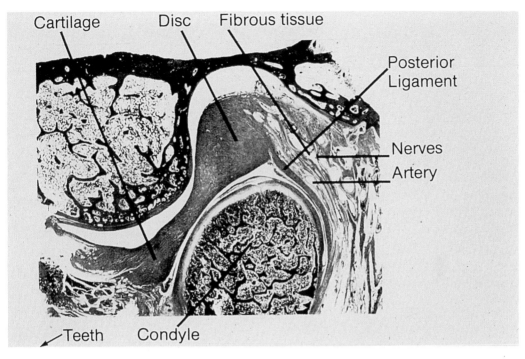

Cartilage   Disc   Fibrous tissue
Posterior
Ligament
Nerves
Artery
Teeth   Condyle

(A)

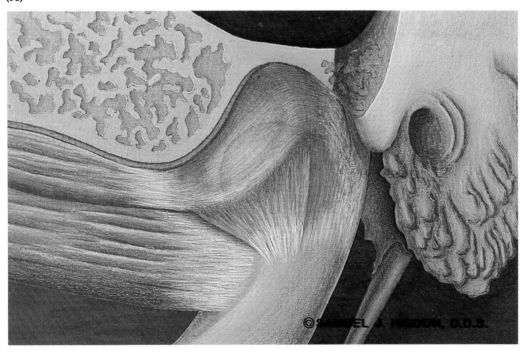

©SAMUEL J. HIGDON, D.D.S.

(B)

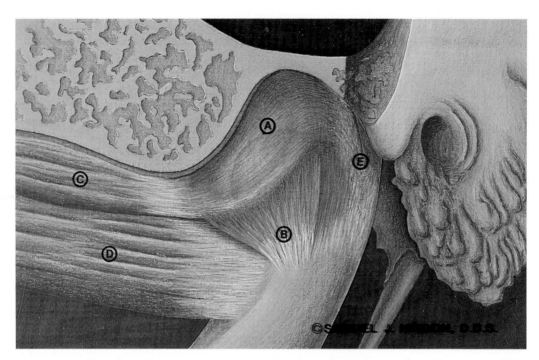

(C)

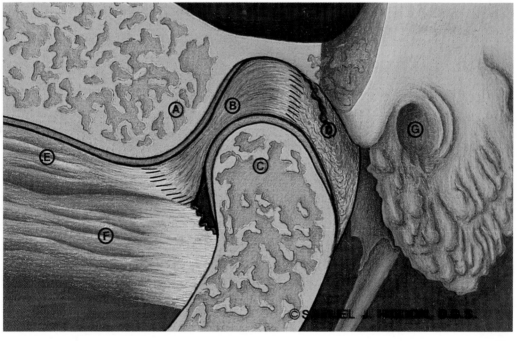

(D)

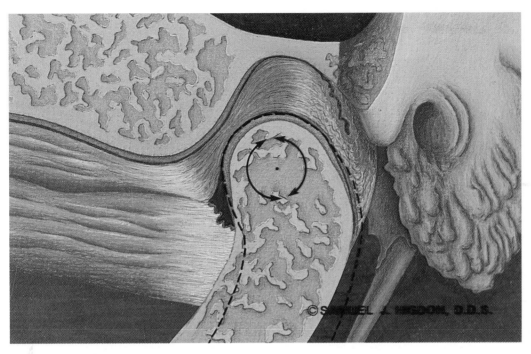

(E)

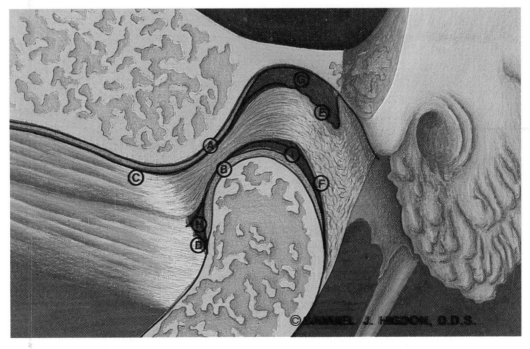

(F)

membered that the temporomandibular joint was originally defined as a "compression movement articulation" and the selection of the word "compression" in that definition is no accident. Due to the tension provided by the muscles and especially the extremely tough and fibrous joint capsule, there is always a compressing force exerted by the condylar head on the intra-articular disc, even upon opening and during rest positions. Thus the

---

Figure 3-9 **(G)** Condyle/disc assembly at point of full translation. Posterior attachment is fully extended. This posterior ligamentous attachment contains elastin, a highly elastic "rubber band-like" material that exerts tension on posterior "heel" of disc. During translation, inferior belly of lateral ptyergoid contracts, but surprisingly, superior belly of lateral pterygoid attached to anterior "toe" of disc does not! **(H–L)** TMJ anatomy during dysfunction. **(H)** During pathofunction, condyle is displaced superiorly and posteriorly with respect to its proper anatomically and structurally balanced position (dotted line). This results in impingement of condylar head into highly sensitive bilaminar zone. Note narrowed posterior joint space. **(I)** Anteriorly displaced disc. Anterior and medial displacement of intra-articular disc is most common form of joint dysfunction. This results from chronic displacement of condylar head superiorly and posteriorly past thickened posterior heel of disc and possible stretching and/or tearing of collateral ligamentous attachments of disc to condyle. **(J)** Clicking upon opening results as condyle regains concave position of disc during translation and in so doing must force its way past thickened heel. Quickly snapping "back into joint," the audible click is heard (follow line). **(K)** Posterior disc "ironing." Sometimes, joints that at one time clicked loudly upon opening and closing lose some of the sharp quality of the click, or it may even disappear entirely. This is due to the fact that discs do not always retain their biconcave form. With chronic loading and deformation of heel of disc by condylar head, previously thicker posterior border of heel of disc becomes progressively thinner in an ironing effect. Hence, audibility of click lessens as condylar head regains center of disc during initiation of translation. Conversely some joints, rather than suffering thinning of heel of disc, suffer from folding of disc in thin central portion due to chronic superior posterior condylar displacement. In such circumstances, condyle may sometimes be able to recapture center of disc and at other times it may not **(I)**. Thus there may be periods of intermittent clicking or intermittent catching or locking. In locking, condyle cannot regain disc but rather pushes it ahead (black line) until translation movement is prematurely halted due to anterior disc jamming within joint. **(L)** Ultimate degeneration of joint, tearing of disc or posterior attachment, remodeling of articular surfaces with eburnation and lipping of condyle. (*Illustrations courtesy of Dr Samuel J. Higdon, Portland, OR.*)

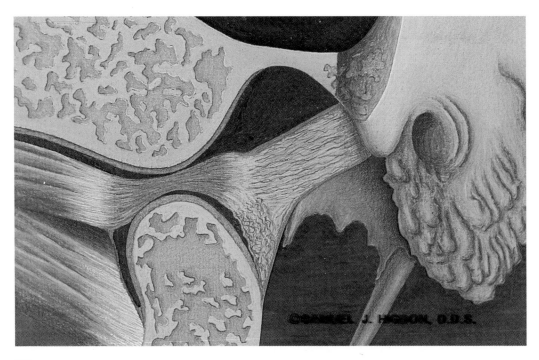

(G)

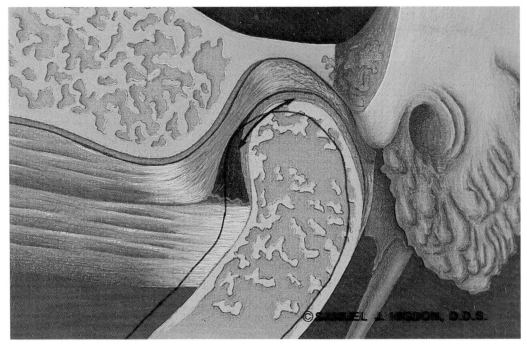

(H)

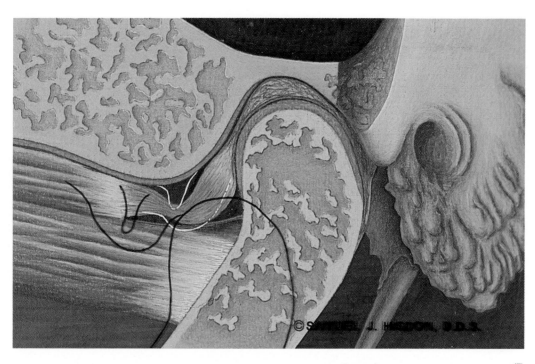

(I)

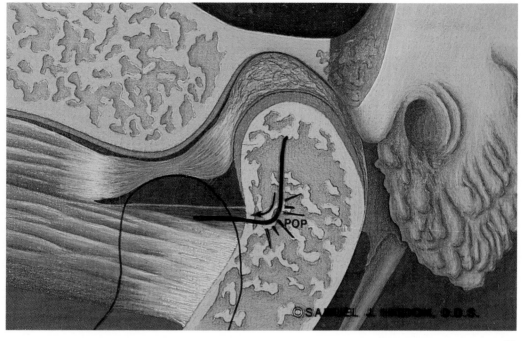

(J)

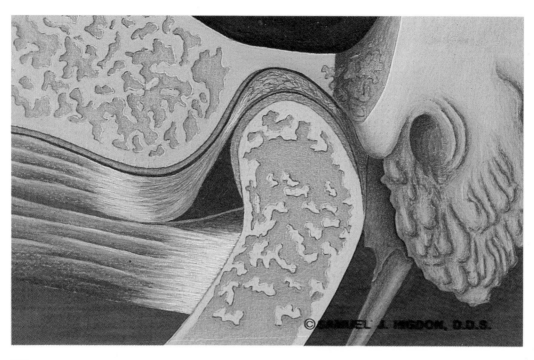

(K)

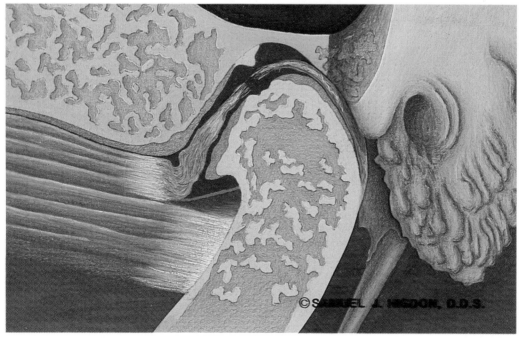

(L)

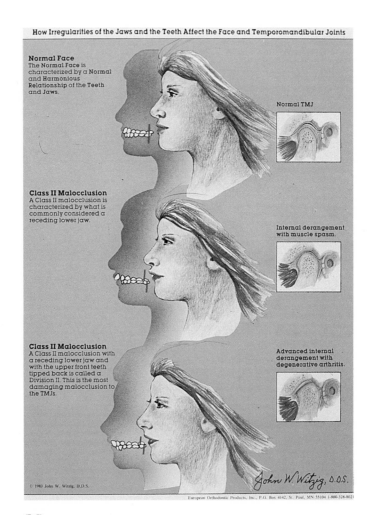

(M)

disc and its upper and lower synovial compartments must serve not only in a lubricating and stabilizing capacity, but must also act as a perpetual absorber of the compressing forces of the condylar head. These forces of "compression" are, of course, extremely intense during occlusion as in mastication and bruxism. But, they are also present, albeit to a far lesser degree, continually during opening and rest positions. Nature's selection of cartilage as the tissue of choice to serve in this capacity between the two opposing bony surfaces of the temporal bone and the condylar head bears mute testimony to Her wisdom. Cartilage, with its resilient, elastic, almost "Teflonlike" qualities, makes a perfect natural-made shock absorber! Due to the biconcave shape of the disc, it is trapped between the convex head of the condyle and the slightly convex eminence of bone forming the slope of the tuberculum. Due to tension created by the muscles and other factors, it moves smoothly down the slope of the glenoid fossa, keeping between the two articular components during the entire range of normal motion. Oddly, the superior head of the lateral pterygoid muscle, which is attached to the anterior portion of the disc, does not constrict during this opening action to pull the disc down the slope of the eminence, as one might think. This muscle serves a much different function during closing! During opening the tension on the elastic ligaments of the bilaminar zone becomes greater and greater as the condyle and disc travel together farther and farther down the slope of the tuberculum. Upon closing, the opposite action happens to the condyle, but something a little different goes on with the disc. The superior head of the lateral pterygoid plays a very important role here. By constricting in a coordinated fashion during closure, it provides the tension that keeps the disc interposed between the condyle and the fossa at just the right spot, counteracting the tension of the stretched posterior ligament. This pulling, or more correctly "restraining," action anteroposteriorly must be coordinated properly at both ends of the disc to keep it in the right place with respect to the condylar head. If something is wrong at either end, ie, an overstretched or torn posterior ligament with little or no elastic power, or a spasmodic superior head of the lateral pterygoid muscle unable to coordinate contraction at just the right rate, the disc-condyle relationship becomes compromised and that's when the patient starts "riding off the disc." Simplistically, it might be thought of as occurring in either one of a combination of two basic stereoscopic ways. The condyle may return to its "normal" rest or full occlusion position within the joint, while the disc, due to a foreshortening of the superior head of the lateral pterygoid due to spasm, might not fully return. The disc does not ascend the complete path all the way back up to its correct position of being poised between the capitulum and tuberculum, but stops, or is restrained, a little short. In the act of closure as the condyle keeps going up and back, it slides past the thickened posterior edge of the restrained disc as the mandibular teeth reach full occlusion.

Alternatively, the superior head of the lateral pterygoid may be functioning perfectly normally, exhibiting no signs of spasm at all. It may just possibly let the disc travel as far posteriorly and superiorly as its own individual anatomical length will allow. But this proves insufficient, as due to the commonly seen skeletal Class II retruded or insufficient mandibular deep bite situation. The occlusion in such cases demands that the mandible must be *overclosed* and retruded posteriorly, resulting in superior posterior displacement of the condyle within the joint capsule, in order to effect full occlusion of the posterior teeth. The net effect is the same: The disc stops ascending during the closure movement within the joint while the condylar head keeps right on going posteriorly and superiorly until it "falls off the back edge of the disc." When this happens, the only place that the condyle can anatomically impinge upon is on the posterior ligament, or highly sensitive bilaminar zone. The disc can't make it all the way back up to provide its interposing, shock-absorbing effect. Thus it stays a little lower down in the anterior portion of the fossa and when the opening motion begins again, the condylar head, which is still being held tightly in the joint capsule by ligaments and muscles, will begin to push the disc ahead of it a little until the reserve elasticity of the now somewhat weakened and slightly overstretched posterior ligament comes into play again. When the tension imported to the disc by the weakened but still unruptured posterior ligament becomes great enough, its tension causes the disc to remain just stationary enough and stable enough to let the condyle hop back up onto it again into its proper concavity; and in so doing, a slight audible "click" is heard. A closing click may often be heard in such cases also, as the condyle returns to its superior "retrodiscal" position again. Due to lateral pterygoid spasm, posterior ligament elasticity weakness, or both, the disc fails to make the trip with its companion condyle completely all the way back. During closure, when the tension of the lateral pterygoid becomes great enough (it is oblivious of the antagonist posterior ligament's noncompensating elasticity), it halts the ascent of the disc, but not the condyle. Halted in its path "prematurely," there the disc stays; and as the condyle keeps right on going toward its final superior position within the joint during centric occlusion, it "falls off" the trailing or stationary disc and the usually less audible closing click is heard once again. Hence what is known as "reciprocal clicking" during opening and closing.

Pain and discomfort many times associate themselves with this process and are usually expressed by the patient in terms of chronic muscle soreness or TMJ-type headaches of varying degrees. Often, unfortunately, the TMJ-related headache is misdiagnosed. These headaches and facial pains result from essentially two sources: intracapsular and extracapsular problems.

The intracapsular problems denote advanced forms of TMJ malarthrosis and degeneration. Clicking is usually the first stage of these degenerative processes. Not every patient that has clicking or is "riding off the disc" is slated for severe degeneration of the joint, but many will continue to suffer and slowly worsen in their state and some will digress to the point of torn posterior ligaments, perforated discs, or the infamous "clinical closed lock" condition which represents the end stage of the process that some feel is amenable only to surgery. Clicking is a common finding (50% to over 60% in various studies!) in patients presenting for treatment of malocclusions; as the Class II variety with its retruded mandible (and therefore condyles) is the most common variety. Therefore, always examine for it!

Some of the most commonly seen problems are those of extracapsular involvement, and that means muscles.

Muscles have to work at an optimum length to function at peak efficiency. Whenever they have to overwork, or work in a way for which they are not designed, pain and fatigue usually result.

A severe loss of vertical, causing muscles to overclose and therefore work inefficiently, or a severely retruded mandible, causing muscles to work inefficiently bioarchitecturally, can bring about circumstances that result in muscles of the masticatory system working *improperly*, and that usually means pain.

Concomitantly, these same problems of a loss of vertical and a severely retruded mandible that are so hard on the musculature can also lead to superior, posterior displacement of the condyle (SPDC) and cause condylar impingement on the bilaminar zone. This could in turn lead to intracapsular problems. Condyles should ride on cartilage, not on vascular bilaminar tissues!

This oversimplified, and sometimes slightly inexact, accounting of TMJ function and pathofunction brings us back to the orthopedic considerations of bicuspid extractions for orthodontic relief of crowding.

We see by the above that we should strive not to do anything in the mouth that would cause the muscles to overwork during functional occlusion of the teeth or to work in a manner in which they were not designed. We would not want to precipitate a loss of vertical dimension of occlusion nor perpetuate retrusive mandibular situations. These are often unwanted side effects of improperly treated four-bicuspid extraction cases.

The entire thrust of the growth and development of the face is down and forward in a direction away from the calvarium.[30-38] We should not do anything orthodontically to go against this biological flow of growth.[39-40] We should not excessively retract premaxillas back, forcing mandibles and their resultant condyles back. We should not be precipitating loss in vertical. When indicated, we should aid in the body's effort to bring the mandible down and forward to meet the premaxilla[41] orthopedically and endeavor to increase the diminished, improper vertical dimension of occlusion.[42] Then proper angulation of the anteriors and proper alignment of the posteriors will result in a well-balanced stable occlusion that is physiologically acceptable to the biological criteria of nature and socially acceptable to the critical eye of the world.

When relief of crowding requires extractions, it's not the bicuspids that should be considered, but rather teeth further back in the arch.

A pleasing full face and healthy temporomandibular joint should also be the goals of every orthodontic case as well as the usual "straight teeth" and functional occlusion.

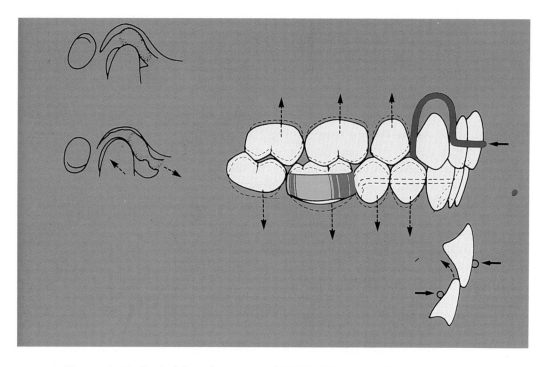

Figure 3-10   Incisal interference and TMJ. Schematic illustration of one of the most drastic combinations of arch interdigitation and its untoward effects on TMJ. In a case where upper arch only is foreshortened by bicuspid extraction to couple anteriors with lower nonextracted mandibular arch, the upper anteriors act as guiding planes as they are struck by lowers in mandibular arc of closure. Premaxillary anterior arch is, in effect, retracted to meet mandibular incisors which can lock the mandible permanently in its pretreatment skeletal Class II retruded position. Upon full closure, lower incisors travel up guiding lingual surfaces of upper anteriors and in so doing can force entire mandible, and as a result its condyles too, posteriorly. This forces condyle off back end of disc into bilaminar zone. Intensified by retention (labial bow on uppers and lingual wire on lowers) upon full occlusion the biting forces are not only absorbed vertically by teeth in posterior quadrants but also superiorly and posteriorly in TMJ due to incisal guidance or interference that is exaggerated anteriorly! Such interferences can also result naturally in pretreatment conditions, the most classic example of which is the Class II, Division 2 deep bite situation!

"You are a clever man, friend John; you
reason well, and your wit is bold; but you
are too prejudiced! You do not let your eyes
see nor your ears hear, and that which is
outside your daily life is of no account to
you. Do you not think there are things
which you cannot understand and yet
which are; that some people see things that
others cannot? . . . Ah, it is the fault of
our science that it wants to explain all, and
if it explain not, then it says there is
nothing to explain. But yet we see around
us every day the growth of new beliefs,
which think themselves new; and which are
yet but the old, which pretend to be young;
like the fine ladies of the opera."

Professor Abram Van Helsing to Dr John
Seward
Chapter 14 of Bram Stoker's novel—
Dracula, 1897

ORTHODONTIC CONSIDERATIONS

When one considers the orthodontic implications of bicuspid extractions to relieve crowding, many factors come into play. The first is so totally elementary that it can be easily forgotten by the clinician more concerned with more immediate problems of diagnosis and treatment planning, and that is: How many teeth are going to be left after the extractions? This is not as easy a question to answer as it first appears. Certainly in a four-bicuspid extraction case, four teeth will be removed, but will that be all? What will become of the third molars in that patient? Extracting bicuspids gains approximately 6 to 7 mm at each extraction site. Since the reason for the extractions in the first place is to relieve crowding, the 6- to 7-mm space is often easily used up in severe cases and although it aids in the relief of such crowding, the space gained in the premaxillary area does little to aid in the relief of crowding in the posterior segments. Here is where the third molar is often struggling to gain enough of its own space to erupt on a full and uninhibited path of entry. Most third molars that are predestined to impact, especially lowers, impact regardless of what happens further forward in the arches.[43-45]

In a severely crowded case of true bimaxillary protrusion, the space gained by the loss of the first bicuspid is entirely used up by the realignment of the remaining teeth. This situation, though rare, may be acceptable. The third molar, however, is often unaffected by the gain of arch length of the other teeth in the anterior segments and is still left on its own, unaided, to shift for itself. In a case where crowding is not quite as severe,

CHART #2

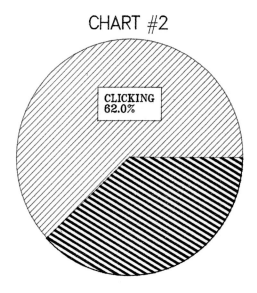

CLICKING
62.0%

CHART SHOWING 62% OF PATIENTS PRESENTING FOR
TREATMENT OF MALOCCLUSIONS SHOWED CLICKING IN
ONE OR BOTH TEMPOROMANDIBULAR JOINTS.

Figure 3-11

yet serious enough to require extraction, there may be an excess of space
gained by removing the premolars thus requiring the anterior movement
(often tilting) of the first and second molars. This may be just enough to
give the slightly crowded lower third molar the necessary room in which
to erupt. Yet the chances are not statistically in favor of a complete and correct eruption. This is due to several reasons. First, the availability of 6 to
7 mm extra space in a given quadrant does not automatically translate to
6 to 7 mm more space for the third molar farther back, as much of this space
is spent in the anterior segment satisfying the arch length demands of the
anterior teeth and remaining premolars. This leaves only a reduced amount,
if any, to be spent by means of moving first and second molars forward
to aid in the delivery of the third molar. Most lower third molar crowns are
more than 6 to 7 mm wide mesiodistally, and require more than that much
mesial displacement of the second molar ahead of them to allow eruption
if completely impacted.

Secondly, the age at which bicuspids are extracted is a factor that does
not lend to aiding in relief of posterior crowding. Patients are usually treated
in their early teens for orthodontic problems and by the time many of them
have had their bicuspids extracted and any "leftover" space made available
for impacted third molars through the use of fixed appliances, not only the
crowns, but often the roots of developing lower third molars have begun
to form and calcify. This compounds the problem of impaction if the lower

CHART #3

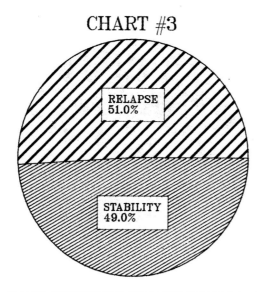

CHART SHOWING 51% OF CASES SURVEYED IN ONE
SAMPLE 7 YEARS OUT OF TREATMENT EXHIBITED
RELAPSE TO SUCH A LEVEL AS TO BE CONSIDERED
UNACCEPTABLE AS FINISHED CASES.

Figure 3-12

third molar is mesially inclined to a moderate or severe degree. If a great amount of space was made available early in the development of this tooth, the crown, regardless of its degree of mesial inclination, would have not only the space but also the time available to right itself and erupt vertically. But once a mesially inclined lower third molar is caught behind a crowded second and the roots have begun to form past the bifurcation, slight relief by means of mesial movement of the teeth in front of it will not usually be enough to prevent impaction. This process often resolves itself to a case of too little too late.

From the above, it is clear to see that if a case is treated by means of extraction of four bicuspids and it is suffering from mild to severe anterior crowding and severe posterior crowding also, the impaction of the third molars seems quite likely. This then answers our initial question. Not only will the four premolars be sacrificed, but very often the four third molars will also require removal.[46] This results in eight teeth being lost with double the surgical insult to the patient. This in itself is a formidable issue, for though the postextraction sequelae of bicuspid removal is universally minimal, the same is not always true of third-molar surgery.

Modern-day oral surgeons have developed excellent techniques for third molar removal, but they will be the first to admit that no surgical procedure is totally free of some degree of risk. Postsurgical infection, paresthesia, dry sockets, and TMJ trauma are all possible complications of difficult lower third molar impaction removal. Though the incidence of these complications is quite minimal due to the excellent state of the modern-day surgeon's methods and skills, certain percentages of these sequelae persist. It must be remembered that for the unfortunate patient who succumbs to one of these complications, the incidence is 100%. Statistics are of little comfort to him. Even if no problems arise, postsurgical healing can be slow and painful for some patients. This only contributes to the ever-present equation of "dentist = pain syndrome" in the minds of the general public. The fear of such procedures weighs on the minds of most patients, and many will postpone third-molar removal for as long as possible, only complicating the problem and intensifying the risk factors. The expense borne by the patient is also a factor to consider. The fees for the extraction of eight teeth are always more than double what they would be for bicuspids alone. The third molar is a far more difficult tooth to remove and therefore justifies a correspondingly higher fee.

Another problem that arises in extraction cases where crowding is not severe is that often teeth must be moved a considerable distance. This requires a great deal of expenditure of time and effort. Stability then becomes an issue and is usually managed with long periods of retention. Yet studies have shown as high as 50% of all orthodontic cases suffer some obvious degree of relapse.[47-49] It has been a nagging problem for both doctors and patients, for nearly a century.

Also, if the posteriors are moved forward, the upper first molar often becomes tilted with its mesial tip leaving it in less than ideal occlusion with the lower. Moving molars forward into extraction spaces often represents a loss in vertical. The lower jaw is a hinge with an arc of closure. The farther out on this arc the molars are, the farther they are from the axis of rotation, the temporomandibular joint. Mesializing molars in "high angle" cases (clockwise growers) may be favorable for the vertical; but in low angle cases (counterclockwise growers) or in cases where the vertical is already compromised, it will only close the bite more which would not be desirable (high-angle case: Y-axis greater than 69 degrees; low-angle case: Y-axis less than 63 degrees). Many Class II malocclusions suffer from a loss of vertical to begin with; mesializing molars worsens this condition. If excessive space remains after the extraction of bicuspids, the lower cuspids and incisors may wind up retroclined to such a degree of interincisal angle as to perpetuate, or over the long run, even intensify the loss of vertical in deep bite problem cases.

Figures 3-13 (A–C), 3-14 (A–C), 3-15 (A–C), 3-16 (A–C) Panographic X-rays showing eruption of third molars into position vacated by extracted second molars. **(A)** Pretreatment condition. **(B)** Third molars partially erupted. **(C)** Third molars fully erupted. Note: all third molars erupted to position without need of orthodontic intervention. (*Courtesy of Dr Merle Bean, Des Moine, Iowa.*)

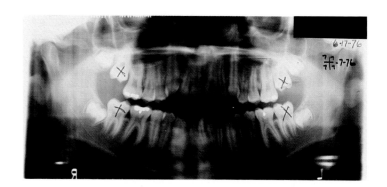

Figure 3-13(A)

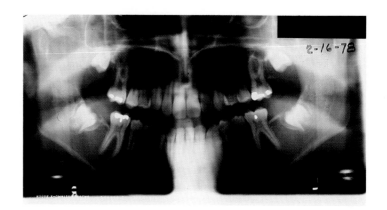

(B)

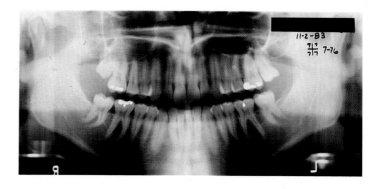

(C)

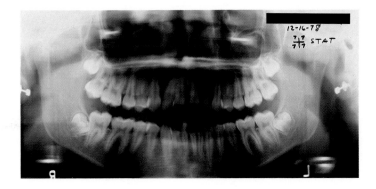

Figure 3-14(A)

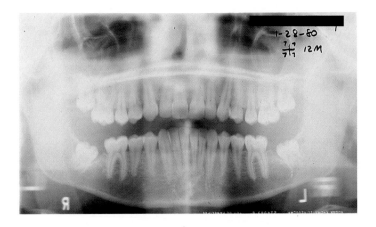

(B)

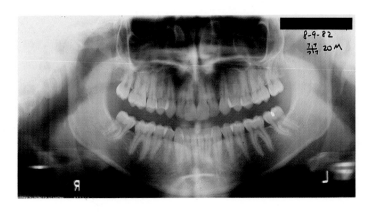

(C)

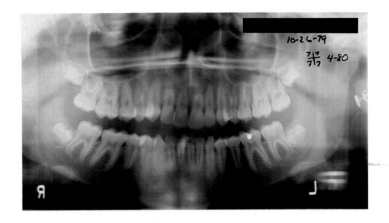

Figure 3-15(A)

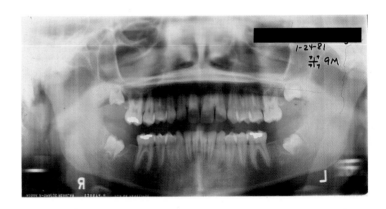

(B)

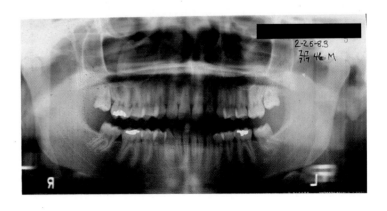

(C)

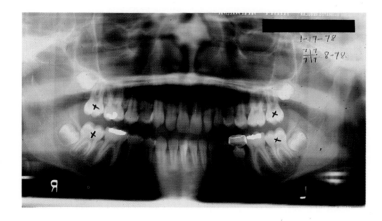

Figure 3-16(A)

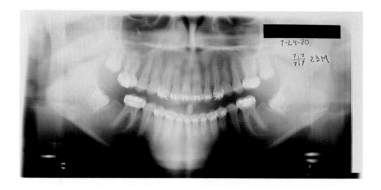

(B)

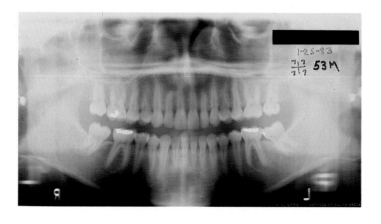

(C)

In four-bicuspid extraction cases, maintenance of the contact points, complicated by the desire for relapse, may be difficult when a case is completed. The contact between the upper cuspid against the mesial of the second bicuspid is not always the picture of correct dental anatomy. This site may be prone to chronic food impaction, especially from stringy meats and fibrous foodstuffs. The protective mesiolingual slope of the mesial marginal ridge of the upper first bicuspid is not present on the second bicuspid, and if the second bicuspid is the tooth that remains, this area may be compromised periodontally. If the upper second bicuspid is sacrificed and the first premolar remains, contact points fare little better. Upper first bicuspids are usually more "bell-crowned" than seconds and when the distal surface of the more effeminate first bicuspid is butted against the large broad flat surface of the mesial of the upper first molar, a less than perfect contact for the protection of the interdental tissues might result.

These issues, as well as others, were never more clearly spelled out than in the study by the eminent periodontist John F. Prichard of Fort Worth, Texas.[50] Concerned over the effects of bicuspid extractions on the dental arches from a periodontal standpoint, Prichard studied 100 former orthodontic patients who had four bicuspids extracted and carefully scrutinized the dental ramifications of this type of treatment on the teeth and oral tissues. Being a periodontist, he owed no particular allegiance to one form of orthodontic technique or another. The list of findings he compiled comes down rather hard against the four-bicuspid extraction system from a dental standpoint. Of the 400 teeth removed and 400 spaces created, the results were as follows:

33.5% of the spaces still had open contacts.
48.5% of the teeth adjacent to the spaces had tilted roots.
55.0% of the patients exhibited some degree of root resorption.
11.0% still had remaining anterior open bites.

Other untoward effects observed were gingival recession; tipping of cuspids, second bicuspids, and molars; periodontal pockets by the cuspids, bicuspids, and molars; end-to-end occlusion of molars; altered occlusion in the molar regions; assorted open contacts in various places in the arches; deep overbites or loss of vertical dimension of occlusion; anterior and even posterior open bites; retroclined lower anteriors; enamel decalcification due to bands; loss of lower anteriors due to periodontal disease; alveolar bone loss of a sufficient level as to require surgery; root resorptions; pulp degenerations due to extreme orthodontic pressures on teeth; and roots of adjacent teeth positioned so as to be in contact with one another, which according to Prichard always results in a periodontal problem (bone resorption) that is amenable only to surgical removal of one of the adjoining roots and subsequent endodontic therapy! To add to this, Dr Prichard reports that the chief complaint of the patients concerning their treatment was a "dished-in face" or "flattened smile." Maintenance of proper contacts and correct dental interdigitation around the corner of the arc from anterior to posterior segments appears to be critical.

The transition between the thin, sharp, incising anterior teeth and the stout, square, grinding posterior teeth is effectuated by the *paired* bicuspids. First appears the more delicate and shapely first bicuspid, a model of form and function. Then the slightly more sturdy second bicuspid, with its more square, husky appearance and thicker base. Like a man and a woman, they appear side by side in the graceful and flowing change anteroposterior of the dental arch, from tall and thin to short and thick. It is a beautifully designed system that has taken Nature millions of years to perfect. Nothing in this favored anterior area is haphazard nor redundant. However, in the posterior areas behind this "chorus line" of teeth is the "spare parts bin." Here extra molars *are* redundant! If extractions are indicated, it would be far better to carry them out in an area where Nature is more forgiving.

"And now I hear your warning voice
across the years of grief and pain,
At night I read your testament
and rouse myself to life again."

Boris Pasternak
"Daybreak" from
The Poems of Dr. Zhivago

THE ADVANTAGES OF SECOND-MOLAR EXTRACTION

At about the same time Wilson in England was seeking alternatives to four-bicuspid-extraction-oriented orthodontics for primarily *orthopedic reasons*, great strides were also being made in this country in the evolution of the second molar extraction concept for primarily *orthodontic reasons* by one of the great American pioneers in this method, Dr D. W. Liddle of Warren, Ohio. As an orthodontist, he became dissatisfied with the results he saw obtained by the techniques of his day, not the least of which was the problem of overexpansion and resultant relapse. He was one of the first to define the formidable combined forward thrust of the second and third molars as etiological factors of both posterior and anterior segment crowding.

Figure 3-17 Uprighting inhibited third molars. **(A)** Schematic representation of uprighting third molars with brass separating rings. **(B)** Separating wires trimmed and in place.

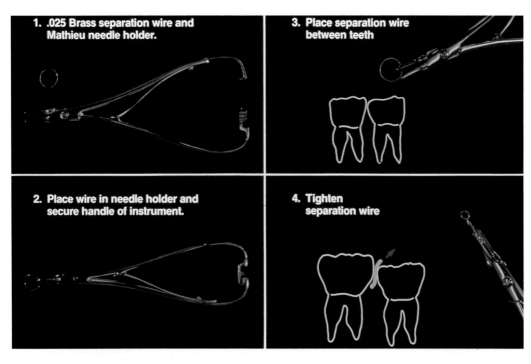

1. .025 Brass separation wire and Mathieu needle holder.

2. Place wire in needle holder and secure handle of instrument.

3. Place separation wire between teeth

4. Tighten separation wire

(A)

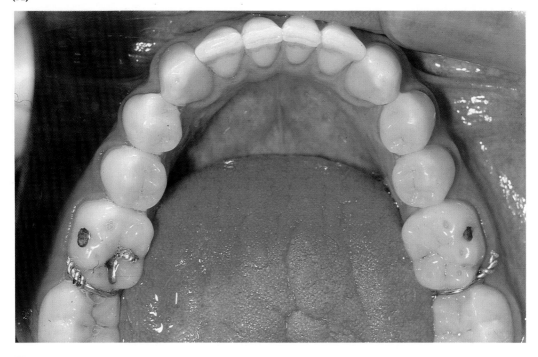

(B)

These and other important concepts were laid down by him in what has now become a classic monograph.[51] He states that extracting bicuspids that have become crowded due to the gigantic forward thrust of the second and third molars is merely "treating the effect," not the cause of of the malocclusion. He goes on to point out that merely extracting the upper second molars while retaining the lower second molars, even in the face of developing third-molar impactions, a procedure explored by some in past years, is also a suspect approach. He states that it results in an "unnatural" occlusion and that retaining the lower seconds level with the occlusal plane while waiting for the upper thirds to erupt is a difficult task at best. Where indicated, he believed the four second-molar extraction method is best.

Orthodontic Significance

Orthodontically speaking, the second-molar extraction concept has many advantages.[52] One advantage is that it offers relief of crowding in both the anterior as well as the posterior segments simultaneously. Rather than the mere 6- to 7-mm space gained by the extraction of a bicuspid, the removal of a second molar delivers almost double that space since they average 10 to 12 mm in mesiodistal length. This is usually more than enough to satisfy the most demanding arch length discrepancies. What space is not used by rearrangement of anterior teeth and bicuspids is simply used up as the third molar erupts and moves forward to close the contact with the first molar.[53-62]

Removal of the second molars also allows for the distalization of the first molars, bicuspids, and even cuspids, if necessary. This, along with relieving crowding, also aids in the increase in vertical when desired. As the first molar and bicuspids are distalized, they move closer to the hinge axis of rotation of the TMJ and come into occlusal contact sooner with the opposing teeth during the arc of closure, thereby increasing the vertical dimension of occlusion. This is the complete opposite phenomenon that takes place in four-bicuspid extraction methods when first molars are mesialized in techniques that do not stabilize them with headgear. Since in the second molar extraction method, there is no excess of space to have to close adjacent teeth into, there is no tipping or tilting of the upper first molars or any other teeth. The contacts also remain intact throughout the arch as there is no drifting back from these overclosed bicuspid extraction spaces. In fact, if any drifting occurs, it is usually of the lower first molars and bicuspids distally! The lower bicuspids and cuspids have a natural tendency to drift distally[63,64] as evidenced by huge open contacts between these teeth observed in patients who have had lower first molars removed due to abscess, excessive decay,

Figure 3-18 **(A)** Separation elastics may also be used in similar fashion to brass separating rings. **(B)** Elastics in place.

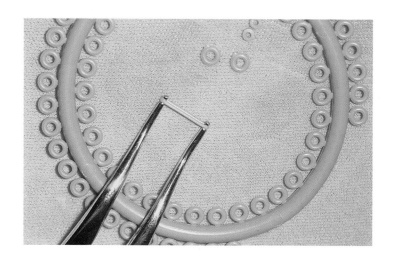

(A)

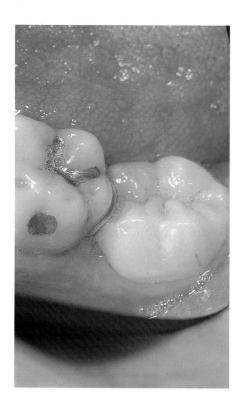

(B)

CHART #4

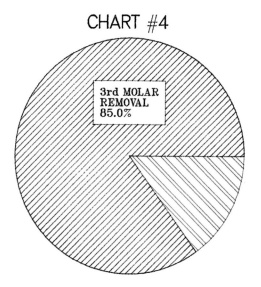

CHART SHOWING RESULTS OF A PUBLIC HEALTH
DEPARTMENT STUDY OF OVER 400 HIGH SCHOOL
SENIORS SHOWING 85% OF THEM REQUIRED 3rd
MOLAR REMOVAL DUE TO IMPACTION.

Figure 3-19

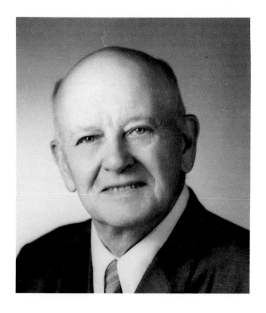

Figure 3-20   David W. Liddle

etc, without the benefit of replacement by means of fixed or removable prosthesis. After second-molar extraction, the natural drift of these teeth in this direction is sometimes enough to correct cases of minor crowding without the use of any appliance at all.[65] This phenomenon is more often observed in the mandible than the maxilla.

With only four teeth removed, 28 teeth remain. This means that more posterior teeth are available for chewing: two bicuspids and two molars per quadrant. The occlusion of these teeth is excellent since no tipping or tilting occurs; therefore prematurities and occlusal imbalances are uncommon.

Of course, being spared the discomfort and inconvenience of third-molar surgery, as these teeth are left to erupt in place of the seconds, is a notion popular with most patients. Also, the reduced fees represented by only relatively simple four extractions as opposed to eight, some of which are not so simple, is a notion always popular with the individuals responsible for the patient's account.

Orthopedic Considerations

Orthopedically speaking, the advantages of second-molar extraction are also numerous. One of the more significant of these is its effect on the face. Since the arch is not constricted by the removal of teeth on a curve, the smile that is dispayed with all the bicuspids present is broad and full. More tooth material is present in this region and it is positioned in a physically larger area. The lips are full and more esthetic since the premaxilla is left in its proper place. It does not have to be retracted to close in a bicuspid gap. If maxillary anterior teeth are protruding, they may be torqued lingually without retracting the premaxillary bone base. This allows the bony support to remain for the upper lip and prevents the artificial lengthening of the nose and the "dished-in" appearance to the face represented by premaxillary dental arch retraction. Some authorities believe that a true maxillary basal bone protrusion never exists, or is at least extremely rare. They feel the maxillary protrusion is simply a matter of labial crown torque of the maxillary anteriors. In any event, without having to retract the anterior segments, the face remains full and well developed, as then the lower jaw, in retruded skeletal Class II cases, may be brought *forward* to meet the cephalometrically correct premaxilla by means of the Bionator. This, in combination with the physically larger arches, prevents constriction of the tongue and improves airway space in addition to the aforementioned benefits derived relative to facial contours.

The temporomandibular joint is also aided by the second-molar extraction method. As the first molars and bicuspids are distalized into the second-molar extraction site to relieve crowding, they correspondingly open the bite and increase the vertical which is so often compromised in severe Class II cases with deep overbite. This aids the oral musculature in attaining a more physiologically acceptable muscle-length-to-work ratio which prevents their overconstriction and imbalance, a cause of discomfort to many patients suffering from deep bites and retruded mandibles. By developing the lower face in a downward and forward direction to meet the *nonretracted* premaxilla, the condyles of the mandible are brought down and forward also. This prevents the superior, posterior displacement of the condyle in the glenoid fossa (SPDC), a condition often associated with severe deep bite Class II cases with retruded mandibles. This mandibular advancement acts as a protective mechanism for the joint. Proper vertical and condyle-disc-fossa relationships are vital to maintaining the health of the TMJ.

THE INTERRELATIONSHIP OF THE NRDM-SPDC PHENOMENON

Anterior incisal interference is one of the concepts that is vital to a correct understanding of how the function of the jaws and teeth may be abnormal to the point of affecting the TMJ. The importance of this relationship cannot be overemphasized in the correct diagnosis of the needs of a given malocclusion. It is best described as that of the NRDM-SPDC phenomenon (NRDM: neuromuscular reflexive displacement of the mandible). Mastication is both a voluntary and reflexive activity. That is, we may perform extremely precise masticatory functions at will, such as biting open a cellophane bag, chewing fingernails, cutting fishing line, etc; or we may "reflexively" chew away habitually while our concentration is diverted to other more distracting events, eg, gum chewing during heated athletic competition or eating popcorn at the movies. Though these muscle motor functions may not be 100% autonomic, such as other bodily functions like digestion, peristalsis, vasoconstriction, etc, certain myofunctional reflexive processes do exist. One of the more important ones comes directly into play in both orthodontic and temporomandibular joint diagnosis.

As the mandible closes and the teeth come into contact, an extremely sensitive set of proprioceptive fibers in the periodontal ligament of each of the teeth feed back stereoscopic information to the brain. The value of this is multifold. First, it prevents any serious and harmful collisions of the teeth with unforeseen hard objects in the food such as unexpected cherry pits, bullet fragments in venison, "old maids" in popcorn, etc. Upon suddenly

---

Figure 3-21 **(A)** University of Osaka study. Erupting second molars pushed teeth in maxillary arch forward an average of 1.6 mm per quadrant. **(B)** Lowers were pushed forward 2.5 mm per quadrant on average. Children studied were 12 to 17 years of age with all deciduous teeth exfoliated, all permanent teeth present and second molars unerupted. **(C)** Amsterdam study. Fifty children were studied after having their second molars removed. Cephalometric analysis 2 years after extraction showed that molars regressed, and lower incisors uprighted slightly!

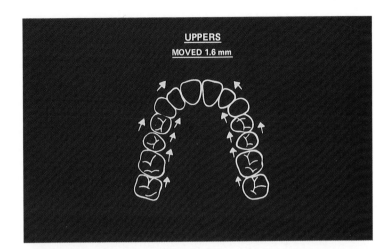

(A)

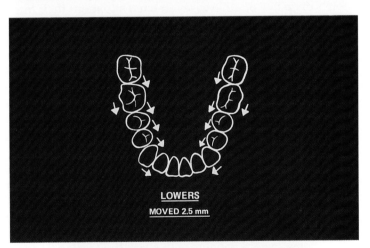

(B)

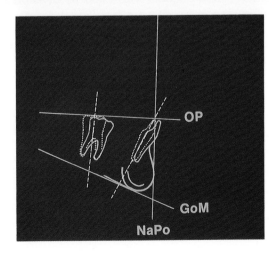

(C)

striking such an object unawares, the individual will reflexively and quite quickly pull the mandible down. This is the exhibition of simple muscle reflex activity due to periodontal ligament feedback on a very primitive and elemental level.

But there is another reflexive jaw-closing movement in which the diagnostician is far more interested, that of anterior incisal guidance. When the mandible closes, especially in deep bite situations, as the lower incisors strike the inclined planes of the upper incisors the neuromuscular reflexive feedback phenomenon causes the three main pairs of closing muscles to guide the arc of closure of the mandible in a more *posterior* direction so as to gracefully coordinate the act of closing. This brings the lower jaws into maximum dental interdigitation while at the same time preventing the lower incisors from "crashing" into the interfering lingual surfaces of the stationary upper incisors. If there were no upper anterior incisors, the mandible could close to its normal orthopedically balanced position (barring posterior occlusal inclined plane problems). But with the presence of the upper anteriors in a deep bite or otherwise retracted situation, their interfering inclined lingual surfaces result, through the reflexive muscle-guiding processes of the proprioceptive fibers of the respective periodontal ligaments of the lower anteriors, in the arc of closure being habitually modified so as to bring the mandible up and back upon full closure. This is done reflexively to avoid the anterior incisal inclined plane interferences. If severe enough over a long enough period of time, this neuromuscular reflexive displacement of the mandible can result in the condyle being forced in a superior, posterior displaced condition within the joint capsule. This in turn would bring it off the posterior end of the disc and allow it to impinge on the extremely sensitive bilaminar zone. Thus we see that what happens as far forward in the dental arches as an improperly angulated upper anterior interfering with a lower incisor in the mandibular arc of closure affects something as far back at the other end of the mandible as the temporomandibular joint! This is why there is an extremely high incidence of temporomandibular joint problems seen in patients with Class II, Division 2, deep bite malocclusions, *or patients with overretracted maxillary anteriors due to bicuspid extraction!* Thus neuromuscular reflexive displacement of the mandible (NRDM) results in superior posterior displacement of the condyle (SPDC).

Figure 3-22   What at first appears as a normal Class I occlusion is in fact a bimaxillary protrusion of ample vertical, as divulged by both **(A)** lateral profile facial view and **(B)** cephalometric evaluation. After carefully planned and executed four bicuspid extraction, fixed-appliance therapy, note improved facial profile **(C)** and also note how much closer the anteriors are to the molars **(D)** in the posttreatment cephalogram. (*Courtesy of Dr Waldemar Brehm, Encinitas, CA.*)

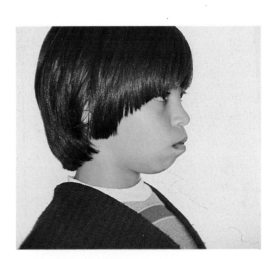

(A)

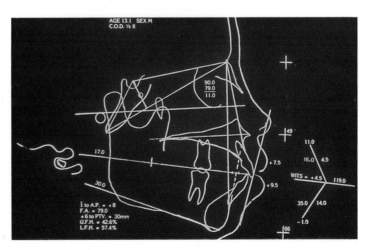

(B)

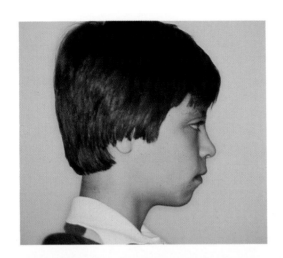

(C)

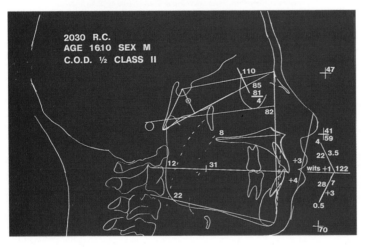

(D)

From the above it may be seen that not only overly retracted maxillary anteriors or overly retroclined maxillary anteriors can act as agents in initiating the NRDM-SPCD phenomenon with its resultant TMJ damage, but also even merely crowded and misaligned anteriors may prove equally guilty of causing trouble. If the maxillary anteriors should be crowded such that *rotations* cause a lingual line angle of an upper front tooth to become lingually displaced enough to be the first surface contacted by the lower anteriors, the mandibular closing arc will be modified so as to force the mandible back to clear it. Blocked-in upper anteriors are also culprits in this regard with the laterals being the most common offenders. Equally, the lower anteriors may also come into play. Should crowding be such that a particular lower front tooth, usually a central incisor, be crowded out labially so as to strike the lingual surfaces of the upper anteriors prematurely during the arc of closure, the same retruded arc of closure will result, reflexively driving the mandible back. These processes are greatly intensified in *deep bite* situations where the mandible is already overclosed and the anterior lower face height or vertical dimension of occlusion is already diminished. In these types of cases, extracting bicuspids and retracting upper anterior teeth even further would be disastrous for the TMJ. Alternative routes to the solving of arch length problems and crowding must be sought. The only viable alternative is the second-molar "replacement" principle.

Lastly, yet another orthopedic advantage of the second-molar extraction method is that the joint is protected from possible damage due to difficult or protracted lower third-molar surgery since these teeth are left alone to erupt in place of the seconds. Such difficult surgery may be all that is needed in a patient whose joints are already compromised due to bicuspid extraction technique to precipitate a "TMJ attack."

Of course, one can never say "never." Obviously, there are the occasional exceptions to almost every rule, and this truism holds for the world of orthodontics. There are cases where bicuspids may be extracted with impunity to gain arch length. But the list of qualifying signs and circumstances that must be met to justify bicuspid extractions is long; and their coincidental and simultaneous existence all at once, all in the same patient, are statistically infrequent. First, the patient must suffer from both severe crowding in the anterior segments and simultaneously exhibit a severe bimaxillary protrusion. Second, the patient's arches must exhibit nearly standard lateral width, being at or very close to the relative Schwarz or Pont's indices. Thirdly, the skeletal development must be equal to or greater than normal, relative to the lower face height, such that if molars were distalized, the bite would be opened beyond a satisfactory cephalometric or esthetic level. In addition to this, some patients will exhibit a legitimate tooth size to jaw size discrepancy beyond the limits of orthopedically correctable tolerances of basal bone. These factors combined with, or without, congenitally missing third molars, combine to produce circumstances under which four-bicuspid extraction is perfectly acceptable. One must always remember to treat the needs of the patient, not the demands of a concept.

"Some circumstantial evidence is very strong, as when you find a trout in the milk."

Henry David Thoreau (1817–1862)
Journal, *November 11, 1850*

SPECIAL CONSIDERATIONS—RELAPSE

One facet affected by the extraction of second molars is so important that it truly deserves special attention, that of relapse. The bane of orthodontists since the days of Edward Angle, relapse has inspired more research, conjecture, countermethods, patient disappointment, and doctor exasperation than almost any other aspect of orthodontics. Many things have been blamed for it: improper technique, removing the appliance too soon, incorrect angulation of anterior teeth, incorrect angulation of posterior teeth, lack of patient cooperation in wearing retainers, failure to employ transeptal fibrotomy, bruxism, mesial drift, anatomical memory, and a host of others. What is especially disconcerting is that some cases remain beautifully stable over long periods of time regardless of the above. Two factors almost never considered are improper or imbalanced muscle function, and the enormous forward thrust of the second molar. Routinely, the third molar is often mistakenly implicated as the culprit. Many a patient has had fixed appliances removed after several years of treatment only to be told to immediately report to the oral surgeon's office to have "wisdom teeth" removed so they "don't push everything crooked again."

Careful examination of certain well-known facts causes a different picture to emerge. The incidence is presently unavailable; yet most clinicians have observed relapse, or recurrence of crowding to be more specific, occurring in patients even after third-molar removal. Yet one never observes the previously mentioned distal drift of the bicuspids or first or second molars after such surgery. This slight distal drifting *is* a phenomenon observed after second molar removal however, provided it is timed properly. This would imply that the mesial thrust of the second molar is far greater than the third molar. There may be a theoretically sound histologic reason for this. Consider the case where a first and second molar have been extracted for reasons of dental pathology. One observes the third molar, if fully erupted, will be both mesially tilted and drifted forward, but only so far. One never observes a third molar migrating mesially all the way to the second bicuspid. It appears that the farther away a tooth moves from its embryonic development site, the weaker its mesial drift becomes. Cell lineage may be responsible for this, ie, the propensity for cells to remain and reproduce in the correct anatomical location. Basement membrane direction may also be a factor. This is why a cut lip heals with dermis on the outside and oral mucosa on the inside as it should. One never observes dermis healing in the cut and migrating up past the vermillion border of the lip to the inner part of the vestibule, nor the opposite, intraoral mucosa healing and migrating out over the outer surface of the lip. Embryonic cell lineage gives everything to know just the right place to develop. One never sees a bicuspid develop between two molars, nor an incisor between two bicuspids. Might it not be possible that, if you pardon the pun, teeth know where their roots are and can sense in some mysterious way on a cellular level when they have drifted too far from their origins? If so, this would explain the strength of the second molar and the weakness of the third molar in the posterior segment. First, if the second molar is left in place, it must help make room for the developing third. Maybe the third stimulates it to hyperactivity in this regard.[66] Being right over the spot where it developed embryonically, the second molar's mesial thrust is at its peak, possibly even intensified by the still unerupted third. If, for some reason, the first molar were to be removed, the second would drift forward into its place.[67] But were a first molar and the two bicuspids to be removed, due to some reason of dental pathology, the second molar would never close the gap to the cuspid! But if the second molar is removed, the third does not have to travel far to come into its place. In the meantime, the crowded and improper arch form has been corrected and a naturally strong stable arch awaits the third's arrival. But when it arrives, its mesial drift is pretty well spent due to its distance from its bed. The forced crowding of the already correctly positioned teeth ahead of it, which are already in a strong and stable arch form, is next to impossible. It has simply traveled too far forward from its embryonic development site to have much drive left.

Another phenomenon lends credence to this theory. When cases are treated for diminished arch width by means of transverse expansion, the relapse after such cases are completed and appliances are removed is always *mesio*lingual if the second molars remain. But oddly when they have been removed and the case has been expanded transversely, the relapse is *disto*-lingual. One long-term study by Schwarze[68] showed that relapse of transversely expanded cases where second molars remained in the mouth resulted in worse crowding after relapse than before the cases received treatment. This implies it was either solely the fault of the retained second molar or the second molar in combination with the third, that was responsible for the cases with retained second molars relapsing mesiolingually.

Cases correctly treated by second-molar removal do in fact show overwhelmingly consistent stability, but there is one other factor to consider. All the credit cannot be vested upon the removal of the second molar. Since this "avant garde" technique is usually associated with individuals who also use functional appliances, the cases treated by second-molar extraction are also usually recipients of functional appliance treatment during some phase of the treatment plan. Therein lies the key. The stability is greatly enhanced, if not guaranteed, by the fact that the other major cause of the malocclusion, improper muscle function, has been corrected by means of the functional appliance. With correct tooth position and correct muscle function, the maxillofacial complex acts as its own retainer. The teeth and alveolar bone then occupy a neutral zone which is the equilibrium point between the muscular forces pushing in (the orofacial musculature, lips, cheeks, etc), and the muscular forces pushing out (the tongue). Correct function around correctly positioned teeth and alveolar bone in correctly formed, unrestrained arches that are properly biomechanically aligned results in that perpetually elusive goal – stability! Everything is back to normal and Nature is satisfied. It's what She had originally intended all along.

Thus, correct muscle function, orthopedic and orthodontic balance, and second-molar removal, where indicated, are theorized to be the keys to successful cases and stability. One has to trust the basic conclusions his mind presents to him after careful deliberation and consideration of what he has observed. Thus the *causes*, and not the effects, of relapse can be treated and eliminated. In support of this theory is the enormous weight of clinical evidence observed by the many who have employed this combination of techniques throughout the years on two continents. Though the theories proposed were initially a result of empiricism, and some of the evidence concerning the powerful thrust of the second molars is truly circumstantial,[69-75] the direct observation of certain clinically observable facts gives the mind the freedom to draw its own natural conclusions. When one stands back and considers the entire gamut of events, trusting in what may be seen, it becomes obvious as to when "the milk has been laced with creek water."

"To strive, to seek to find, and not to yield"

"Ulysses"
Alfred Lord Tennyson (1809–1892)

THE SECOND MOLAR REPLACEMENT ALTERNATIVE – A THERAPEUTIC MANDATE

We have made a number of points quite clear:

1. One of the most critical components of orthodontic therapeutics is the need to correct arch length discrepancies and relieve dental crowding in an effort to obtain proper arch form.

Figure 3-23 Case study. Spontaneous correction of crowding by removal of second molars. Views of 11½-year-old patient with moderately crowded cuspids in all four quadrants. **(A) (B) (C)** Pretreatment study models show crowding of cuspids and remaining anterior teeth. **(D) (E) (F)** Final occlusion showing spontaneous correction of crowding without aid of appliances but by second molar removal alone. **(G)** Unilateral radiographs of right and left posterior quadrants show both second and third molars present. **(H)** Panographic X-ray shows third molars fully erupted in place behind first molars.

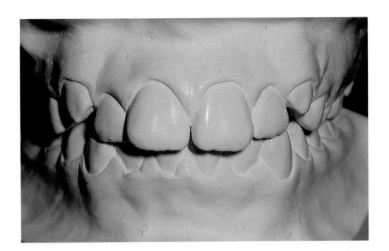

(A)

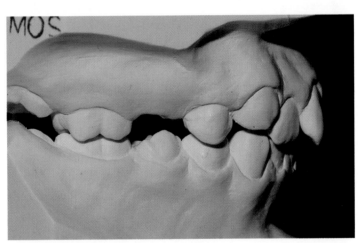

(B)

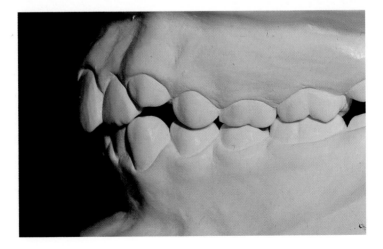

(C)

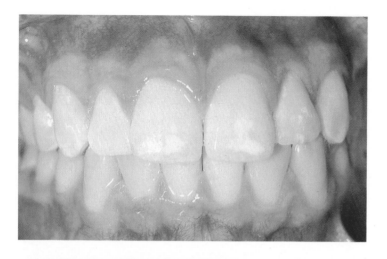

(D)

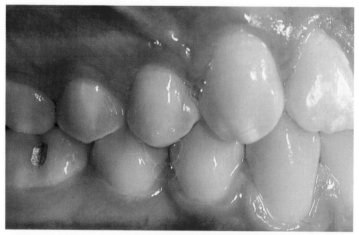

(E)

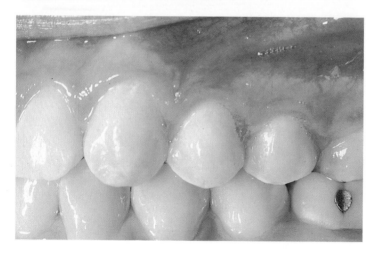

(F)

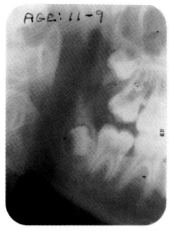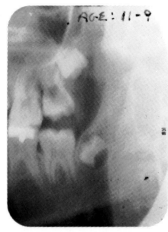

(G)

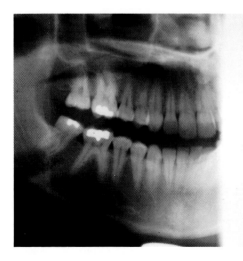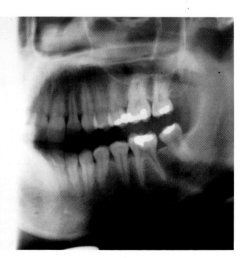

(H)

2. The American orthodontic community has traditionally embraced the four-bicuspid extraction method as the *only* method of treatment where extractions are indicated.
3. The therapeutic mechanics that follow bicuspid extractions often leave the patients with dished-in faces, flattened smiles, unstable occlusions, and retracted maxillary anteriors, all of which cause the mandibular arc of closure to be retruded, often to the point of causing severe TMJ problems.
4. Correction of such TMJ problems always consists of reverse tooth movement labially in the anterior area followed by repositioning and "realignment" of the mandible down and forward with Bionator therapy!
5. Even with bicuspid extraction to relieve crowding anteriorly, there is often still not enough room provided posteriorly to allow third molars (usually lowers) to erupt, which often results in impaction.
6. Removal of impacted third molars increases surgical insult and risk to the patient and carries the possibility of postsurgical complications such as infection, pain and discomfort, TMJ damage (for difficult extractions), and paresthesias. Expense is also increased to the patient.
7. As a result of the above, eight teeth are removed, leaving the patient with only 24 teeth.

The alternative of second-molar replacement with thirds avoids these problems and exhibits the following advantages.

1. It prevents the retraction of maxillary anteriors as there are no bicuspid spaces to close. This allows the mandible to be developed down and forward, which is compatible with the TMJ.
2. Faces are fuller, and smile lines are broader and not flattened.
3. Stability is greatly enhanced as the gigantic forward thrust of the second molars is replaced by the thirds.
4. Treatment time is made easier, shorter, and far more dependable.
5. Treatment methods using this technique avoid the use of elastics and prolonged use of fixed appliances or retainers, and eliminate the need for headgear, a notion *very popular* with most patients.
6. It leaves the patient with 28 teeth and a low surgical insult and risk.

On an even more basic level, it is inefficient and reflects lack of overall control of the case to take out bicuspids and "wait and see" if the third molars are going to be able to have the room to erupt or not. Extracting them years later when they become impacted is like therapeutically "sweeping up the loose ends." If extractions are indicated, it is far more professional to perform them once, and right, the first time.

The highly reputed oral surgeon, Dr John Austin of Saint Paul, Minnesota, advocates the evaluation radiographically of every 11- to 12-year-old, regardless of his or her need for orthodontics, to determine whether second molars should be extracted or not merely for the advantage of the avoidance of the impacted third-molar situation.[76] The careful monitoring of the patient through these critical years of growth and development is justified for the surgical implications alone.

We must continually look at the patient and his second molar–third molar status during this period and continually evaluate his progress, taking the proper steps which are in the best interests of the patient at the proper time. Timing is critical. Second-molar extraction is best between the ages of 10 or 11 up to 15 years in the lower arch or even as late as age 20 years for the uppers. The actual limiting factor for successful eruption to take place seems to be at around the time the bifurcation of the roots of the third molar begin to be clearly seen.[77]

Extracting the second molar in place of the third molar, allowing the third to safely erupt into place, is a viable alternative to the impacted third molar ritual in patients who need no orthodontic therapy. But to avoid dished-in faces, flattened smiles, unstable occlusions, and compromised temporomandibular joints, for the patient needing orthodontic treatment accompanied by dental extractions, *there is no alternative* to second-molar extraction; *there is no debate*.

The second molar replacement technique becomes both for the patient and the treating clinician a therapeutic mandate!

REFERENCES

1. Hawley CA: Treatment of Class II of distoclusion. *Int J Orthod* 1930;16:127–139.
2. Tweed CH: Indications for extraction of teeth in orthodontic procedure. *Am Assoc Orthod Trans* 1944;22–45.
3. Salzmann JA: The rationale of extraction as an adjunct to mechanotherapy and the sequelae of extraction in the absence of orthodontic guidance. *Am J Orthod Oral Surg* 1945;31:181–202.
4. Salzmann JA: Criteria for extraction in orthodontic therapy related to dentofacial development. *Am J Orthod* 1949;35:584–610.
5. Straug RHW, Waugh LM: Advisability of extraction as a therapeutic aid in orthodontics. *Am J Orthod Oral Surg* 1947;33:141–144, 153–160.
6. Herzberg BL: Extraction in orthodontic treatment – cases in which extraction of the first four bicuspids is advisable. *Dent Clin North Am* 1960;789–794.
7. Begg PR: Differential force in orthodontic treatment. *Am J Orthod* 1956;42:481–510.
8. Steiner CC: Power storage and delivery in orthodontic appliances. *Am J Orthod* 1953;39:859–880.
9. Jarabak JR: Development of a treatment plan in light of one's concepts of treatment objectives. *Am J Orthod* 1960;46:481–514.
10. Stoner MM: Force control in clinical practice. *Am J Orthod* 1960;46:163–186.
11. Graber TM: The edgewise appliance in routine practice. *Am J Orthod* 1960;46:1–23.
12. Kloehn SJ: A new approach to analysis and treatment of mixed dentitions. *Am J Orthod* 1953;39:161–183.
13. Brehm W: *The "New" Advanced Straight Wire Diagnosis and Treatment Planning 3-Day Seminar – Course Manual*.
14. Angle EH: *Treatment of Malocclusion of the Teeth*, ed 7. Philadelphia, SS White Dental Manufacturing Co, 1907.

15. Angle EH: The upper first molar as a basis of diagnosis in orthodontia. *Dent Items* 1906;28:421–460.
16. Angle EH: The latest and best in orthodontic mechanism. *Dent Cosmos* 1928; 70:1143–1158.
17. Graber TM: *Orthodontics: Principles and Practice*. Philadelphia, WB Saunders Co, 1961, p 4.
18. Ketcham AH: A preliminary report of an investigation of apical root resorption of permanent teeth. *Int J Orthod* 1927;13:97–125.
19. Ketcham AH: A progress report of an investigation of apical root resorption of vital permanent teeth. *Int J Orthod* 1928;15:310–325.
20. Dickson GC: The natural history of malocclusion. *Dent Pract* 1970;20:216–232.
21. Cole HJ: Certain results of extraction in the treatment of malocclusion, thesis, University of Illinois, 1947, cited in Sleichter CG: Effects of maxillary bite plate therapy. *Am J Orthod* 1954;40:850–870.
22. Eirew HL: An orthodontic challenge. *Int J Orthod* 1976;14:21–25.
23. Wilson HE: The orthodontist and disorders of the mandibular joint. *Int Dent J* 1952;3:235–236.
24. Wilson HE: Etiology of mandibular joint disorders: their correction and prevention by orthodontic treatment. *Trans Eur Orthod Soc* 1953;200–210.
25. Wilson HE: Early recognition of some etiological factors in temporo-mandibular joint disorders. *Trans Br Soc Study Orthod* 1956;88–98.
26. Wilson HE: Extraction of second molars in treatment planning. *Orthod Fr* 1964;25:61–67.
27. Wilson HE: The extraction of second permanent molars as a therapeutic measure. *Trans Eur Orthod Soc* 1966;141–145.
28. Wilson HE: Extraction of second permanent molars in orthodontic treatment. *Orthodontist* 1971;3:1–7.
29. Wilson HE: Long term observation on the extraction of second permanent molars. *Trans Eur Orthod Soc* 1974;50:215–221.
30. Hellman M: The face in its developmental career. *Dent Cosmos* 1935;77:685–699, 777–787.
31. Atkinson SR: Changing dynamics of the growing face. *Am J Orthod* 1949;35: 815–836.
32. Gilda EJ: Analysis of linear facial growth. *Angle Orthod* 1974;44:1–14.
33. Nanda RS: The rates of growth of several facial components measured from serial cephalometric roentgenograms. *Am J Orthod* 1955;41:658–673.
34. Knott VB: Growth of the mandible relative to a cranial base line. *Angle Orthod* 1973;43:305–313.
35. Bjork A: The significance of growth changes in facial pattern and their relationship to changes in occlusion. *Dent Rec* 1951;71:197–208.
36. Bjork A: Variability and age changes in overbite and overjet. *Am J Orthod* 1953; 39:779–801.
37. Bjork A: Variations in the growth pattern of the human mandible: Longitudinal radiographic study by the implant method. *J Dent Res* 1963;42:400–411.
38. Bjork A: Sutural growth of the upper face, studied by the implant method. *Acta Odontol Scand* 1966;24:109–127.
39. Luzi V: CV value in analysis of sagittal malocclusions. *Am J Orthod* 1982;81:478.
40. Mills CM, Holman G, Graber TM: Heavy intermittent cervical traction in Class II treatment: A longitudinal cephalometric assessment. *Am J Orthod* 1978;74: 361–379.

41. Moore AW: Orthodontic treatment factors in Class II malocclusion. *Am J Orthod* 1959;45:323–352.
42. Weinberg L: Posterior bilateral condylar displacement: its diagnosis and treatment. *J Prosthet Dent* 1976;36:426–440.
43. Williams R, Hosila FJ: The effects of different extraction sites upon incisor retraction. *Am J Orthod* 1976;69:388–410.
44. Faubion B: The effects of the extraction of premolars on the eruption of mandibular third molars. *J Am Dent Assoc* 1968;76:316–320.
45. Richardson M: The relative effects of the extraction of various teeth on the development of mandibular third molars. *Trans Eur Orthod Soc* 1975;79–85.
46. Hinds CE, Frey KF: Hazards of retained third molars in older persons. *J Am Dent Assoc* 1980;101:246–250.
47. Little RM, Waller TR, Riedel RA: Stability and relapse of mandibular anterior alignment—first premolar extraction cases treated by edgewise orthodontics. *Am J Orthod* 1981;80:349–365.
48. Uhole MD: Long term stability of the static occlusion after orthodontic treatment. *Am J Orthod* 1981;80:228.
49. Wilkinson LC: Some things to keep in mind when treating a four bicuspid extraction case. *Angle Orthod* 1952;22:47–52.
50. Prichard JF: Four bicuspid extractions in orthodontic treatment—is it the treatment of choice? Recorded notes of a lecture given before the annual meeting of the American Academy of Gnathologic Orthopedics, Fort Worth, Texas, Sept 18–21, 1974.
51. Liddle DW: Second molar extraction in orthodontic treatment. *Am J Orthod* 1977;72:599–616.
52. McBride LJ, Huggins DG: A cephalometric study of the eruption of lower third molars following loss of lower second molars. *Trans Br Soc Stud Orthod* 1970;42–47.
53. Huggins DG: Eruption of lower third molars following orthodontic treatment. *Dent Pract* 1963;13:209–215.
54. Henry CB, Morrant GM: *Biometrica* 1936;28:378–427.
55. Cryer BS: Third molar eruption: The effect of extraction of adjacent teeth. *Dent Pract* 1967;17:405–418.
56. Breakspear EK: Indications for extraction of the lower second permanent molars. *Trans Br Soc Stud Orthod* 1966;122–124.
57. Richardson ME: The early developmental position of lower third molars relative to certain jaw dimensions. *Angle Orthod* 1970;40:226–230.
58. Smith D: The eruption of lower third molars following extraction of second molars. *Trans Br Soc Stud Orthod* 1957;55–57.
59. Lawlor J: The effects on the lower third molar of the extraction of the lower second molar. *Br J Orthod* 1978;5:99–103.
60. Halderson H: Early second permanent molar extractions in orthodontics. *Am J Orthod* 1961;47:706–707.
61. Lehman R: A consideration of the advantages of second molar extractions in orthodontics. *Eur J Orthod* 1979;1:119–124.
62. Rindler A: Effects on lower third molars after extraction of second molars. *Angle Orthod* 1977;47:55–58.
63. Berg R, Gebauer U: Spontaneous changes in the mandibular arch following first premolar extractions. *Eur J Orthod* 1982;4:93–98.
64. Mills JRE: The effect on the lower incisors of uncontrolled extraction of lower premolars. *Trans Eur Orthod Soc* 1964;357–370.

65. Huggins DG, McBride LJ: The eruption of lower third molars following the loss of lower second molars: a longitudinal cephalometric study. *Br J Orthod* 1978;5:13-20.

66. Vego L: A longitudinal study of mandibular arch perimeters. *Angle Orthod* 1962;32:187-192.

67. Mitchell W: The extraction of the first permanent molars: a beneficent conservative operation. *Dent Cosmos* 1899;41:524-533.

68. Schwarze CW: Expansion and relapse in long follow-up studies. *Trans Eur Orthod Soc* 1972;263-274.

69. Sakuda M, Kuroda Y, Wada K, et al: Changes in crowding of teeth during adolescence and their relation to the growth of the facial skeleton. *Trans Eur Orthod Soc* 1976;93-104.

70. Bjork A, Skeiller V: Facial development and tooth eruption, an implant study at the age of puberty. *Am J Orthod* 1972;62:339-383.

71. Kaplan RG: Mandibular third molars and postretention crowding. *Am J Orthod* 1974;66:411-430.

72. Chapman H: The normal dental arch and its changes from birth to adult. *Br Dent J* 1935;58:201-229.

73. Sillman JH: Dimensional changes of the dental arches: a longitudinal study from birth to 25 years. *Am J Orthod* 1964;50:824-842.

74. Lundstrom A: Changes in crowding and spacing of teeth with age. *Dent Pract* 1969;19:218-223.

75. Humerfelt A, Stagsvold O: Changes in occlusion and craniofacial pattern between 11 and 25 years of age. *Trans Eur Orthod Soc* 1972;113-122.

76. Austin J: Personal communication, July 1985.

77. Ahlin JH, White GE, Tsamtsouris A, et al: *Maxillofacial Orthopedics*. Chicago, Quintessence Publishing Co, 1980, p 278.

Additional References of Interest

78. Allen WJ: Mandibular stability with the twin-wire appliance. *Am J Orthod* 1966; 52:483-494.

79. Chipman MR: Aims and methodology of treatment according to age groups. Permanent dentition age group. *Am J Orthod* 1957;43:661-678.

80. Coben SE: Growth and Class II treatment. *Am J Orthod* 1966;52:5-26.

81. Dougherty HL: Failures in orthodontics. *Trans Eur Orthod Soc.*

82. Gaber TM: Maxillary second molar extraction in Class II, malocclusion. *Am J Orthod* 1969;56:331-353.

83. Gaber TM: Maxillary second molar extraction in Class II, malocclusion. *Am J Orthod* 1970;58:401.

84. Henry BC: Prophylactic odentectomy of the developing mandibular third molar.

85. Martinek CE: Treatment planning. *Am J Orthod* 1960;46:253-269.

CHAPTER 4
The Sagittal Appliance

The Sagittal active plate is an arch-*lengthening* appliance. It may be used to develop arches by actively moving teeth, in groups or singly, in an antero-posterior direction along the crest of the alveolar ridges. By means of proper design and active screw selection, it may be used to move teeth on either side of the arch unilaterally or bilaterally. It may be used to relieve crowding in the posterior segments, develop immature premaxillas, and also relieve anterior crowding. The upper Sagittal appliance, by virtue of having acrylic plates covering the occlusal surfaces of the maxillary teeth, can double over as an excellent intraoral splint to relieve temporomandibular joint and muscle discomfort often associated with certain severe malocclusions. It is economical to construct, durable in performance, and comfortable and esthetic for the patient to wear. When properly used, it produces excellent results, while allowing the clinician to continually maintain a positive form of orthodontic control.

In the overall picture of orthodontic treatment, the importance of the Sagittal appliance cannot be overestimated. Active forces are necessary to move teeth into their proper positions on the arch in crowded cases.[1] Fixed appliances have been utilized for this purpose extensively in the past, but the Sagittal can also provide this force while at the same time providing all the benefits of a removable active plate.

217

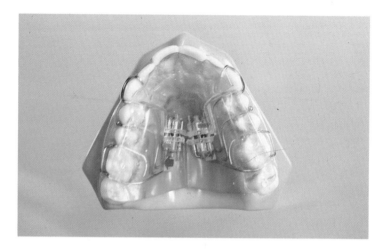

Figure 4-1 Basic maxillary Sagittal I appliance. (*Courtesy of Ohlendorf Co., St Louis, MO.*)

Active arch preparation is the keystone to allowing the Bionator to be used to its full and proper potential. As stated in a previous chapter, the Bionator is an arch-aligning appliance. If you don't have arches, you are not ready for the Bionator. Sagittal active plates help get the arches ready by helping obtain proper anteroposterior arch form. The early-model European functional appliances (Andresen-Häupl Activator, Bionator, etc) were referred to as "miracle appliances." Well, the real miracle is in finding a case where the teeth are not crowded out of position and are sufficiently arch-shaped in arrangement to require only the jaw-to-jaw alignment of a functional appliance without the benefit of previous arch preparation. Single appliance cases of this type are infrequent. Active plate arch preparation goes hand in hand with functional appliance therapy to allow the practitioner to use these two modalities to treat a large assortment of malocclusions.

Active plates in general go back as far as Robin, who in 1902 described a split plate he had designed that made use of an active screw for expanding the component parts. The British also experimented with removable active plates in the first decade of the century.[2] But active plate popularity was minimal, most likely due to the fact that they had to be constructed out of vulcanite, a material not well suited for the abuse screws and spring

Figure 4-2 **(A)** Saggital I appliance as it appears at insertion prior to expansion screw activation. Note that unlike older "Y-plates" that preceded it, modern Sagittal appliance covers occlusal surfaces of maxillary posterior teeth with acrylic. Appliance may be used to distalize posterior quadrants either **(B)** unilaterally or **(C)** bilaterally and to any varying degree of each as is required by the case. (*Courtesy of Ohlendorf Co., St Louis, MO.*)

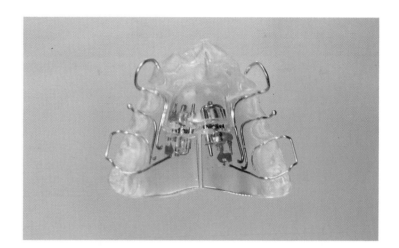

(A)

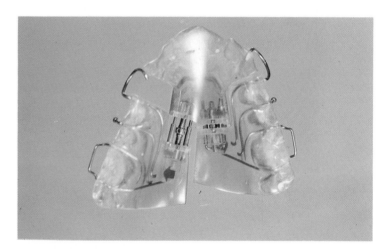

(B)

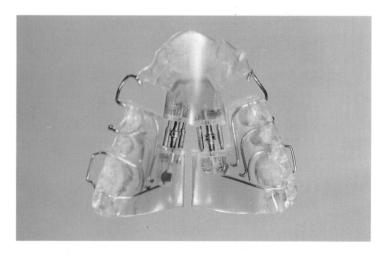

(C)

wires could exert on an appliance. Also, fixed appliances were coming into their own at this time in America and enjoyed immense popularity.

Men like Nord and Tischler advanced the science of active plates further in the 1930s in Europe, but the real founding father of active plate technique has always been considered to be the legendary A. M. Schwarz of Vienna, Austria. He published a book in 1938 devoted entirely to the design and use of these appliances.[3]

Many variations of active plates were described and experimented with, and some proved more practical than others. Since the basic elements are so simple (a base plate of acrylic; retention clasps; and active screws, wires, and springs of one sort or another), the various combinations possible are limited only by the type of derangement and collapse of teeth in the arch and the clinician's own imagination. Admittedly, certain combinations of rotations and malpositions of teeth are easier to correct with modern-day fixed appliances, but the ability to carry out orthopedic and bulk movements of entire segments of teeth endows the active plate with a value and permanence in total orthodontic care that has allowed them to justifiably survive down to this day.

An early forerunner of the Sagittal appliance was referred to as the Y-plate because of the shape of the cuts on the base plate separating the plate into its component parts. Most of the early model Y-plates or lateral expansion active plates of that era had a labial bow, and ones which are constructed that way today still bear the name of "Schwarz plate" after the man who brought their use to such a high level of proficiency. The earlier models also made much greater use of springs and wires for the movement of teeth. While this is still true of more modern designs to a certain extent, the development of highly refined and precision-machined screws has changed the general use of these appliances a great deal.

Figure 4-3 Palatal view discloses position of clasping wires relative to teeth. Note middle portion over palatal rugae area which should be kept as thin as possible to provide tongue room to aid in speech and patient comfort. Clear plastic model reveals location of two expansion screws relative to their position with respect to roots of teeth and alveolar crests.

Figure 4-4 Expansion screws are designed to be activated by inserting key into central cylinder from the tissue side and levering the key upward or towards midline of appliances. One such 90-degree turn of cylinder expands jackscrew by 0.25 mm. Maximum expansion of screw itself is 8 mm. The famous Scheu designed 714 expansion screw is used in the configuration in this maxillary Sagittal. Directional activation indicator arrows are processed directly into acrylic of appliance to insure the operator (either patient or doctor) levers key in proper direction. Smaller mandibular appliance requires a proportionally smaller screw, the E.O.P. Forestadent 01-134-1315. Its smaller size causes it to open only 0.12 mm per quarter turn, ie eight turns will open it 1.0 mm.

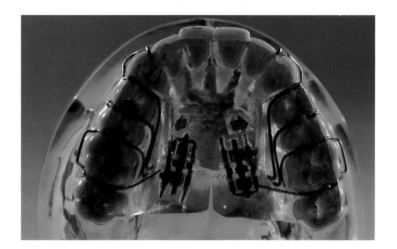

Figure 4-3

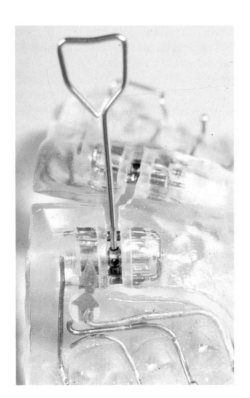

Figure 4-4

In present-day usage, the expansion screw is relied upon to a far greater extent, while the fine-tuning of tooth positioning after bulk movements of the active plates are accomplished is often left to more manageable methods such as the fixed appliances.

As the name implies, the Sagittal appliance develops the arches in primarily an anteroposterior direction. Some slight oblique development is possible, but this is a function of the offset placement of the expansion screws. But generally screws are placed parallel to the anteroposterior plane or parallel to the crest of the alveolar ridges. The direction of the main component of force delivered by the appliance both in the maxilla and the mandible, and as a result in the direction of the main part of the expansion, is dependent primarily upon one all-important factor—the status of the second molar. If the second molar is intact, the primary direction of the development of the arch will be of the anteriors in an *anterior* direction. This is especially useful in the development and expansion of a crowded or retruded premaxilla as in a Class II, Division 2, case.

However, if the second molars have been removed, the primary direction of movement of the teeth will be of the posterior segments in a *distal* direction. This is exceptionally useful in cases of severe anterior crowding where it has been determined cephalometrically and by other diagnostic aids that the premaxilla is in the correct position, but the posterior segments have drifted forward, a direct cause of the anterior crowding.

Of course, the appliance itself expands in both directions at once. It is just that with the second molars *in*, the expansion is about 80% anteriorly, and with the second molars *out*, the expansion is about 80% posteriorly.

Though the primary direction of expansion is on the anteroposterior plane, when a Sagittal is used to distalize posterior segments with the second molars out, there will be a moderate arch width increase realized. This is due to the fact that as the first molar and bicuspids travel distally, they occupy a naturally wider position on the arch, which widens as it goes posteriorly. However, it must be emphasized that this increase in arch width is not great, although it is extremely stable.

Figure 4-5 Lower Sagittal appliance. Note that no acrylic covers occlusal surfaces of lower posterior teeth. Special note: lower Forestadent expansion screws are smaller to accommodate overall smaller appliance used in mandibular arch and are engineered to require two 90-degree turns of central cylinder to obtain same physical expansion (0.25 mm) as larger Scheu 714 used in upper. Therefore, they must be turned twice to obtain same linear distance of expansion. (Lower screw type: Forestadent 01-134-1315)

Figure 4-6 Early prototype Sagittal appliances developed by Voss derived their lineage from basic designs referred to as "Y-plates" developed by Schwarz. Witzig added the acrylic occlusal pads, redesigned expansion screw location and as a result, became responsible for the appearance of the appliance as we know it today.

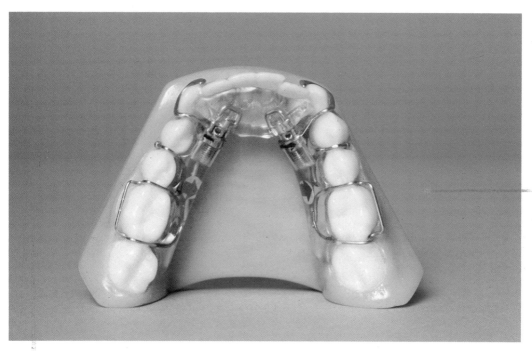

Figure 4-5

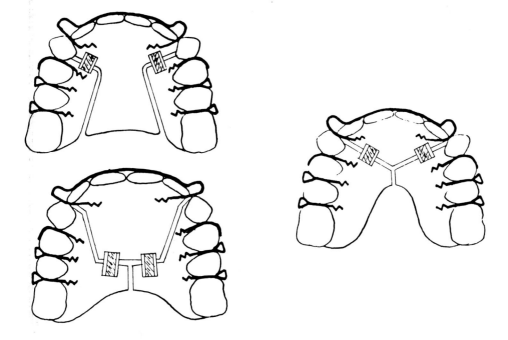

Figure 4-6

Venienti occurrite morbo.
"Meet the disease as it approaches."

Perius, Roman Poet (AD 34–62)

APPLIANCE DESIGN, FUNCTION, AND ADJUSTMENT

The design of the Sagittal appliance is essentially dependent upon the type of distortion present in the dental arch for which it is to be utilized.

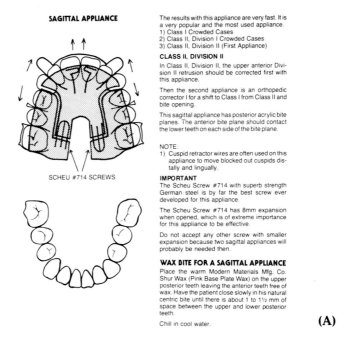

SAGITTAL APPLIANCE

SCHEU #714 SCREWS

The results with this appliance are very fast. It is a very popular and the most used appliance.
1) Class I Crowded Cases
2) Class II, Division I Crowded Cases
3) Class II, Division II (First Appliance)

CLASS II, DIVISION II

In Class II, Division II, the upper anterior Division II retrusion should be corrected first with this appliance.

Then the second appliance is an orthopedic corrector I for a shift to Class I from Class II and bite opening.

This sagittal appliance has posterior acrylic bite planes. The anterior bite plane should contact the lower teeth on each side of the bite plane.

NOTE:
1) Cuspid retractor wires are often used on this appliance to move blocked out cuspids distally and lingually.

IMPORTANT
The Scheu Screw #714 with superb strength German steel is by far the best screw ever developed for this appliance.

The Scheu Screw #714 has 8mm expansion when opened, which is of extreme importance for this appliance to be effective.

Do not accept any other screw with smaller expansion because two sagittal appliances will probably be needed then.

WAX BITE FOR A SAGITTAL APPLIANCE
Place the warm Modern Materials Mfg. Co. Shur Wax (Pink Base Plate Wax) on the upper posterior teeth leaving the anterior teeth free of wax. Have the patient close slowly in his natural centric bite until there is about 1 to 1½ mm of space between the upper and lower posterior teeth.

Chill in cool water.

(A)

Figure 4-7 **(A)** Sagittal appliance. **(B)** With second molars in, action of the Sagittal is primarily anterior, with second molars out, action is primarily in posterior direction.

Figure 4-8 Construction bite for Sagittal appliance. Thickness of wax should be no more than 1 to 2 mm between posterior teeth when registering construction bite. Greater thickness produces appliance with acrylic bite pads too thick for patient comfort and function.

Figure 4-9 Sagittal I appliance operates on the principle that there is only one set of molars (upper first) left in the mouth to which it is attached, as second molars have been extracted. This results in an action that produces approximately 80% to 85% distalization to only 15% to 20% development anteriorly. When second molars (depicted in drawing) are removed, forces of expanding plate will be primarily in distal direction.

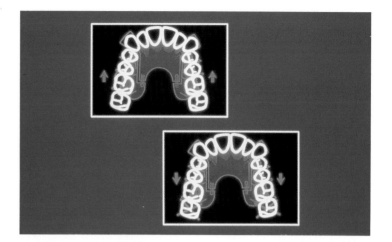

Figure 4-7(B)

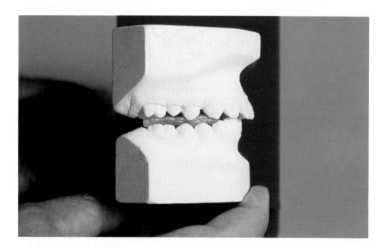

Figure 4-8

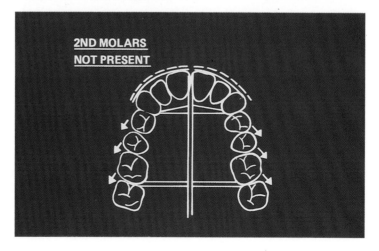

Figure 4-9

But all these types of appliances have certain general components in common.

First, for the maxillary appliance, there is the palatal portion or base plate. It extends out over the occlusal surfaces of all the posterior teeth at a thickness of 1.5 to 2.0 mm. This represents an addition developed by Dr Witzig to the old Y-plates of Dr Herman Voss and A. M. Schwarz. The appliance is sectioned into three component parts: one braced against the anterior premaxilla and midpalatal area, and two braced against the posterior teeth and lingual gingival areas along the posterior teeth on each side. The sectioning cut travels from the posterior edge of the appliance at the halfway point between the palatal midline and the lingual occlusal crest where it runs forward parallel to the midline of the midpalatal suture to a point level with the maxillary first molar, then turns 90 degrees for a distance slightly greater than the width of the expansion screw to be used, then turns 90 degrees anteriorly again and runs to a point distolingual to the maxillary cuspids where it turns at about a 45-degree angle toward the labial surface where the section travels just distal to the distal edge of each respective cuspid. In unilateral situations only one section appears on the side to be moved and the appliance is subsequently divided into only two parts.

The posterior segments contain the claps which retain the appliance. An Adams clasp on the first molar and an Adams clasp or ball clasp in the bicuspid area are usually the standard fare.[4] The cuspid may or may not be clasped with a simple C-type clasp depending on whether or not it is to be moved. The base of the cuspid clasp is also placed in the posterior section. Sometimes a labial bow is used in specific design cases to manage a protruding incisor or in other anterior tooth control–type problems. Also, on occasion, labial retaining clasps are used to retain protruding lateral incisors when premaxillary development is required as in a Class II, Division 2 case.

Though the Sagittal appliance is designed to be worn at all times, and especially while eating, this does not qualify it as a functional appliance, a misnomer prevalent in the profession today. Its action is strictly *active* by means of opening the expansion screws or manipulating any of the various wires that might be added. It makes use of the old adage: "Teeth will move through bone, but they won't move through acrylic." Its action, biologically, is the same as that of a fixed appliance. The forces used to move teeth are generated by the appliance itself. Although eating with the appliance in the mouth may be considered "functioning" on it, it has nothing in common with the actions of truly functional appliances such as the Bionator, Frankel, Bimler, Activator, etc. One can understand the confusion generated in the minds of those unfamiliar with removable appliances when active plates such as the Sagittal are referred to incorrectly as "functional appliances."

It is a very important aspect of active plate action that they be worn while eating. Even the action of biting on the appliance when not eating helps seat the appliance and helps it carry out its designed orthodontic movement. Wearing the appliance during eating is so advantageous in helping it carry out its action that it is estimated by some that the treatment time for a given case may be reduced by as much as 50% if this is done. This, of course, necessitates that the appliance be made as thin and comfortable as the physical demands of the situation will allow.

When the teeth occlude on the acrylic occlusal pads of the maxillary Sagittal appliance, it helps drive the plate into firm contact with both the maxillary teeth and palatal tissues. When the screws have been activated, the appliance is expanded just enough that when it is driven to place, it exerts a gentle pressure on the teeth and tissues causing the orthodontic movement to take place.[5-11] This action exists once the screws are opened by virtue of the fit of the appliance and the action of the clasps alone, even in the absence of the increased pressures of occlusion. However, the action of the appliance is futher intensified and is far more thorough and efficient when the jaws close on it and the contacting lower teeth drive it firmly into place against the maxillary teeth, attached gingivae, and palate. Thus the appliance produces change in tooth position and also in the surrounding bone by converting mechanical pressures into biological energy. As the mechanical pressures generated by the action of the appliance stimulate the cells in the socket area on a bone crystalline level, minute electrical potentials are generated that act to stimulate bone and collagen cells to remodel to a more favorable stress level around the root of the tooth being acted upon. This phenomenon might be referred to as a form of piezoelectric effect and is hypothesized to be the biological principle behind all forms of orthodontic and orthopedic change, as well as bone healing.[12-21]

It has been known for years that certain types of crystals, most commonly quartz, Rochelle salt, and ammonium dihydrogen phosphate change their shape when placed in a magnetic field.[22] The reverse is also true. When placed under external mechanical stress, these same crystals will generate minute electrical voltages. Thus is hypothesized the theory that electricity is produced by pressure on bone relative to tooth movement through bone, and the belief that the bone crystals act in a similar manner. The theoretical minute voltages stimulate bone remodeling to take place, reshaping the bone to adapt to the pressures generated by the tooth root.

Regardless of how the biology takes place, the orthodontics definitely takes place and with proper design, management, and patient compliance, excellent results can be obtained.

We will now look at the various general actions for which Sagittal appliances may be used. As with all removable appliances, both functional and active, the proper clinical management, which means proper diagnosis, appliance selection, design and adjustment, and patient cooperation are what determine the degree of success obtained with the case. For the purposes of convenience we shall refer to the two main types of Sagittals as (1) Sagittal I, for the purposes of distalizing the posterior segment after second molars have been removed; and (2) Sagittal II, for the purposes of moving and developing a retruded premaxilla forward with the second molars intact to serve as anchorage. The appearance of the two appliances is almost identical. It is the difference in their resultant actions that makes specific nomenclature handy. One of modern-day man's most persistent problems is communication. A third type, the Sagittal III, is nothing more than a modified Sagittal II with "Frankel pads." These pads assist in holding the upper lip forward. The tension thereby imparted to the periosteum over the maxillary labial plate of bone aids in "pulling" the premaxilla forward in pseudo-Class III corrections.

THE SAGITTAL I

The Sagittal I appliance is designed to distalize one or both posterior segments to varying degrees as necessary to relieve anterior crowding, which usually expresses itself in the form of blocked-out cuspids, in Class I crowded cases. It also may be used for the same purpose in Class II, Division 1, cases so that after the posterior segments have been distalized, the protruded premaxilla, which may or may not have crowded anteriors, may be rotated down into correct position with the insertion of the Bionator (necessary in Class II cases). Of course, the distalization of the posterior segments implies that the second molars have been removed.

The distalization of the posterior segments is a result of several factors. First, with the second molars removed, there is much less molar-induced mesial force present against which the distalizing component of the appliance must push. Actually, in both arches, but especially the mandible, only the force of the first molar offers more than the usual static resistance, for if the first molar were not present, the bicuspids and even the cuspids can have a tendency to drift distally if not locked in by occlusion.[23,24] This natural "distal-drifting" force in the bicuspid area is inconsequential compared to the enormous power generated by the mechanical pressures of the plate itself. Yet at least it is not a force in the undesired opposite direction which the appliance must combat.

Figure 4-10 Case study of Sagittal I technique. Classic example of sagittal or A-P crowding of maxillary arch exhibiting labially blocked out cuspids. **(A)** Constructed Sagittal I appliance on pretreatment model. All four second molars were extracted prior to insertion of appliance. **(B)** The appearance of appliance after activation of expansion screws. Observe the amount of expansion present in the plate. Occlusion on posterior acrylic occlusal pads is slightly reduced in Sagittal I technique to assist in distal displacement of posterior segments, while occlusion on anterior bite plate portion of appliance is kept heavy. No cuspid retraction wires were required in this particular case. **(C)** Note final results with space for crowded cuspids to "drop in" and complete their normal eruption sequence now that posterior segments have been distalized. Lower arch was less crowded and "self-corrected" after removal of second molars without use of any appliances!

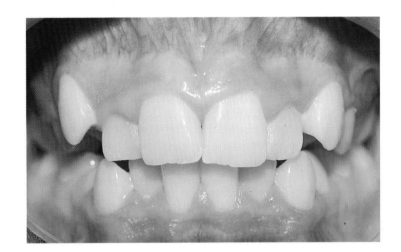

(A)

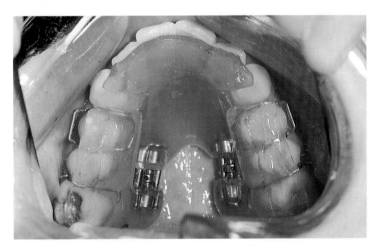

(B)

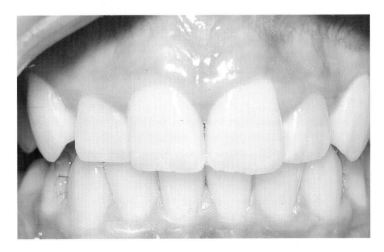

(C)

If the cuspids are blocked out labially due to anterior crowding, cuspid retraction clasps may be added to help pull them into place once the molar and bicuspids are distalized and arch length increases.

The palatal portion of the maxillary Sagittal must be thick enough in the premaxillary area to allow contact upon closure with the lower cuspids, or the lower laterals if the cuspids are out of occlusion. This will serve as the anchorage for the appliance. But the area of acrylic over the rugae area should not be too thick, so as to allow for as much tongue room as possible to facilitate speech. As the lowers articulate with this "bite-plate" area upon closure, they seat the appliance firmly against the soft tissues of the anterior palatal area and the six upper anterior teeth. This allows for the "gang-up" phenomenon to take place, whereby the middle portion of the appliance is braced by the premaxilla and six anterior teeth. As the screws are opened and the appliance expanded, this combination forms an anchorage base that serves to push the remaining two sections of the appliance against the remaining six posterior teeth. The balance of force is tipped in favor of the premaxillary area, and the posteriors are forced to yield to a distal movement. Some clinicians are fond of expanding the screws alternately instead of both on the same day so as to intensify this effect. This takes advantage of the phenomenon of cross-arch anchorage. Usually the screws may be given one 90-degree turn every three to four days depending on patient age, cooperation, etc. For some it can only be once every five to seven days! But if the screws are only turned alternately every fourth day, one utilizes the force of nine teeth ganged up cross-arch-anchorage–wise against three. Clinical experience and personal preference usually dictate the choice of either the bilateral (simultaneous) or unilateral (alternating) method for distalizing posterior segments of a given case. The alternating unilateral method is a technique more common for lower Sagittals. Lower Sagittal expansion screws are also smaller than those used on uppers. As a result they must

---

Figure 4-11 Sagittal I technique acrylic reduction. To aid in proper distalization of maxillary posterior quadrants into space created by missing second molar, articulating paper is used to register heavy occlusal contact points, which are then reduced slightly on posterior acrylic pads. This keeps occlusion heavy on anterior bite plane portion of plate, but light on posterior portion. In this example, markings of articulating paper are heavy on left side of plate but on right side have been reduced in posterior segments, only keeping occlusion heavy on cuspid area congruent with proper Sagittal I technique.

Figure 4-12 Once expansion screws reach their expansion limit of 8 mm, the plate becomes weak at point of insertion of screws into acrylic. This space may be filled in to fortify plate by placing common clear plastic tape behind the screw to act as a matrix, and flowing quick-cure acrylic into the space. After hardening in warm water, it may be trimmed and polished.

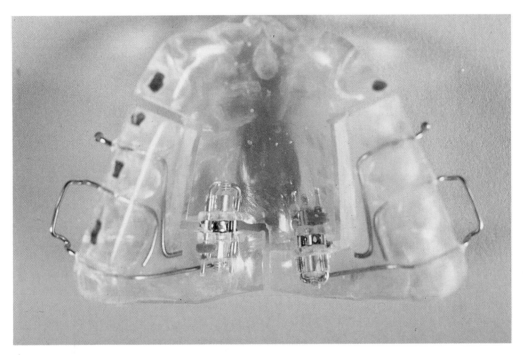

Figure 4-11

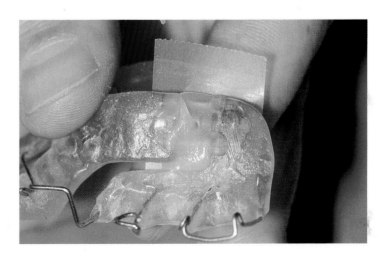

Figure 4-12

be turned twice as often, as one 90-degree turn only expands the appliance 0.125 mm, ie, one turn may be imparted every other day.

Adjustments

Adjusting the acrylic on an upper Sagittal is another important factor which facilitates treatment. When distalizing posterior teeth, it is important to keep the occlusion *solid on the premaxillary portion,* ie, lower cuspids or laterals contacting the upper acrylic bite plate area. Yet it is desirable to have only *light* contact on the posterior acrylic pads covering the occlusal portions of the posteriors. This allows the posterior segments to be distalized more easily without the interferences against the acrylic pads of firm occlusion with the lowers, which act to retard their movement. The appliance is checked with common articulating paper, and heavy marks indicating firm contact posteriorly are noted and relieved with common acrylic burs. This process may be performed every 3 or 4 weeks during the patient's treatment or as is necessary at their routine checking appointments. Of course, as the acrylic is relieved, the lower teeth will erupt slightly[25-28] and increase the vertical to a small degree, but this is not a significant problem and may even be desirable in cases of deep overbite where a Bionator will be called upon eventually to finish the case.

The occlusion must not be completely ground away on the posterior part of these appliances as this will cause tipping and loosening of the appliance during mastication and deglutition. This makes for a frustrated patient who will usually cease wearing the appliance during eating, decreasing its efficiency and increasing the length of treatment.

Treatment Time Line

When the appliance is inserted in the mouth for the first time, the routine checks are made for possible sore spots due to excessive impingement of acrylic or clasps on the tissues. Sometimes a small bubble of acrylic will appear in the cusp fossa of the acrylic occlusal pad causing the appliance to rock a little upon application of digital pressure from front to rear. Careful inspection and reduction of such areas with round burs insures a stable, comfortable fit for the patient.

As with all removable appliances, allow about a week for the appliance to "settle in" before instructing the patient to activate the expansion screws. Inform the patient that his mouth will water for a day or so until he gets used to the new gadget and that his speech will improve rapidly as the tongue accommodates to the new acrylic surface. The sibilant sounds, especially the (s) seems to be the last to give in to correct pronunciation.

However, most patients, children especially, accommodate to the appliance fairly quickly, provided it is not too thick. The acrylic pads should not be more than 2 mm thick and the appliance should allow for as much tongue room as possible, especially in the anterior area. Inform the patient that he may gradually work into eating with the appliance in place and he may start out with easier foods or snacks rather than the full-fledged meals. But stress the point that the more he chews with his appliance in place, the quicker he will see favorable results. Some clinicians only refer to the Sagittal as an "eating appliance" when discussing it with the patient in order to stress the importance of this factor. Good patient-doctor rapport is important in obtaining the cooperation necessary to carry this out. One might choose to remind the patient of what musing Valentine, one of Shakespeare's *Two Gentlemen of Verona* once said: "How use doth breed habit in a man!"

If cuspids have been blocked out labially and anteriorly, as is common in many malocclusions, cuspid retraction wires may be added to the appliance so that once the expansion takes place and the bicuspids and first molar are distalized, the retraction wire, attached to the section moving posteriorly, may be used to pull the cuspid distally into place. This adds extra drag to the motion of the lateral sections of the plate as they move distally, thereby requiring more treatment time to obtain movement. This means using every fourth or fifth day as a time to turn the expansion screws. One may wish to create room for the cuspids first, then "tease" them down into place by sequential activation of the cuspid retraction wires.

As the teeth in the posterior segments distalize, several things happen. First, they are being moved to a wider position on the dental arch, so the arch width increases slightly. Crowding begins to be relieved and space starts appearing into which the cuspid may be correctly positioned. If a great deal of *rotation* or malalignment still exists as this process takes place, fixed appliances may be called upon to more readily facilitate proper tooth positioning. This works extremely well once sufficient space is gained through the distalization of the posterior segments. The Straight Wire or similar type appliance utilizing bonded brackets is especially efficient here. Some clinicians on rare occasion may even use the two techniques in combination on certain cases. Special care must be used in designing the clasps of the Sagittal when it is to be used in conjunction with fixed appliances at the same time so that the clasps do not interfere with the arch wires or brackets.

Another observation that will be made is that as the posterior segments distalize, the vertical will open.[29-30] This is often helpful in cases of Class II malocclusions suffering from deep overbite and will help make the Bionator's job, once it is employed, all the easier.

Occasionally, if the teeth have to be distalized a long way, the interproximal marginal ridges will become uneven due to the backward tipping of the teeth. This usually rights itself with function in due time as the roots upright themselves to a more correct angulation. If this process is lagging behind for some reason and is a concern to the clinician, simple Straight Wiretype mechanics quickly and easily corrects the angulation problem and evens up the marginal ridges. But it must be remembered that this phenomenon is a minor complication that arises only in cases where teeth must be distalized a great distance and is easily corrected if spontaneous correction does not occur. However, this is not a particularly important problem compared to the alternatives of either no treatment or bicuspid extractions.

One of the beauties of Sagittal appliance therapy is that once the teeth have been moved into their proper position in the arch, retention is never a problem. Sagittal expansion results in an *extremely stable* situation. All the teeth are in their natural positions and with the enormous mesial driving force of the second molars absent, relapse is almost nonexistent.

Another point of interest in Sagittal I technique is that since the second molars are out, movement of the teeth in a distal direction occurs rather easily and rapidly. At the rate of one 90-degree turn of the expansion screw every four days, in little over a month a full 2 mm of expansion of the appliance has taken place, and in 2 months almost 4 mm! This is extremely rewarding and motivating to both the patient and doctor. Even if the 2- to 4-mm space gain that is obtained during the first several months of treatment is not discernible to the untrained eye of the patient or parent, the gaps that open up in the appliance as it is expanded are easily seen as a sign of progress by anyone.

The screws most commonly used in modern-day appliances open to 8 mm. When they approach this limit, the appliance becomes quite flexible. If more movement is required, new impressions must be taken along with a new construction bite, and a second appliance must be made. The first appliance can act as a brief retainer until the second one is delivered, since there may be just enough minor relapse to prevent the second appliance from easily going to place. During the interim, while waiting for the second appliance to be constructed, the first appliance may be strengthened by adding quick-cure acrylic into the gap spaces. This also makes the appliance a bit more comfortable to wear for the patient. It is a simple procedure that can easily be done in the office and requires little time for curing, trimming, and polishing.

In the event a slight arch asymmetry exists whereby one of the maxillary posterior segments needs minor lateral expansion, the expansion screw on that side may be processed into the appliance at an oblique angle to the area in question such as to not only produce a distalizing effect but also some minor arch expansion in a lateral direction. As the teeth are distalized, they also are forced to a more buccal direction on the arch. However, these techniques are only for slight deviations; if a substantial change in arch width is needed, one is better off using appliances designed specifically for that purpose.

Figure 4-13   Basic Sagittal II appliance. **(A)** Note the Sagittal II braces itself against two sets of molars, firsts and seconds. **(B)** Lateral view shows posterior bite pad thickness and clasping identical to Sagittal I. **(C)** Close-up view of lateral retraction, or stabilization wires, used in classic Class II, Division 2 anterior arrangements.

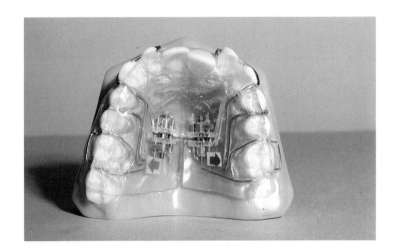

(A)

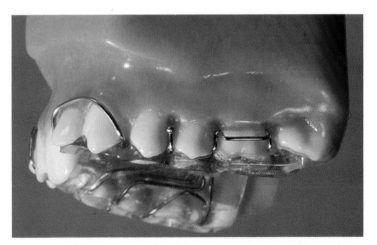

(B)

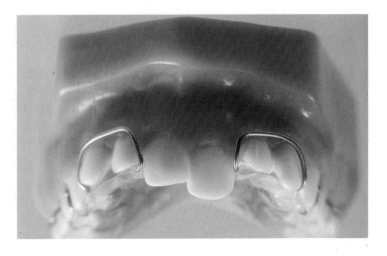

(C)

In certain cases where the upper second molars have been removed but the lowers retained, as when the lower thirds are congenitally missing, acrylic may be extended beyond the occlusal of the upper first molar to act as a stop to prevent the supraeruption of the lower second molar during treatment.

THE SAGITTAL II

All but identical in appearance to the Sagittal I, the Sagittal II appliance is used for expansion of the arch in the completely opposite direction. Instead of distalizing teeth posteriorly, it develops them *anteriorly*. Using the second molars as anchorage and by means of the appropriate adjustments, the Sagittal II can be used to apply labial crown torque to the anterior teeth or even be used to open up the premaxillary sutures, thereby developing the entire premaxilla as in Class II, Division 2, cases, or even pseudo-Class III situations.

The two major factors affecting the action of the appliance in the upper arch are the anchorage offered by the second molars and the adjustments of the acrylic.

The anchorage of the second molars is of itself a formidable force. But in addition to this, it complies with the gang-up concept giving eight teeth, or as many as ten if the third molars are sufficiently developed, to act against six teeth, or usually only four as the cuspids seldom, if ever, need to be pushed forward.[31] When the plate is expanded by means of the jackscrews, the pressure generated will cause the teeth to move in the direction of least resistance. Eight or ten teeth against six, or actually only four, is hardly an even contest. Especially so when one considers that the eight or ten teeth are almost all multirooted or large and the four are single-rooted and

---

Figure 4-14 Sagittal II appliance operates on the principle that it must act against first and second molars. This results in an action that is approximately 80% anterior. This is symbolized by labial flaring of dashed lines across front of the six anterior teeth.

Figure 4-15 **(A)** Premaxillary sutures may be opened in order to gain true orthopedic development of premaxillary area in Class II, Division 2 cases that require more than just labial crown torque. This is due to keeping occlusion of the lowers heavy on both anterior and posterior portions of the appliance, retention of second molars as anchorage, and placing of the "cut" of anterior portion of appliance distal to the cuspid. Only in cases where labial crown torque of anterior centrals and/or laterals alone is required may the cut be altered to mesial to the cuspid. **(B)** When developing the premaxilla forward and upward in Sagittal II technique, if a labial bow is used as part of the appliance, it must be kept clear of anterior teeth.

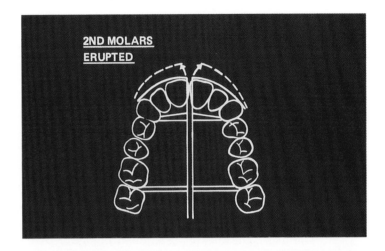

Figure 4-14

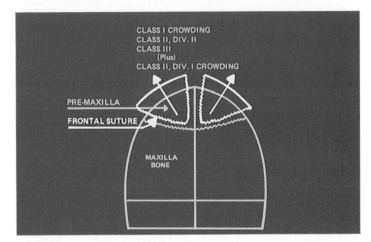

Figure 4-15(A)

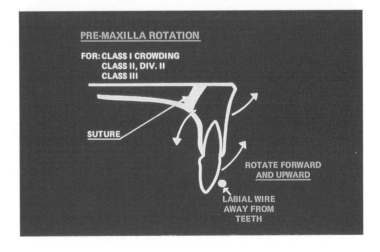

(B)

sometimes quite a bit smaller, as in the case of the upper laterals. However, it must be remembered that the anterior palate can also act as a form of anchorage. This is why it is imperative that to counter this resistance the second molars remain intact to obtain this anterior protrusive action. Otherwise, in the event of their removal, the action would be primarily distal. The status of the second molar is actually the prime factor in determining what the ultimate effect of Sagittal appliances on the arches will be.

In many Class II, Division 2 cases, the gang-up principle is intensified by the addition of the maxillary cuspids as allies to the posterior group, by means of cuspid retraction clasps. Often the cuspids in Division 2 cases are in satisfactory position, and only the laterals and/or centrals suffer from excessive lingual crown torque. In this case the cut through the anterior flange may be altered in its position so as to be placed distal to the laterals rather than distal to the cuspids as is normally done. (Cut on mesial when "mesializing" as in Sagittal II; cut on distal of cuspid when distalizing as in Sagittal I.) This makes the ratio of posterior anchorage teeth to anterior movement teeth 12 to 4, a gross mismatch! Torquing the maxillary anteriors forward to their proper interincisal angle again in such situations often is simply a matter of wearing the appliance and turning the screws every 3 or 4 days.

Adjustments

Adjusting the Sagittal II for the purpose of developing the premaxilla is an important factor in increasing the efficiency of the appliance. As with the Bionator, adjustments make the difference between a case that utilizes the full advantages of what the appliance has to give and a case where the end goal is accomplished only after a certain amount of struggle on the part of both the patient and clinician.

For labial crown torque, the appliance is adjusted so that the *posterior acrylic pads* covering the occlusal surfaces of the maxillary posteriors make *firm contact* with the lower posteriors. In addition, and this is a point of some confusion among clinicians, the *anterior bite plane* area should also make *solid contact* with the lower cuspids (or laterals if the cuspids are out of occlusion). There are several reasons for this. First, by hitting solidly on the anterior section, more force is applied to the upper anterior teeth, increasing the efficiency of the appliance. Secondly, as the appliance expands, a certain amount of flexion occurs across the open space of the screws reducing the force this anterior section of the plate can produce in the premaxilla. Firm contact by the lower cuspids helps compensate for this factor and drives the acrylic to place against the resisting lingual surfaces of the upper teeth. Some practitioners feel the appliance should have firm contact in the posterior area for anchorage and only light contact in the anterior bite plane area (the complete opposite of the Saggittal I). This is not so much incorrect as it is merely inefficient. They feel, possibly, that the firm contact in the anterior area also would only cause some distalization of the posterior segments as with the Sagittal I. However, this is quite unlikely due to the simple fact that the second molars are still in place and contribute to the gang-up principle preventing any appreciable distalization. This, combined with the extra anchorage provided by the firm contact of the lower posteriors on the acrylic occlusal pads, makes for expansion to the front the only feasible result. Nature always takes the easy way out.

Also, firm contact on the anterior as well as posterior part of the plate is more efficient because it helps combat the phenomenon of the front edge of the anterior bite plate section from "walking out" from under the incisal edges of the upper anteriors. This effect is observed when the appliance is opened faster than the teeth or bones can keep up or if insufficient pressure is being applied by the anterior section of the plate to move the teeth. The same observation is made when the patient turns the expansion screws at regular intervals but fails to wear the appliance for an adequate amount of time each day. Even with firm contact on the anterior part and correct wearing and opening sequences, a certain amount of this may take place, requiring reduction of the edge of acrylic that protrudes past the incisal edges of the upper anterior teeth for the sake of esthetics. If contact from the lowers is only light in this area, the chances of the palatal section's anterior edge walking out from under the front teeth are increased and the treatment time will only be unnecessarily lengthened.

Another adjustment that must be made to effect correct labial crown torque to the upper centrals and laterals is to reduce the acrylic adjacent to the lingual surface of the palate behind the roots of the teeth being torqued forward. This procedure must be carried out approximately once every 3 to 4 weeks at the regular checking appointment. As the anterior section of the plate advances with the opening of the expansion screws, the plate must be steadily reduced behind the palatal gingivae of the teeth being moved so as to only contact the lingual surfaces of the teeth concerned at the cingulum area. The acrylic must be adjusted clear up to what would be the apex area of the roots of the teeth being torqued labially. This allows for proper torquing of the crowns of the teeth labially without causing the palatal acrylic to hang up as a result of contact with the palatal tissues and rugae. It also helps prevent the aforementioned walking-out phenomenon.

With the combined action of firm contact on both anterior and posterior bite planes and the reduction of acrylic behind the roots of the teeth being moved, controlled and effective positioning of the teeth can be carried out. If one tooth requires more individualized movement, the acrylic may be reduced or increased in the cingulum area of that particular tooth to either retard or increase its movement as is needed. A labial bow may also be added to provide an extra source of force from the labial to help control individual tooth movements, such as rotations, more effectively.

In cases where the laterals are blocked forward and already sufficiently labially torqued but the centrals only are retroclined, lateral retraction clasps may be added to hold them firmly while the centrals are moved forward. Of course, the acrylic abutting the lingual surfaces of the laterals must be reduced to remain free and clear of contact as the plate is expanded.

240 240   The Sagittal Appliance

When total premaxillary development is required, the occlusal adjustments are the same except that the acrylic is *not* reduced on the palatal and rugae areas so as to maintain firm contact across the entire soft tissue surface. This complete surface area contact is useful for opening up the premaxillary sutures to push the premaxilla up and forward when necessary. If both actions are required, labial crown torque and premaxillary rotation, the latter may be accomplished until the orthopedic development is adequate, and then after adjusting the acrylic behind the teeth, the same appliance is put to continued use to torque the teeth alone even farther labially.

Since opening the premaxillary sutures for the purposes of orthopedic development provides a great increase in resistance, more time is required between turning of the expansion screws. The screws should be turned only once every five to seven days. This allows the appliance more time to do the increased work required to perform this action. This is another reason solid contact on the anterior bite plane by the lower cuspids and/or anteriors is important.

In cases where the premaxillary immaturity is severe, as in a pseudo-Class III situation, the anterior bite plane may be extended over the incisal edges of the upper anterior teeth to aid in jumping the bite if any anterior crossbite situation exists.

Lower Sagittals operate on the same principle as the uppers except there are no adjustments required during expansion, and the direction of the expansion is solely dependent on the status of the second molars. Usually lower Sagittals are used only to distalize posterior segments after second molar removal. Since there are no acrylic pads covering the occlusal surface, the only adjustments needed during treatment are the turning of the expansion screws and an occasional tightening of the clasps. Occasionally, a sore spot will appear under the acrylic on the lingual gingivae. Simple adjustment with acrylic burs is all that is necessary to alleviate the problem.

Figure 4-16 In proper Sagittal II technique, occlusion (indicated by markings left by articulating paper) is kept heavy on both anterior and posterior portions of plate.

Figure 4-17 Reduction of palatal portion of appliance on tissue side in rugae area allows forces of expansion to be delivered solely to lingual surfaces of anteriors. This results in labial crown torque (tipping) without any orthopedic development. Note unilateral stabilization wire designed to prevent further advancement of maxillary left lateral. Acrylic lingual to this tooth would then be reduced by corresponding amount. When both laterals are to be restrained, wires are used bilaterally.

Figure 4-18 Class III Sagittal appliance. Note anterior bite cap protrudes fully past incisal edges of upper anterior teeth to aid in "unlocking" anteriors and facilitate jumping the bite forward past the lowers.

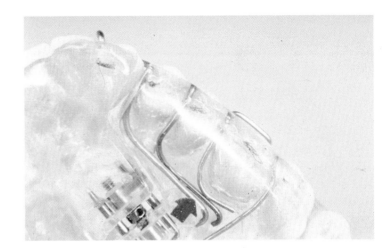

Figure 4-16

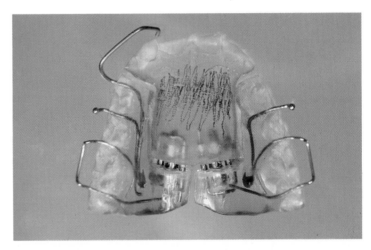

Figure 4-17

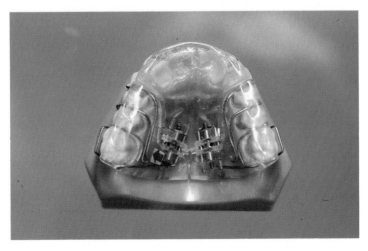

Figure 4-18

CLASS III SAGITTAL APPLIANCE

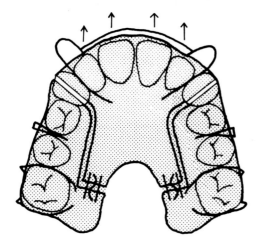

The anterior bite plane should extend slightly forward of the upper incisors, so as to contact the lower incisors in bite occlusion.

This is an excellent appliance for Pseudo Class III cases with a reverse overbite.

Do not treat an open bite skeletal Class III case with this appliance.

SCHEU #714 SCREWS

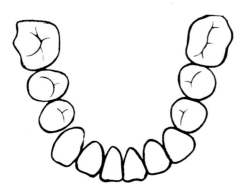

Figure 4-19 Class III Sagittal appliance.

Figure 4-20 **(A)** Clasps for cuspids on upper Sagittals act to stabilize plate and may be used to "tease" cuspid down into proper position once space has been created for it. **(B)** Adjusting cuspid clasp with three-pronged plier. **(C)** Adjusting Adams clasp with three-pronged plier across the horizontal bar to bend peaks into interproximal undercut. Wire may also be bent as it exits the acrylic to roll entire clasp assembly into the interproximal spaces.

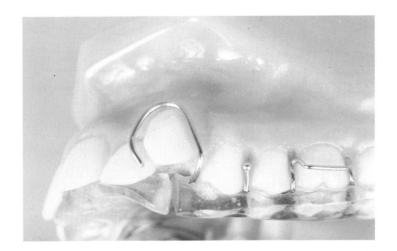

(A)

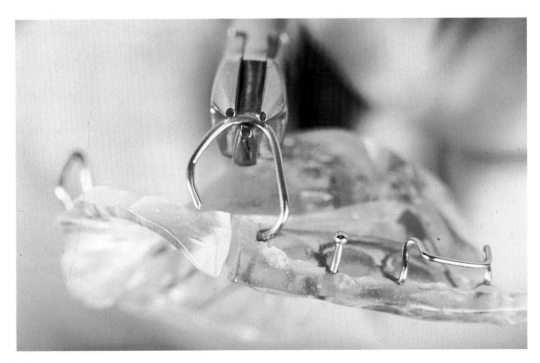

(B)

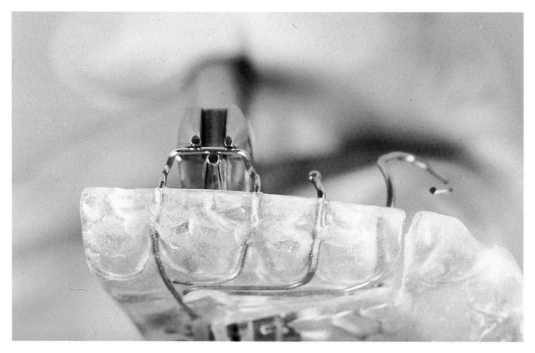

(C)

Clasps

There are two basic ways of tightening the Adams clasps on these appliances to increase the retention. One is to place the middle prong of a three-prong pliers inside the horizontal bar of the clasp coming from the lingual, with the other two prongs coming from the buccal, and to crimp the horizontal bar slightly so it is bowed out to the buccal. This will cause the peaks of the bends at the mesial and distal of the Adams clasp to toe-in more toward the undercut of the crown. If there is insufficient "bell shape" to the crown so that there is very little undercut area, a second method is to use a fine-nosed pliers to grip the clasp wire as it exits from the acrylic and, holding the appliance firmly, gently bend the wire a very slight amount in an arch to the interproximal. This places the peaks of the bends in a deeper position in the interproximal spaces as the horizontal bar and peaks of the clasp are rolled gingivally. Care must be exercised so as not to "roll" the clasp into the interproximal areas too deeply, as tissue irritation and soreness will result. However, this technique requires that the wire exit the acrylic at a steep enough angle such that the acrylic will be thick enough to prevent splitting as the clasp wire is torqued upward from the occlusal surface.

Construction Bite

Warm the special pink base-plate wax in a water bath of 140°F and roll or fold the sheet until it is of sufficient shape and thickness so as to fit nicely over the posterior segments at a thickness of at least 6 to 10 mm. The wax block should be free of the anterior teeth and be inserted and pressed into place against the maxillary posteriors. Then the patient should be instructed to slowly close into his normal habitual bite until there is a space of about 1.5 to 2 mm between the occlusal surfaces of the posterior teeth. Remove the wax bite and cool so that it is firm enough to be trimmed. Trim off the excess wax at the occlusobuccal edge of the imprints and reinsert into the mouth so that the accuracy and thickness may be checked. If satisfactory, double-check against an accurate set of models that will be used for appliance construction. Send upper and lower models to the laboratory along with the wax bite for appliance construction.

Treatment Time Line

The length of time required for correction of crowding or lingual inclination of anterior teeth, or the opening of upper premaxillary sutures depends on the severity of the problem, patient age, cooperation, etc. But generally these appliances work rather quickly and a 6- to 7-month treatment time is common. In cases requiring double appliance therapy, upper and lower, the maxilla usually proceeds more rapidly than the mandible. This is most likely due to the differences in bone densities. Cases requiring two appliances for the same arch will naturally take longer. Periodic routine checking appointments determine the point at which the treatment is sufficient. In cases where the premaxilla is expanded forward or the upper anteriors torqued labially, as always, overcorrect slightly. This often takes the form of several millimeters past desired end position. If spaces open up, they may easily be closed when the second phase of treatment is initiated, ie, Bionator for Class II cases.

In Sagittal I technique retention of the posterior segments is unnecessary, as once the teeth have been distalized after the extraction of the

---

Figure 4-21 Case study of Sagittal II technique. Pseudo-Class III case that was corrected by a combination of Sagittal II and then unilateral Sagittal I techniques. **(A) (B) (C)** Initial pretreatment pseudo-Class III bite relationship of maxillary anteriors and slightly anteriorly positioned upper-right cuspid, and severely blocked out upper-left cuspid. **(D)** Insertion of first Sagittal II appliance (maxillary second molars remain in place). Occlusion is checked and kept balanced and heavy on both anterior and posterior bite plates of appliance as per dictates of correct Sagittal II technique. **(E)** Appliance after expansion of plate. **(F)** Maxillary arch after treatment with first Sagittal appliance. Note maxillary left lateral and cuspid are still short of arch length and remain slightly crowded. Also, slight over-correction of maxillary anteriors past their present position is desirable. Hence, maxillary left second molar was removed and with maxillary right second molar in place for anchorage to help with the gain of a slight anterior over-correction to the six anteriors, a second Sagittal appliance **(G)** was constructed with cuspid retraction wires bilaterally. **(H)** Upon activation of second appliance, upper-left posterior quadrant is distalized to gain remaining space for maxillary left cuspid and lateral. Upper-right posterior quadrant remains in place due to reinforcing anchorage provided by remaining maxillary right second molar. As right-side screw is expanded, anteriors are pushed slightly farther forward. Once the upper-left quadrant is adequately distalized, cuspid retraction wires are activated to apply gentle pressure to their mesial and labial surfaces to assist in their proper retrieval into correct position in the arch. **(I)** Maxillary arch after second Sagittal appliance. Note distalized upper-left quadrant (maxillary left second molar extracted) and over-correction of six anteriors labially. Lip pressure plus natural relapse forces will settle these teeth back to proper overjet relationships to lower anteriors. **(J)** As they settle they may be aided into proper tooth position with simple Straight Wire technique. (Bracket on maxillary right lateral incisor had "popped off" prior to taking this photograph. It was removed from archwire for this photo and then replaced to complete the case.) **(K)** Retainer placed to aid in stabilizing teeth. **(L)** Final posttreatment correction of case. Note correct maxillary arch form (with retainer in place).

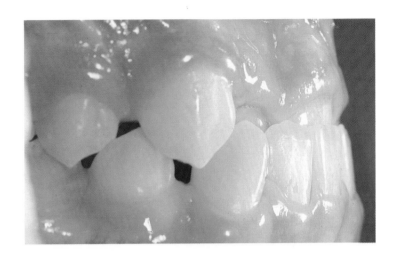

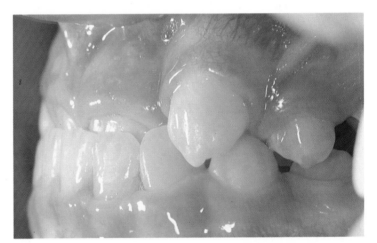

(A)

(B)

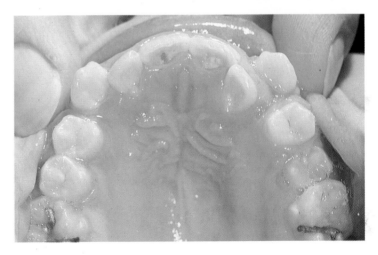

(C)

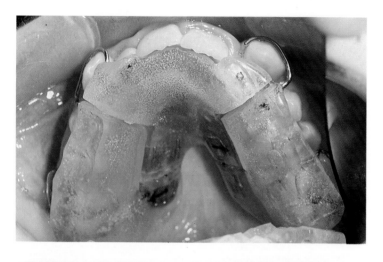

(D)

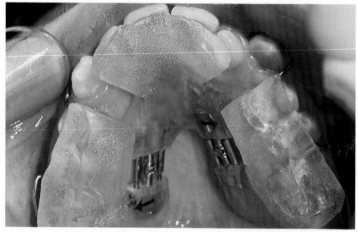

(E)

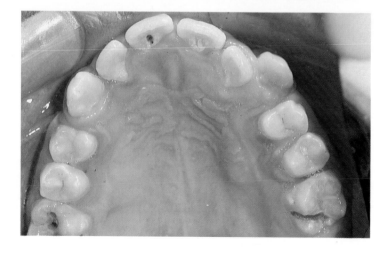

(F)

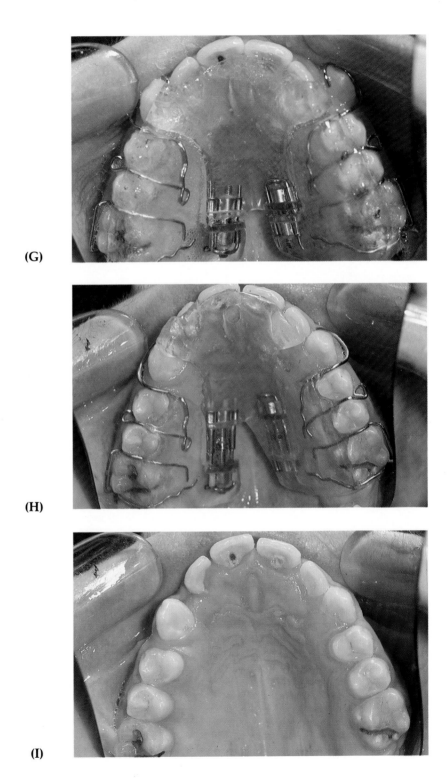

(G)

(H)

(I)

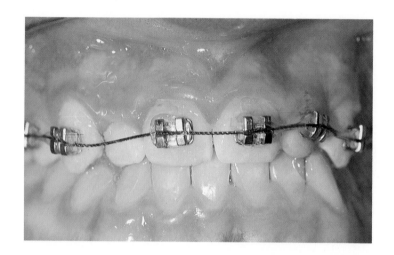

(J)

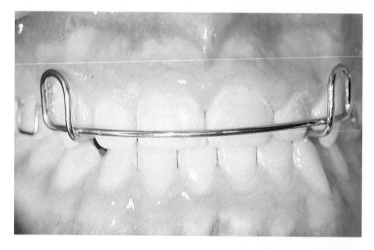

(K)

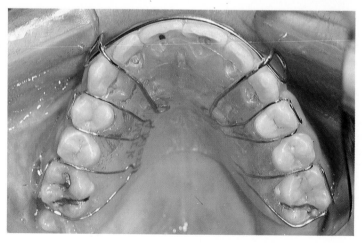

(L)

second molars, they almost always stay put. Again, Sagittal expansion distally is always more stable than lateral expansion.

However, this is not always true of Sagittal II technique. One area of concern should be in the adequate retention of the anterior development of the premaxilla and anterior teeth in severe Class II, Division 2, cases. Once expansion to the correct arch form and proper crown torque is achieved in an anterior direction, retention for a period of time, at least half the treatment time or longer, is advisable. The appliance acts as its own retainer, but simpler, thinner Hawley types may also be used. If retrogression of the upper anteriors back to their former Division II angulation appears to be taking place, the appliance may be closed a little until it fits snugly once again and reinserted to push the regressing anteriors back out again. This regaining of lost anterior development will occur much more rapidly the second time. Follow this by longer and more active periods of retention.

"You must look where it is not,
as well as where it is."

Gnomologia, 1732
T. Fuller, Editor

INDICATIONS FOR USE

It is of utmost importance for the clinician to understand when the use of the Sagittal appliance is indicated. Not every case of arch crowding is an indication for either developing premaxillas forward or distalizing posterior segments backward. The key to determining when such appliances are best utilized is through the use of the various model analysis systems available as an aid to diagnosis.

The word "sagittal" is derived from the original Latin root *sagitta* which means "arrow." It is also the etymological basis for the name of the southern constellation Sagittarius, "the Archer," the ninth sign of the Zodiac. It must be remembered that, like an arrow, the Sagittal appliance is designed primarily for front-to-back expansion of the dental arch in a linear direction. This implies that if it is used to correct a narrow, short arch of crowded teeth, the end result will be a narrow, longer arch of uncrowded teeth. True, as posterior segments are distalized, they occupy a spot at a wider portion of the arch; but this lateral component of arch width gain is slight and only in the most posterior area around the first molars. In the bicuspid area, this effect is very near nonexistent. Even if the expansion screws are offset at an angle instead of their usual setting parallel to the midsagittal plane, simple geometry shows the lateral component of expansion is to be very slight compared to that of the distal (a direct function of the sine of the angle the long axis of the screw is offset from the linear sagittal plane). Regardless of efforts to modify its action, a Sagittal's development is still primarily anteroposterior.

This will serve well if proper diagnosis indicates the need for this type of development. But it must be ascertained ahead of time that sufficient arch width exists to allow anteroposterior development only. If such methods as the Schwarz or Pont's analysis systems (discussed later) indicate a need for lateral development, the appropriate appliances (also discussed later) should be utilized for this purpose *first* before eliciting the services of the Sagittal. But once this lateral dimension has been developed therapeutically, or if it exists naturally prior to treatment, and there still exists either anterior premaxillary insufficiency or crowding of the posterior segments forward with blocked-out cuspids, the Sagittal appliance is indicated.

The first and most obvious indication for a Sagittal appliance is the classic Class II, Division 2, malocclusion. This particular condition takes precedence over any other as far as selecting the Sagittal as an initial appliance, even in the face of arch width insufficiencies, for one simple and very important reason: the preservation and protection of the temporomandibular joint. It is a rare case where a moderate to severe Class II, Division 2, malocclusion does not imply a compressed or strained temporomandibular joint. As described earlier, anything that causes the condyle of the mandible to ride up off the posterior limit of the disc onto the bilaminar zone is potentially harmful to the joint. Anything that causes the muscles of the mastication to overwork in an inefficient manner, or in a condition of unstable or poor biomechanical advantage can, if severe enough, result in pain, deformity, and degeneration of the musculoskeletal complex of this anatomical region. Class II, Division 2, malocclusions with concomitant deep overbite and loss of vertical run an extremely high risk of such conditions arising.[32] The more severe the Division 2 tendency, the higher the risk of joint involvement. Some clinicians refer to this type of malocclusion as "untreatable," meaning that premaxillary development with a Sagittal II to correct the Division II angulation, thus unlocking the mandible, is the only way to successfully alter the case to a point where it is amenable to other forms of therapy. The other methods commonly used in orthodontics such as bicuspid extraction techniques applied to this type of case are merely a means of courting disaster in the form of almost certain posttreatment temporomandibular joint involvement.

The Sagittal II, used to treat Class II, Division 2, cases not only develops the premaxilla forward, allowing the trapped mandible to grow down and forward, but also acts as a TMJ splint to instantly increase the vertical and free up the condylar fossa articulation, thus immediately decompressing the joint. This allows the mandible to resume its normal growth rate which, up until the time of the insertion of the appliance, has been retarded due to the locking of the lower incisors behind the retroclined upper incisors upon closure. This "splinting effect" will often relieve relatively quickly some of the symptoms of headache-type pain and discomfort associated with Class II, Division 2, deep bite cases. Mandibles that are "unlocked" by such treatment often quickly resume normal growth rates in the growing child and often assume an accelerated growth rate![33]

Cephalometric analysis will divulge whether the premaxillary sutures should be developed forward followed by labial crown torque or whether labial crown torque alone is sufficient to correct the problem. This, of course, determines the appropriate type of appliance adjustments to be used.

VERTICAL MOVEMENTS OF THE PREMAXILLA WITH THE SAGITTAL APPLIANCE

There are occasions when the premaxillary orthopedic development of a given individual may be excessive in the vertical plane. This would result in a smile line where all of the clinical crowns of the maxillary teeth are revealed upon smiling along with a substantial portion of the attached gingivae. This excessive premaxillary vertical development is often referred to as the "gummy smile" effect. Some clinicians such as Dr James Evans of Rapid City, South Dakota, have developed a technique as an adjunct to Sagittal appliance usage that they feel corrects this condition to some degree. At the conclusion of Sagittal appliance active treatment, while the patient is wearing the appliance in the retentive phase to allow for functional uprighting of the roots, the appliance may be adjusted such that the anterior portion of the plate receives maximum contact from the lower incisors. The posterior segments are reduced on their occlusal surfaces so that the acrylic of this portion of the plate barely touches the lower posterior teeth, if at all. This imparts the maximum amount of the forces of occlusion on the anterior mushroom-shaped middle section of the plate, which in turn imparts these vertically directed forces to the premaxillary bone section itself. With heavy function, persistent wear, and periodic reduction of the posterior occlusal acrylic to keep the upward forces at their maximum, it is felt that in the growing child, such circumstances generate enough force to disengage

Case Study Illustrations—Following Pages

Figure 4-22   Case study of combined Sagittal I and Sagittal II technique. Class II, Division 2 case of extreme anteroposterior arch length loss completely corrected by combined Sagittal II/Sagittal I technique without the aid of any other type of appliance! Initially, due to premature loss of all four deciduous cuspids, there was severe A-P arch length loss with only 2 mm remaining for each permanent cuspid. Deep overbite locked the occlusion in skeletal Class II mandibular retrusion. First, an upper Sagittal II appliance was inserted to develop the upper Division 2 anteriors forward. Then, both upper and lower Sagittal II appliances were used. After their employment, all four second molars were removed and the case was allowed to correct spontaneously for one year, during which each cuspid gained an additional 3 mm on average. This is done so the next set of Sagittal I appliances

Figure 4-22 continued

would not have to work so hard. After a year, extraction sites have healed to the point where subsequent Sagittal appliance therapy produces A-P development in about a 50/50 ratio front to back.

(A) (B) (C) Pretreatment appearance of arches intraorally. Note extremely small space remaining for each permanent cuspid.

(D) (E) (F) During treatment with first Sagittal II appliance, maxillary permanent cuspids erupt. **(G)** Note that occlusion is kept heavy on both anterior and posterior bite plate portions of the plate as is desirable with proper Sagittal II technique. **(H)** After full expansion of first Sagittal II appliance expansion screws, open spaces may be filled in with quick-cure acrylic to prevent back turning of screws and to also strengthen appliance. Appliance is worn in this manner as its own retainer to prevent lingual relapse of labially torqued anterior teeth.

(I) Maxillary arch after initial period of Sagittal II development. Note that this is after use of second upper Sagittal II appliance. During its use, a lower Sagittal II was also employed. Important: the maxillary anteriors are expected to rebound from this over-corrected position to their proper position in the arch, and when they do, there will be a slight increase in crowding because posterior quadrants themselves are still in their pretreatment forward position as evidenced by initial severity of pretreatment crowding. Therefore, at this point all four second molars are removed in first steps of converting the case to Sagittal I technique to distalize these posterior quadrants. **(J)** Occlusal views of freshly inserted new upper Sagittal I appliance. **(K)** Labially displaced cuspids being "teased" into place with cuspid retraction wires. **(L)** Mandibular arch upon insertion of last Sagittal I appliance. **(M)** Maxillary appliance after expansion increasing A-P arch length further. Note broken portion of left front side of bite plate. **(N)** Appearance of maxillary and mandibular arches after posterior quadrants have been slightly distalized and anteriors slightly mesialized (50/50 due to healed sockets of extracted second molars) creating enough room to bring cuspids into place. **(O)** Lower appliance in mandibular arch effecting slight overcorrection. (This required two lower appliances.)

(P) (Q) (R) (S) Final appearance of maxillary and mandibular arches before and after eruption of third molars into perfect position behind firsts. **(T) (U) (V)** Coalescence (settling in) of over-expansion of arches into proper position of final Class I interdigitation. Notice that all bicuspids are present! Increased mandibular growth made possible naturally by unlocking of the restraining and interfering Class II, Division 2 deep bite. **(W) (X) (Y)** Before and after facial appearance of patient. Notice improved facial profile due to correct, advanced mandibular position. Mandible grew naturally to correct position once occlusion was "unlockd." This is one of reasons why Sagittal is considered true orthopedic appliance. To repeat, no other appliances were used; entire case completed with Sagittal II/Sagittal I overcorrection and second molar replacement techniques. "Nice going!" to all involved.

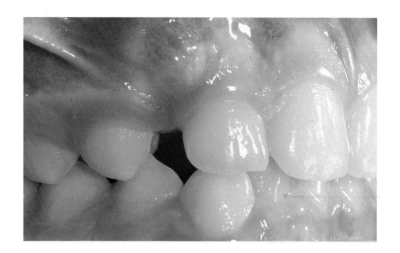

(A)

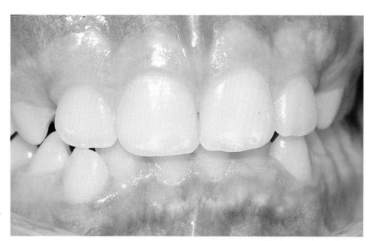

(B)

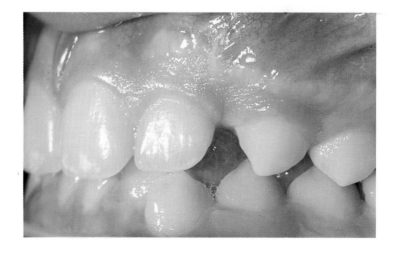

(C)

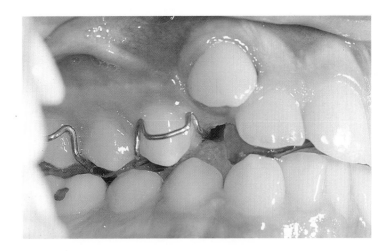

(D)

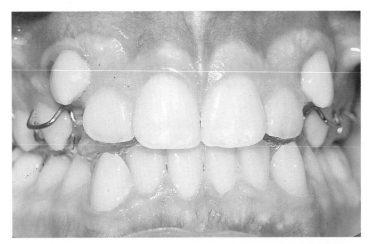

(E)

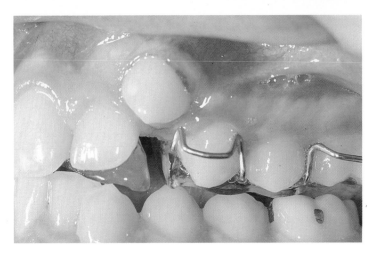

(F)

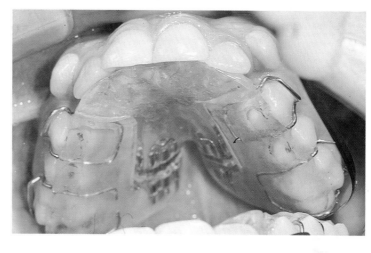

(G)

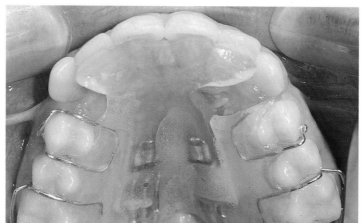

(H)

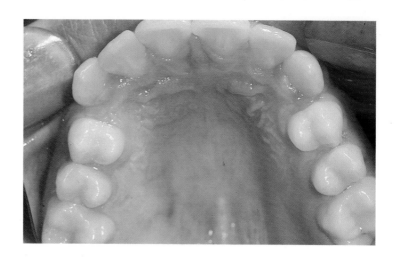

(I)

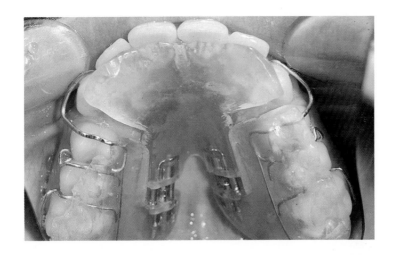

(J)

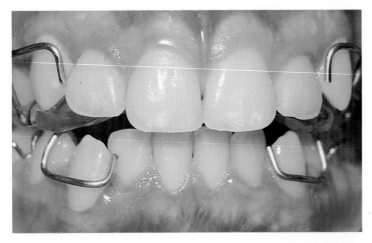

(K)

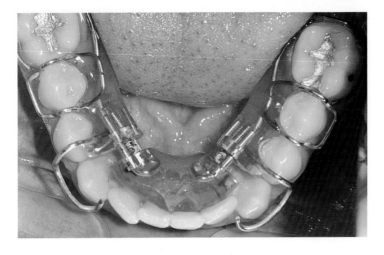

(L)

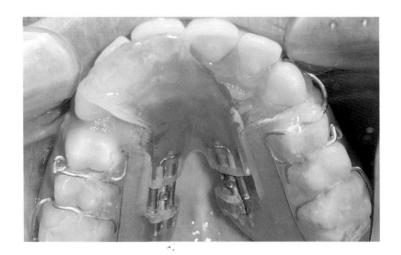

(M)

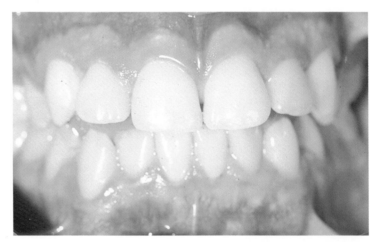

(N)

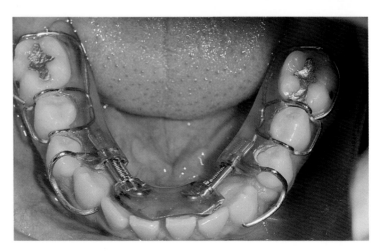

(O)

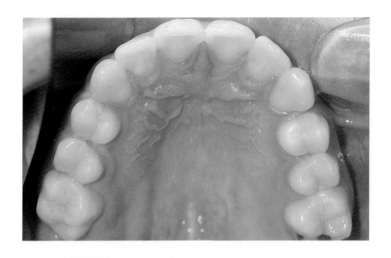

(P)

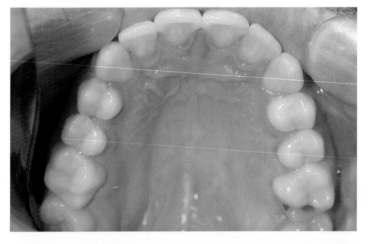

(Q)

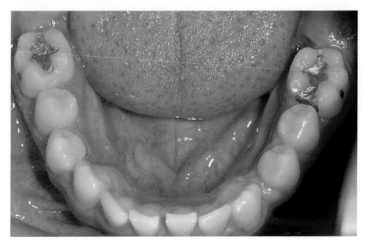

(R)

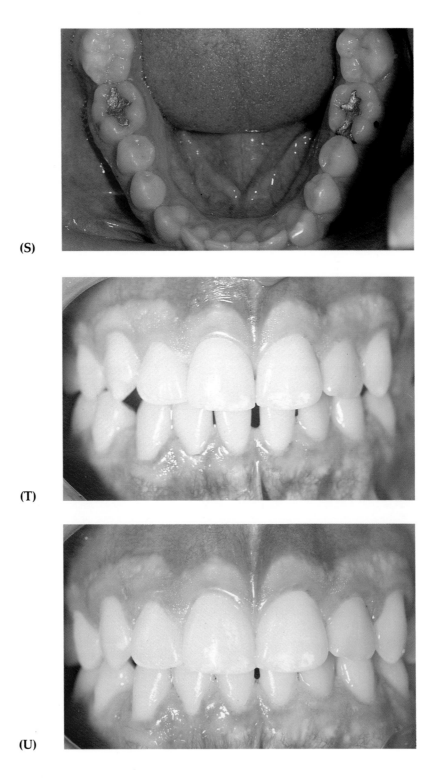

(S)

(T)

(U)

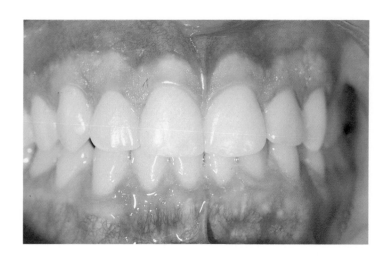

(V)

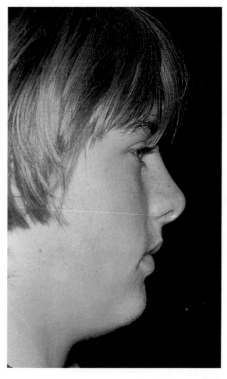

(W)

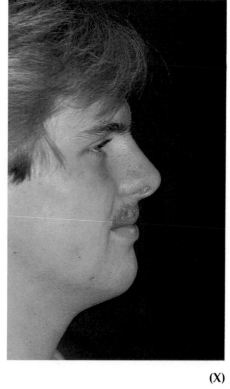

(X)

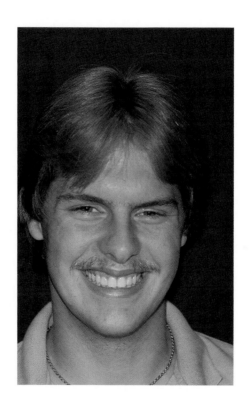

(Y)

the entire premaxilla along its suture lines and drive it superiorly as a whole. There may also be some slight intrusion of the anterior teeth, but this is speculative.

Whether the premaxilla is actually intruded, or merely held vertically stable while the rest of the growing face and maxillofacial complex grows and develops down and around it, or both, is also subject to speculation. This technique is not recommended for cases of severe premaxillary osteogenic hyperplasia or cases where the ANS-PNS palatal plane is canted severely downward. These types of exaggerated problems are amenable only to surgery.

SYMMETROSCOPE

As stated previously, once the arch width has been determined to be adequate by means of one model analysis method or another, and crowding still exists in Class I or Class II, Division 1, cases, the Sagittal I may be called upon to treat the case. But that brings up the question of arch symmetry. We are confining ourselves, for now, to symmetry in an anteroposterior direction. One posterior quadrant may be crowded farther forward than the other and require more distalization than the other. A simple and straightforward way of detecting this is by means of the use of a symmetroscope.

The symmetroscope is nothing more than an acrylic grid with lines demarking millimeter increments. It is placed over a model of the dental arch on a line directly over the midline of the arch (the midpalatal suture of the maxilla). By aligning the midline of the grid with the midline of the model and a baseline perpendicular to one of the first molars, a simple and relatively accurate approximation of the number of millimeters of relative advancement of one side of the arch over the other is obtained. Actually, what we in America refer to as a symmetroscope is not a true symmetroscope at all. Its correct name is an "orthodontic cross," (sounds like another form of constellation that should appear in the Southern sky). The actual symmetroscopes were designed in Europe during the late 1930s and early 1940s by men like Phillips, Korkhaus, and Schwarz.[34] The orthodontic cross is of European lineage also, having been developed by Kantorowitz and improved by Korkhaus. But the term "symmetroscope," signifying the little plastic grid,

---

Figure 4-23 **(A)** Symmetroscope. Sometimes referred to as an "orthodontic cross," symmetroscope can be used to determine relative anteroposterior movements of adjacent posterior quadrants. In this example, note how horizontal line touches mesial of upper-left first molar, yet with vertical lines parallel to mid-palatal suture, the upper-right first molar (and as a result the entire posterior segment) is drifted forward. They may have **(A)** either 10 mm grid demarcations only or **(B)** 1 mm grid demarcations in addition. (*Courtesy of Johns Dental Laboratories, Terra Haute, IN.*)

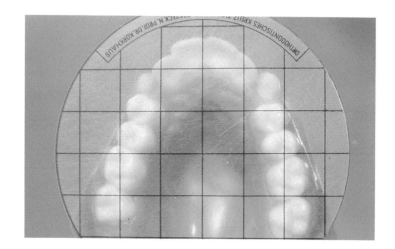

(A)

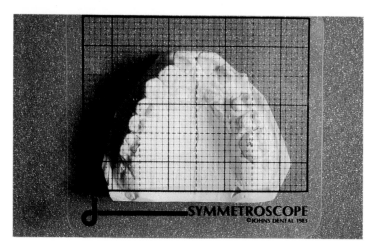

(B)

is so entrenched in the daily usage of American orthodontics that it seems it is here to stay.

Of course, the primary advantage of the symmetroscope comes into play when the arches are asymmetrical in an anteroposterior direction. Should the anterior teeth occupy a correct cephalometric position, but both posterior segments be crowded forward blocking out the cuspids equally on both sides, the symmetroscope may still be used to give an approximation of the amount of distalization necessary to correct the crowding. By again placing the grid over the model with the center line parallel to the midpalatal suture, align the baseline perpendicular to the tip of the cuspid rugae. These rugae ideally should bisect the lingual surface of the maxillary cuspids and may be used as a general guide to the correct position of the tooth in the maxillary arch. After alignment, check the number of millimeters forward of the baseline perpendicular that the tip of the cuspid crown sets. This will give a reasonable approximation of the distance the posterior segment must be distalized. Of course, if the cuspid is rotated besides, additional arch length will be needed as rotated teeth in the anterior segment give up space. Additional space will also be needed if one of the bicuspids is blocked out or in, labially or lingually. When the number of millimeters of distance needed is estimated in this way, it gives the clinician a rough idea of the amount of time necessary for completion of the movement. This, of course, is also a function of patient age, cooperation, screw-turning frequency, etc.

CAREY ANALYSIS

Another method of determining arch length discrepancy is by means of a Carey analysis.[35] This method consists of measuring the linear distance from the mesial of the first molar on one side of the arch to the mesial of the first molar on the other side of the arch. This measurement, SA, is then subtracted from the summation of all the mesiodistal widths of all the teeth in the arch, ST, the four bicuspids, two cuspids, and four incisors. The difference is the extra arch length needed to round out the crowded arch. Thus SA − ST = D equals the arch length discrepancy. A fine jewelry chain, the type used for women's necklaces, works well in this method for measuring a model of the arch from the mesial of one first molar around to the mesial of the opposite first molar. If a tooth is unerupted, measurements may be approximated from an x-ray film or the following chart of statistical average mesial/distal widths of teeth.

	Upper Width	Lower Width
Central incisor	8.5 mm	5.3 mm
Lateral incisor	6.6 mm	5.9 mm
Cuspid	7.8 mm	6.6 mm
First bicuspid	6.9 mm	7.0 mm
Second bicuspid	6.6 mm	7.0 mm

Once the value of D is calculated, a ratio must be computed between it and the two posterior segments, as seldom, if ever, can all the arch length discrepancy be made up by simply distalizing one segment unilaterally. Also, one must consider whether it is not actually the anterior premaxilla that is at fault. If so, one would be remiss to extract second molars and use a Sagittal I to gain space by distal-driving when the posterior segments are only partially to blame or completely unresponsible for the discrepancy. One must determine if the action should be Sagittal I totally (posterior), Sagittal II totally (anterior), or a combination of both. This is done cephalometrically and by direct clinical observation.

If a combination of treatment is desired, then the Sagittal II technique *must* be used first, as this employs the use of intact second molars as anchorage against which the appliance can brace itself to push the premaxilla and/or maxillary anterior teeth forward. Then, when proper premaxillary development is secure and stable, one may extract the second molars and convert the Sagittal II to a Sagittal I by means of the appropriate adjustments and start to distalize the posterior segments to obtain the desired effect. If the first appliance has been opened an appreciable amount, one might be better off using it as a retainer while a new Sagittal is constructed on fresh models of the mouth in its present expanded condition. This is usually the case in arches needing both types of appliances.

If only a Sagittal I is required to relieve the crowding and gain arch length, the question is then posed, "What do you do with the value D obtained from the Carey analysis?" The discrepancy only acts as a guide to correction, but it may not always be simply divided in half with each segment being expected to be distalized a distance represented by D/2. The arch may be collapsed asymmetrically. This problem is solved once again with the use of the symmetroscope. Direct clinical observation during treatment is the ultimate determinant of when the expansion is adequate, but having the case properly analyzed prior to treatment will make things much more predictable and secure in the clinician's mind. This analytical preparation in turn reflects itself in a positive attitude that the patient can sense and makes for easier acceptance of the various facets of wearing the appliance. Forewarned is truly forearmed. Proper symmetrical arch form is the ultimate goal. The appliance is merely activated front to back, one side to the other, until it is obtained.

In the event one segment requires more distalization than another, the plate is eventually expanded unevenly. When the shorter segment's distalization is complete, the screw may be tied to its reinforcing rods through the holes in the central rotating cylinder to prevent back-turning. This mechanical action may happen on occasion as the pressures generated on the appliance during use are great enough to force the expansion screws to close on themselves. Tying the screw with a piece of brass separating wire or wire ligature is a handy way to prevent this unwanted action. This acts to retain and preserve the space gained through the action of that particular segment of the plate while the other segment is still being distalized. It is best to avoid filling in the opened screw area with quick-cure acrylic until one is certain expansion on that side is complete, as this prevents ever using the screw again should more expansion be desired.

In the lower dentition the same diagnostic rules apply. If crowding exists, first and foremost the clinician should check the arch for width discrepancies. If these also exist, they should be treated first, as on the upper arch, with the appropriate appliances. Only then should the arch-lengthening appliances be called upon to finish. This is due to the commonly observed fact that lateral development is always much more prone to relapse than anteroposterior development. Thus the Sagittal appliance acts as a retainer to hold the newfound lateral development while it is going about its business of expanding front to back.

In the event a lower Sagittal appliance is indicated, it will operate on the same principle as the uppers. The status of the second molars indicates the direction the expansion will take once the appliance is activated. The appliance will *distalize* posterior segments, first molar and all, right through the alveolar bone of the mandible without "dumping" the lower anteriors forward, provided the second molars have been removed. If they are intact, the main thrust will be in an *anterior* direction. This would result in labial crown torque being exerted on the mandibular incisors. Again, the expansion screws on the lower appliances are half the size of those on the uppers with threads half as big. Therefore, they must be turned twice as often to effect the same linear distance of expansion.

As appearance goes, lower Sagittal appliances look like modified Schwarz plates (discussed in a later chapter) with the screws in the lingual side plates rather than at the lingual midline area. Like the Schwarz plate, lower Sagittals have no occlusal coverings of acrylic. In the lower arch they are merely redundant and unnecessary.

For the purpose of clarity in communication, lower Sagittal appliances may be named in an identical manner to the upper Sagittals, ie, Sagittal I to distalize posterior segments and Sagittal II to develop the lower anterior arch forward. Actually the nomenclature is quite simple and very logical. The names Sagittal I and II imply the number of molars erupted and present and therefore the ultimate direction of expansion: one (I) molar present equals posterior movement of bicuspids and molars; two (II) molars present equals anterior movement of incisors.

In the rare case of retroclined lower anteriors requiring a Sagittal II to flare them forward, several factors must be considered. First, these types of arches are usually a result of being forced into such a circumstance by severely retroclined upper anteriors as in a severe Class II, Division 2, deep overbite case. These cases indicate that hyperactivity of the orbicularis and mentalis is quite likely. Should the treating clinician suspect such hyperactivity of the muscles, especially the mentalis, the action of Frankel pads may be of some use to retrain the muscles during treatment. These small acrylic pads fit down into the labial vestibule and are attached to the main body of the appliance by means of wires crossing over from the lingual acrylic. These pads must be carefully checked at regular intervals to avoid sore spots and insure proper function.

*"But soft compassion melts my soul to save
a youth so blooming with a mind so brave."*

From the *"Shah Namah" of Firdausi*
(AD 932–1020)
Persian National Epic Poem

Mixed Dentition Usage

In all the areas of orthodontics, no field is more critical to the patient or more satisfying to the clinician than that of interceptive orthodontics in the mixed dentition stage. It is at this time in the child's development that the judicious use of proper preventive and corrective orthodontics may avoid more serious and extensive treatment later on. One instance is the use of a modified Sagittal appliance to regain lost leeway space of Nance.

In the event a deciduous first and/or second molar are lost prematurely with resultant first permanent molar impingement on the leeway space,[36-47] a simple modified Sagittal may be inserted to distal-drive the first permanent molar. The permanent second molar may be left intact. It will usually offer little resistance, as it is developing distal enough and inferior enough to the first molar in the younger patient so as not to act as a deterrent to posterior movement. X-ray examination of the location of the second molar will usually divulge a space behind the first molar into which it may be moved by the distalizing effect of the appliance. Usually the distance required is not great. Once it is obtained, simple space maintainers of the common band/loop variety may be inserted to hold the space.

The appearance of the little appliances used for this purpose varies somewhat from those used in the adult dentition. The lowers are the same, but the uppers look like the Schwarz plates of old with the occlusal coverings missing and the screw running in an anteroposterior direction rather than a transverse direction, as is usually associated with Schwarz plates. Commonly these plates are unilateral as the case dictates. The reason the occlusal bite plates are often not used is that due to the "softness" of the bone in the young growing patient, the first molars may be distalized with relative ease. However, if the patient is suffering from TMJ complaints, chronic headaches, or muscle soreness due to a coexisting deep bite, the occlusal bite plates may be used to help open the vertical and decompress the joint. This action is only due to the "splinting effect" of the interocclusal acrylic and not due to any orthodontic effect of bite opening or mandibular advancement as with a Bionator.

There are clinicians who reside in both camps relative to the occlusal pads. One side says they are necessary to prevent occlusal interferences from inhibiting the movement of the tooth. The other side says they are unnecessary. The individual circumstances of each case should determine whether or not they are used. If the child complains of headaches or any of the other TMJ symptomatology and is exhibiting a deep bite and/or re-truded mandible (determined cephalometrically), the palliative effect of open-ing the vertical with the occlusal bite plates is an advantageous course to pursue until the lost E-space is regained and the appropriate appliance may be used to correct the TMJ problem orthopedically.

There are several basic methods for determining where the final posi-tion of the first molar, upper or lower, should be once distalization is com-plete and the E-space regained and retention initiated. There are the concepts of the flush terminal plane and the mixed dentition analysis and, of course, cephalometrics.

The concept of the flush terminal plane acting as a guide is easy to take advantage of when distalization is required in a quadrant where the

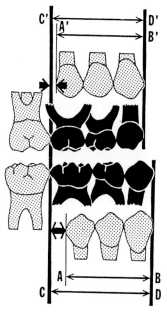

Figure 4-24 Flush terminal plane. In most normally developing mixed dentitions, upper and lower first permanent molars align in an end to end horizontal relationship with their mesial surfaces tangent to perpendicular line referred to as the flush terminal plane. Note the combined widths of the deciduous cuspid and first and second molars in the maxilla, C'−D', is greater than the combined widths of the cor-responding permanent teeth, A'−B'. In the mandible, the difference is even greater, about 2.7 mm on average. When deciduous mandibular cuspid and molars are exfoliated, a "leeway space" causes a gain in space for lower permanent teeth to be realized. This allows the lower first permanent molar to drift farther forward than the upper first per-manent molar effecting the conversion from one-half Class II to full Class I.

opposing quadrant is intact and uncompromised, ie, C's, D's, and E's are present and intact. In a normal healthy mouth in the mixed dentition stage, the upper and lower first permanent molars are directly on top of one another in a slight or half-Class II molar relationship. This is perfectly correct and as it should be. This results in the upper and lower first molars aligning themselves in such a way that their mesial surfaces are both in imaginary contact with a vertical plane running tangential to these mesial surfaces and parallel to the long axis of the teeth. The distance from the mesial of the upper first permanent molar to the distal of the upper permanent lateral incisor is occupied by three teeth: the deciduous cuspid and the deciduous first and second molars respectively. But this space is usually greater than the summation of the mesiodistal widths of the three permanent teeth that will occupy the space once the deciduous teeth are exfoliated. This allows the permanent maxillary first molar to drift forward slightly once the deciduous teeth are lost. The same is true for the lower. However, here the discrepancy between the widths of the three deciduous lower teeth and the three permanent teeth is *even greater* (probably due to the wider deciduous E and narrower permanent cuspid). Upon exfoliation, this allows the lower permanent first molar to drift forward even farther than the upper. This increased mesial drift combined with the function of the inclined plane action of the mesial cusp slopes of the upper molar against the distal cusp slopes of the lower molar gradually and gracefully effect the change from half-Class II to Class I. Nature has thought things out pretty well.

From the above it is easy to see that in a case where an upper deciduous second molar, or E, has been lost prematurely and the first permanent molar has drifted into the space, if the lower opposing quadrant is fully intact, distalization of the offending molar back to the original flush terminal plane is all that is required. Distalizing it farther could possibly result in a Class III molar relationship once the lower deciduous teeth exfoliate and the lower permanent molar is drawn forward. This is not the worst of catastrophies, however, as the eruption of the powerful second molar will usually push everything on top forward again anyway. It merely represents efficiency in time, effort, and concern for both patient and doctor to put the teeth in the nearest to correct position the first time.[48]

MIXED DENTITION ANALYSIS

The second basic analysis system commonly used to determine the extent of arch length discrepancy in the younger patient is the mixed dentition analysis.[49-51] Since not all the permanent teeth are unerupted yet at this stage of the patient's development, certain approximations must be used. It is determined in the following manner.

First, measure the sum total of the arch length anterior to the molars, mesial first permanent molar to the mesial of the opposite first permanent molar. This may be done in two ways. One way is to measure the arch with a lightweight jewelry chain, string, etc, from the mesial of the first molar across the approximate centers of the labial surfaces of the clinical crowns of the teeth to the mesial of the opposite first permanent molar. Another way is to measure with a Bowly gauge from the mesial of the right first permanent molar to the mesial of the right deciduous cuspid. Then measure from the mesial right deciduous cuspid to the mesial of the left deciduous cuspid and then from the mesial of the left deciduous cuspid to the mesial of the left first permanent molar. Add the three measurements together for the sum total of arch length anterior to the molars. Taking the sum total of arch length anterior to the permanent molars represents the actual existing arch length.

To obtain the *predicted* arch length necessary for that particular arch, one must first measure the mesiodistal widths of the lower permanent right or left central and right or left lateral. Adding the two gives the total $S = \overline{2 + 1}$. To obtain the predicted space necessary for the upper permanent cuspid, first bicuspid, and second bicuspid, simply add 11 mm. To obtain the predicted space needed for the lower permanent cuspid, first bicuspid, and second bicuspid, add only 10 mm.

This allows the clinician to compare the predicted total arch length as compared with the actual measured arch length. Or it can be compared in one-third sections, right and left (the middle is usually never analyzed as a single unit using this system). For instance, the space actually measured from the mesial of the first permanent molar to the mesial of the deciduous cuspid in a given upper or lower quadrant may be *less* than the predicted necessary space calculated from the respective formulae for the upper quadrant $(\overline{5,4,3|} = S + 11)$ or lower $(\overline{5,4,3|} = S + 10)$. This would indicate potential crowding. There is an important buffer area involved in this system. The average leeway space is 2 to 3 mm in the maxilla and 3 to 4 mm in the mandible for the total arch. This means that when predicted total space is subtracted from the actual total measured space there should be a surplus of 2 to 3 mm for the upper and 3 to 4 mm for the lower. If measured space minus predicted space results in a number lower than these values, relative to their respective arches, or in a negative number, there will most likely be some crowding when the permanent teeth erupt. This, of course, may

---

Figure 4-25 Case study. Regaining lost "E" space. Regaining lost "E" space in the mixed dentition as a result of first molar impingement on the space created by a prematurely lost deciduous second molar is an important form of interceptive orthodontics. **(A)** Pretreatment study model reveals maxillary first molar has drifted considerably forward into space formerly occupied by deciduous second molar. **(B)** A unilateral Sagittal appliance for the mixed dentition was constructed **(C)** and inserted. **(D)** After only 3½ months of excellent patient compliance, note regained "E" space due to expanded appliance and distalized first molar leaving room **(E)** for upper-right second bicuspid to erupt freely. **(F)** View of expanded appliance on finishing model.

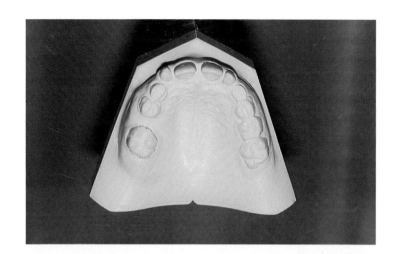

(A)

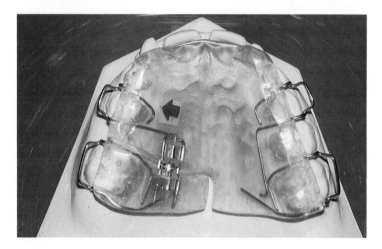

(B)

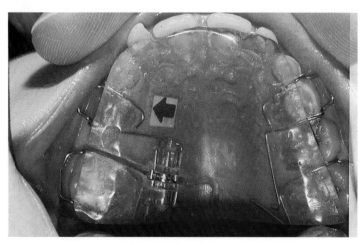

(C)

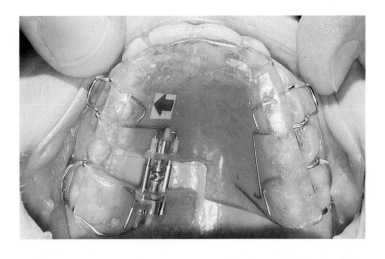

(D)

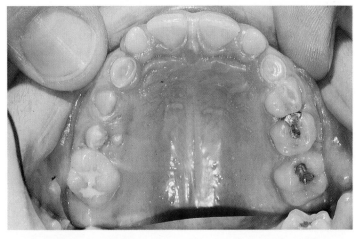

(E)

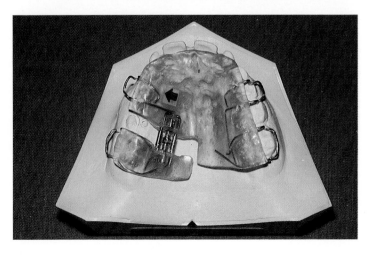

(F)

be due to the mesialization of the first permanent molars and in such cases is an indication for the interceptive use of the aforementioned sagittal appliance to regain proper arch length. Since the quadrant measurement is taken from the mesial of the first permanent molar to the mesial of the deciduous cuspid, it is obvious as to which tooth is the culprit as far as eating up the arch length goes. Deciduous cuspids are seldom, if ever, seen distalized back from their normal position in the arch; therefore, any arch length loss is due to mesial migration of the first permanent molar and not the distal migration of the deciduous cuspid!

SUMMARY

Thus it can be seen from the preceding that the Sagittal appliances may be used to move teeth in both the permanent and mixed dentitions. They may be used to develop immature premaxillas, the only true orthopedic aspect of the appliance, and can apply torque to retroclined maxillary and mandibular incisors labially. They may be used to distalize posterior segments, relieve crowding, and regain lost E-space in the mixed dentition (primarily orthodontic functions). In cases of severe temporomandibular joint and muscle pain, they can even act as a palliative by serving as an intraoral splint to open the vertical and decompress the compromised joint. They are esthetic, economical to construct, and easy to wear and adjust.

The Sagittal's main forte is movement of the teeth along alveolar ridges that are already existing at an adequate arch width. It is true that the appliance has an orthopedic function of opening up the premaxillary sutures and developing the premaxilla, but this is only in Class II, Division 2, cases. In all other cases the primary function of the appliance is, for the most part, orthodontic. Specifically, it is orthodontic movement in an anteroposterior direction. They are not designed for use in cases where arch *width* is a problem. There is another entire family of appliances designed and developed specifically to handle this particular aspect of malocclusion of the dental arches!

REFERENCES

1. Stephens CD, Lloyd TG: Changes in molar occlusion after extraction of all first pre-molars: a follow-up study of Class II, division 1 cases treated with removable appliances. *Br J Orthod* 1980;7:139–144.
2. Badcock JH: The screw expansion plate. *Trans Br Soc Orthod* 1911;3–8.
3. Schwarz AM: *Gebissregelung mit Platten.* Vienna, Urban & Schwarzenberg, 1938.
4. Adams CP: *The Design and Construction of Removable Orthodontic Appliances,* ed 4. Bristol, England, John Wright & Sons Ltd, 1970.
5. Oppenheim A: Tissue changes particularly in bone incident to tooth movement. *Am Orthodontist* 1911;3:57–58.
6. Schwarz AM: Tissue changes incident to tooth movement. *Int J Orthod* 1932; 18:331–352.

7. Stuteville OH: Summary review of tissue changes incident to tooth movement. *Angle Orthod* 1938;8:1–19.

8. Oppenheim A: Possibility for physiologic orthodontic movement. *Am J Orthod* 1944;30:277–328.

9. Moyers RE, Bauer JL: Periodontal response to various tooth movements. *Am J Orthod* 1950;36:572–580.

10. Reitan K: Continuous bodily tooth movement and its histologic significance. *Acta Odontol Scand* 1947;7:115–144.

11. Gianelly AA: Force-induced changes in the vascularity of the periodontal ligament. *Am J Orthod* 1969;55:5–11.

12. Bassett CAL, Becker RO: Generation of electrical potentials in bone in response to mechanical stress. *Science* 1962;137:1063–1064.

13. Bassett CAL, Pawluk RJ, Becker RO: Effects of electrical currents on bone in vivo. *Nature* 1964;204:652–654.

14. Bassett CAL: Electrical effects in bone. *Sci Am* 1965;213:18–25.

15. Becker RO, Bassett CAL, Bachman CH: Bioelectric factors controlling bone structure, in Frost H (ed): *Bone Biodynamics.* Boston, Little, Brown & Co, 1964, p 209.

16. Braden M, Bairstow AG, Beider I, et al: Electrical and piezo-electrical properties of dental hard tissues, *Nature* 1966;212:1565–1566.

17. Cochran GVB, Pawluk RJ, Bassett CAL: Stress generated electric potentials in the mandible and teeth. *Arch Oral Biol* 1967;12:917–920.

18. Epker BN, Frost JM: Correlation of bone resorption and formation with the physical behavior of loaded bone. *J Dent Res* 1965;44:33–41.

19. Reitan K, Kvan E: Comparative behavior of human and animal tissue during experimental tooth movement. *Angle Orthod* 1971;41:1–14.

20. Utley RK: The activity of alveolar bone incident to orthodontic tooth movement as studied by oxytetracycline induced fluorescence. *Am J Orthod* 1968;54:167–201.

21. Zengo AN, Pawluk RJ, Bassett CAL: Stress-induced bioelectric potentials in the dento alveolar complex. *Am J Orthod* 1973;64:17–27.

22. Cady WG: *Piezoelectricity: an Introduction to the Theory and Applications of Electromechanical Phenomena in Crystals.* New York, McGraw-Hill Book Co, 1964.

23. Berg R, Gebauer U: Spontaneous changes in the mandibular arch following first premolar extractions. *Eur J Orthod* 1982;4:93–98.

24. Mills JRE: The effect on the lower incisors of uncontrolled extraction of lower premolars. *Trans Eur Orthod Soc* 1964;357–370.

25. Hemley S: Bite plates, their application and action. *Am J Orthod* 1938;24:721–736.

26. Hopkins SC: Bite planes. *Am J Orthod* 1940;26:107–119.

27. Bahador MA, Higley LB: Bite opening, a cephalometric analysis. *J Am Dent Assoc* 1944;31:343–352.

28. Sleichter CG: Effects of maxillary bite plane therapy in orthodontics. *Am J Orthod* 1954;40:850–870.

29. Klein PL: An evaluation of cervical traction on the maxilla and upper first permanent molar. *Angle Orthod* 1957;27:61–68.

30. Mills CM, Holman RG, Graber TM: Heavy intermittent cervical traction in Class II treatment: A longitudinal cephalometric assessment. *Am J Orthod* 1978;74:361–379.

31. Dewel BF: Clinical observation of the axial inclination of teeth. *Am J Orthod* 1949;35:98–115.

32. Yerkes IM, Witzig J: Functional jaw orthopedics: mastering more than technique, in Gelb H (ed): *The Clinical Management of Head, Neck, and TMJ Pain and Dysfunction,* ed 2, Philadelphia, WB Saunders Co, 1985, pp 598–618.

33. Witzig J: Unpublished case reports of computerized cephalometric analyses of Rocky Mountain Data Systems, Los Angeles.
34. Häupl K, Grossman WJ, Clarkson P: *Textbook of Functional Jaw Orthopaedics*. London, Henry Kimpton, 1950, pp 97–100.
35. Carey CW: Linear arch dimension and tooth size. *Am J Orthod* 1949;35:762–775.
36. Willet RC: Premature loss of deciduous teeth. *Angle Orthod* 1933;3:106–111.
37. Foster CS: Functional space maintenance has its place in dentistry for children, *J Am Dent Assoc* 1936;23:1052–1058.
38. Weber FN: Prophylactic orthodontics. *Am J Orthod* 1949;35:611–635.
39. Brandhorst DW: Promoting normal development by maintaining function of the deciduous teeth. *J Am Dent Assoc* 1932;19:1196–1203.
40. Chapman H: Orthodontics: The necessity of histories to establish etiology; the necessity of extra function in retention; the necessity of preserving spaces closed by premature loss of deciduous teeth. *Int J Orthod* 1927;13:768–775.
41. Conover CS: Deciduous teeth—Effect of too early loss and too long retention. *Int J Orthod* 1928;14:576–583.
42. Curley JE: The deciduous molars—Nature's space retainers. *J Am Dent Assoc* 1931;18:1650–1658.
43. Humphrey WR: Dentist's responsibility in the prevention of malocclusion. *J Am Dent Assoc* 1931;18:1607–1612.
44. Sippy B: Early loss of teeth—a study of effects. *J Am Dent Assoc* 1928;15:2228–2234.
45. Lundstrom A: The significance of early loss of deciduous teeth in the etiology of malocclusion. *Am J Orthod* 1955;41:819–826.
46. Linder-Aronson S: The effect of premature loss of teeth. *Acta Odontol Scand* 1960;18:101–122.
47. Richardson ME: The relationship between the relative amount of space present in the deciduous teeth and the rate of space closure subsequent to the extraction of a deciduous molar. *Dent Pract* 1965;16:111–118.
48. Dewel BF: Objectives of mixed dentition treatment in orthodontics. *Am J Orthod* 1964;50:504–520.
49. Ballard ML, Wylie WL: Mixed dentition case analysis—estimating size of unerupted permanent teeth. *Am J Orthod* 1947;33:754–759.
50. Moyers RE: *Handbook of Orthodontics for the Student and the General Practitioner*, Chicago, Yearbook Medical Publishers, Inc, 1973; pp 369–379.
51. Tanaka MM, Johnson LE: The prediction of the size of unerupted canines and premolars in a contemporary orthodontic population. *J Am Dent Assoc* 1974; 88:798–801.

"They spell it Vinci and pronounce it
Vinchy; foreigners always spell better than
they pronounce."

Mark Twain (Samuel Clemens)

CHAPTER 5
The Transverse Appliance

The Transverse active plate is an arch-widening appliance. However, the word "Transverse" not only describes a particular type of appliance but it is also used as a collective term to denote a whole potpourri of devices used to gain arch width. These range all the way from the delicate, leisurely paced, ballerinalike Crozat appliance (the gnathologist's delight), all the way up to the two-fisted, suture-splitting, high-speed heavyweights like the rapid palatal expanders! The appliances used for arch widening may utilize orthodontic movement, orthopedic movement, or a combination of both. They also may be either fixed or removable. They often sport names derived from a description of the anatomical plane in which they work, the speed at which they operate, the number of coils in the wire used, the screw action used, letters of the alphabet, and surnames of the men who developed them, names both European and American. Names like Transverse, Porter arch, Quad-Helix, split-jack, K-D appliance, specialized lingual arch, Schwarz, and Jackson. (Note: The name Schwarz is often misspelled Schwartz and often mispronounced as Schwartz or Schwartzy. It is spelled and pronounced simply — Schwarz!) Arch widening is a concept that goes back into history equally as far as the other functional appliances and active plates. The appliances used to accomplish this effect have over the years been surrounded by confusion, misunderstanding, and controversy. Therefore, as far as the family of FJO appliances goes, Transverse active plates fit right in.

279

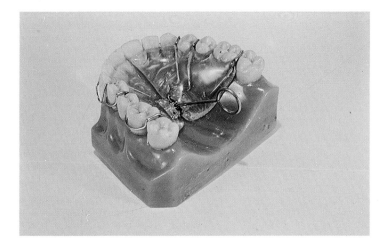

Figure 5-1 Maxillary Schwarz plate, cornerstone of the removable active plate family of appliances is used for developing arches laterally to their naturally tolerable limits of arch width.

The Transverse system of appliances plays an extremely important role in the preparation of the mouth for proper finishing. As stated previously, much of the work of orthodontics is concerned with the skeletal Class II-type patient, and the best functional appliance available for treatment of the Class II deep bite case is the Bionator. But since the Bionator is an arch-aligning appliance, it mandates the dentitions of the upper and lower jaws be reasonably arch-shaped prior to its use. If not, arch preparation is indicated. The real workhorses of the FJO system are the Sagittal and Transverse active plates that act as arch formers and arch preparers for the final step of the arch-aligning Bionator.

One of the most common faults of the Class II, Division 1, malocclusion is the loss of arch width. This may be due to several factors of which some of the most common are habits of improper function like thumb sucking, deviant swallowing, and tongue-thrusting.[1-6] The classic result of such improper function is often an upper arch that has lost its Roman arch shape and has suffered from lateral collapse with concomitant labial flaring of the maxillary anteriors. This in turn results in the change to a more pointed Gothic arch shape of the upper dentition. The functional occlusion during this process usually drags the lower teeth lingually as the inclined plane action of the cusps of the upper teeth act to narrow the lower teeth into an arch of approximately the same proportions.[7,8] This arch-narrowing process only aids in forcing the maxillary anteriors to torque labially and is an ally to the forces of improper function in that direction. If the aforementioned inclined plane action fails to move the lower posteriors lingually, posterior crossbites develop or the entire mandible is locked by the occlusion in a more skeletal Class II retruded position, keeping back where it may interdigitate itself more completely with the upper arch at a point where the upper arch is wider.

Proper arch shape, along with other important factors, is critical to long-term retention. The tongue must be given a proper amount of volume in which to operate. If impinged upon by teeth and bone, the latter will eventually give way. A properly trained tongue, lip seal, and swallow reflex in conjunction with adequately developed, rounded arches should be an ideal goal for every case for the clinician to strive toward. Functional appliances that retrain muscles and active plates that have sufficient power to reshape bone help attain this goal.

What is meant by "proper" arch form? What should the ideal arch form be? Is it the same for every patient? Hardly. There are several excellent analysis systems available to describe numerically what the correct arch shape should be.[9-14] Some systems, more mathematically oriented,[15-20] have described the human dental arch in the form of a catenary curve represented by equations such as:

$$y = 1/2m \ (e^{-mx} + e^{+mx}), \text{ or}$$

$$y = a/2 \ (e^{-bx} + e^{+bx})$$

Though these exotic mathematical equations may provide an accurate medium for computer manipulations and an esoteric fascination for the erudite members of the dental community, they are for all intents and purposes impractical for the common practitioner.

As for comprehending the idea of just what comprises an adequate arch shape, a much more common and accessible method is available to aid the clinician in helping him understand what he sees in his diagnostic study casts. It is basically simple, yet the underlying principle behind it is incredibly profound. It is referred to, somewhat tongue-in-cheek, as the "Leghorn analyzer"—the common chicken egg! Upon studying the shape of the maxillary dental arch, if it seems to assume the shape of the more rounded end of an egg, you may assume that the case is fairly close to normal. But if the outline of the teeth assumes the appearance of the more pointed end of an egg, it is a tip-off that a Pont's or Schwarz analysis is needed. Many clinicians fail to detect these sometimes subtle differences in arch shape and assume they may proceed directly to a Bionator without even measuring the study casts of a case to see if adequate width exists. Keeping this simple comparison in mind while examining study models offers a quick and easy way for the practitioner to "get a feel" of what might be involved in treating a given case that on the surface appears easy. Teeth may be "straight" and well aligned in an upper arch that is actually of itself too pointed, yet not enough so as to blatantly resemble the sharp Gothic arch outline. This simple mental reference method can serve to guard against a practitioner making a hasty decision not to perform the appropriate model analysis system on a given case simply because he was fooled into thinking its width was already adequate. If one can forgive the levity, it's a long way from differential equations; but it's a handy way to think about arches!

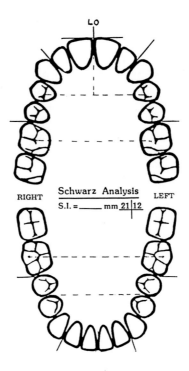

Figure 5-2 Schwarz (Bonn) Analysis. Originally referred to as a modified Pont's Analysis, the Bonn Analysis was developed by Schwarz, Korkhaus, Kantorowicz, and others in the mid-1920s as an alternative to Pont's Analysis which had been used since 1909.

Two more commonly used methods of dealing with arches are the analysis systems of Schwarz and of Pont.

SCHWARZ MODEL ANALYSIS SYSTEM— BONN ANALYSIS

The Schwarz analysis devised by Dr A. M. Schwarz[21] of Vienna is commonly used to determine the amount of discrepancy in millimeters of actual measured arch width versus ideal arch width in the upper and lower dentitions. It is a simple and easy formula to follow and offers a good guideline of how wide an arch for a given case should be. Simply measure the mesiodistal widths of the maxillary central and lateral incisors. Let this total be represented by SI. Now add 8 mm to this figure. This should be the ideal distance measured linearly directly across the arch between the distal pits of the maxillary first bicuspids. Let this number be represented by ub. Therefore SI + 8 = ub. Measure the actual distance across the distal pits of the maxillary first bicuspids and compare it to the calculated ideal distance, ub, and this will give you the discrepancy in millimeters that the arch is deficient as far as development width in the bicuspid area is concerned. For the molar region repeat the calculation, this time substituting 16, such that SI + 16 is equal to the ideal distance across the arch between the central pits of the maxillary first molars. Given this value as um, SI + 16 = um. Now take the actual transverse distance between the distal pits of the maxillary first molars taken from the model and subtract it from the calculated ideal distance for the discrepancy in molar width in millimeters. If ub and um show approximately the same amount of deficiency, then a simple transverse development of equal amounts in both the bicuspid and molar regions will bring the arch to the correct width. If the discrepancy is greater in the anterior region than in the posterior, more development with the appropriate appliance in the bicuspid area than in the molar area will be needed. Conversely, if the discrepancy is greater in the molar area than in the bicuspid region, more development will be needed posteriorly.

Discrepancy ub = discrepancy um → equal development laterally
Discrepancy ub > discrepancy um → more anterior development laterally
Discrepancy ub < discrepancy um → more posterior development laterally

The value SI, the sum of the widths of the *maxillary* centrals and laterals, is also used in the calculations of the lower arch width deficiencies. Again, start by adding SI + 8. In the mandible this value represents the ideal transverse distance between the mesio-labial marginal ridge points of the mandibular second bicuspids, lb, such that SI + 8 = lb. Compare this ideal calculated value with the actual measured value of the distance between the mesiolabial marginal ridge points of the mandibular second bicuspids to get the discrepancy in the bicuspid region. For the mandibular molar area, take the sum of the *maxillary* incisors and add 16, SI + 16. This represents the ideal distance between the central part of the middle buccal cusps of the mandibular first molars, lm: SI + 16 = lm. If only two buccal cusps are present on the lower first molar instead of the customary three, the center of the distobuccal cusp is used for the measurement. Compare this ideal calculated distance with the actual measured distance across the distal grooves of the mandibular first molars for the discrepancy in millimeters in arch width in the molar area.

If the discrepancy in the bicuspid area is equal to the discrepancy in the molar area, simple lateral development with the appropriate appliance will bring the case to correct width. If the discrepancy is greater in the bicuspid region (more collapse anteriorly), more development will be needed in that area than the molar region. If the discrepancy is greater in the posterior area, more development will be needed there than in the bicuspid region.

Schwarz Analysis Corrections by Facial Type

In developing an analysis system for the determination of ideal arch width for a given case, it was decided that a given fixed constant could not be used in one formula that would be applicable to all facial types. With this in mind Schwarz modified the basic ideas of Pont's theories on ideal arch width and, in conjunction with Korkhaus, Kantorowicz, and others, modified the width-determining formulae to allow for correction of the original constant depending on which of the three basic facial-type categories the patient might fall into. These three basic facial types as viewed frontally are as follows:

Mesoprosopic.   This is the average type of individual whose facial outline follows a generally paraboloid pattern. The dental arches tend to develop to a nicely shaped geometric Roman arch form.

Leptoprosopic.   This type of individual when viewed frontally exhibits a long narrow facial outline with greater predominance of vertical dimensions with less influence seen in the lateral dimensions. Correspondingly, the dental arches tend to be longer anteroposteriorly and more narrow.

Euryprosopic.   This type of facial pattern is more dominant in the lateral dimensions than in the vertical dimensions and appears as a more square and stocky facial outline. The dental arches tend to be shorter anteroposteriorly but more square or widened out laterally.

The modifications used to accommodate such variance in facial type are simple. The constants used in the formulae are 6, 7, and 8 for lepto-, meso-, and euryprosopic patterns respectively.

Leptoprosopic: SI + 6 = bicuspid width
SI + 12 = molar width
Mesoprosopic: SI + 7 = bicuspid width
SI + 14 = molar width
Euryprosopic: SI + 8 = bicuspid width
SI + 16 = molar width

As may be seen from the above, a greater range of adaptability is now available using these individualized corrections which allow for differences in skull type. It would be remiss to try to force the development laterally of an extremely narrow set of arches in a very leptoprosopic-type individual trying to make him accommodate the larger SI + 8 bicuspid arch width reserved for the naturally wider-based euryprosopic individuals. This could potentially result in overexpansion of the width of the arches with a concomitant undesirable penchant for instability. In selecting an arch width standard more individualized for a given patient's particular tolerances, the clinician insures a greater chance for long-term stability and success.

Schwarz Arch Height (LO) Calculation (Corrected)

A correction in desired arch height was also developed by Schwarz to go hand in hand with the facial-type width corrections. The arch height, LO, as measured from the imaginary line across the width of the bicuspids to the facial surfaces of the central incisors, should be half the ideal or calculated bicuspid crossarch width, LO = (SI + K)/2. Schwarz uses 34 mm as the magic arbitrary dividing line for the determination of a *corrected* LO as follows:

If SI < 34 mm, then
$$\text{Leptoprosopic} = \text{LO} + \tfrac{1}{2} \text{ mm, and}$$
$$\text{Euryprosopic} = \text{LO} - \tfrac{1}{2} \text{ mm}$$

If SI > 34 mm, then
$$\text{Leptoprosopic} = \text{LO} + 1 \text{ mm, and}$$
$$\text{Euryprosopic} = \text{LO} - 1 \text{ mm}$$

Of course, the individual LOs are calculated using one half the bicuspid ideal widths corrected to facial type. Unfortunately, there is only one problem with this beautiful theory of calculating the arch height expressed in terms of the LO. It's a fantasy! It would be nice if the anterior arch form always followed this formula, but the actual calculated LO values are of only limited clinical value, as their original developers were quick to confess. This is due to several reasons, one orthodontic and one orthopedic, as might be expected. First of all, from an orthodontic standpoint, a particular dental arch in a narrow-faced leptoprosopic-type individual may require a trans-arch width of less than the average SI + 6 in the bicuspid region in order to remain stable to the determined pressures of lateral collapse, if the proper tooth-to-tooth contact points are to be maintained in such a slightly narrowed arch, the anteriors must necessarily arc out farther labially in a slightly more Gothic outline. This is in part due to the laws of the ellipse, which is in part what the arch outline actually is. As the edges of an ellipse approach one another, its focus to apex distance must increase. Similarly, the LO value for such a "pointed and narrowed" arch must in reality be greater than one half the bicuspid transarch width. If such were the case, attempting to create an LO at half the SI + K value would force either gross distortion of the arch outline (making it quite square) or, conversely, force the appearance of rotations, which in the anterior region give up arch length. What is required of a narrower-type arch is a slightly more pointed or Gothic arch outline. This would place the mesial contact of the maxillary centrals considerably beyond the calculated LO point. A narrow-faced individual with disproportionately wide teeth (higher SI values) would fall into this category.

Conversely, in a euryprosopic-type individual with an already wide arch, the actual outline might place the maxillary anteriors short of the calculated LO point in a more Roman or "squared," albeit stable, arch outline.

Orthopedically speaking, the clinician concerned about the temporomandibular joint can throw the LO calculation out the proverbial window. The arc of closure, ie, the position of the condyle within the temporomandibular joint during that arc of closure, will in fact be what determines the ultimate posttreatment position of the maxillary central incisors and hence the ultimate anterior arch form. But this is the subject of an entirely different discussion to be delved into in further detail at a later time. Suffice it to say for now that quite often the actual orthopedically and orthodontically correct anterior arch form frequently will fall quite close to the calculated LO measurement. But remember, in a certain important number of cases it will not! And that is perfectly fine, for we must always remember to treat to harmony, beauty, and function; not to the dictates of theoretical formula. Treat to the patient's needs; not to the numbers.

What this all shows is that what turns out to be not enough for one might well be too much for another. Such corrected formulae allow a greater expression of creativity and clinical judgment for the practitioner and allow him to treat each of his patients on a more individualized basis, thereby increasing his chances for a successful outcome.

PONT'S ANALYSIS—ORIGINAL AND CORRECTED

A second analysis system for determining arch width is the Pont's analysis. Developed just after the turn of the century by the French dentist Dr A. Pont, it is reputed to be more precise than the Schwarz and involves some slightly more intricate calculations. As with the Schwarz, it starts with the summation of the mesiodistal widths of the four maxillary anteriors represented by SI. (Note: In the event a case exhibits sesmoid or "peg" laterals, use a value 2 mm less than that of the central as a substitute for the lateral. It is preferable to expand the case out to the ideal width with gaps between the laterals and other anterior teeth and to restore them with modern-day operative or crown and bridge procedures.) The premolar width is then calculated to be from central point to central point of the middle fissure across the first bicuspids by the following formula. (American authors traditionally use the distal pit instead of the center of the middle fissure. The distance is so close that such discrepancies in all practicality are a moot point.)

$$\text{Pont's premolar index} = \frac{SI \times 100}{80}$$

This gives the calculated, ideal Pont's premolar width for the maxilla relative to the measured value SI of the given case. Subtracting the patient's actual central point to central point upper bicuspid transverse linear distance, or width, taken from the study model from this calculated Pont's width, gives the development needed laterally in millimeters in the premolar region.

Figure 5-3 (A) Pont's analysis is based on the sum of mesiodistal widths of the four maxillary anteriors, SI. (B) From SI, mathematical computations using given constants may be made to determine ideal cross-arch width of the upper first bicuspids and molars. (C) Pont's "P" index determines cross-arch width of lower first bicuspids relative to upper first bicuspids. (D) The Pont's "W" index determines cross-arch width of lower first molars relative to upper first molars.

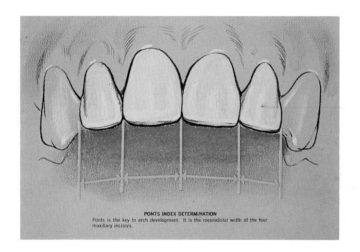

PONTS INDEX DETERMINATION
Ponts is the key to arch development. It is the mesiodistal width of the four maxillary incisors.

(A)

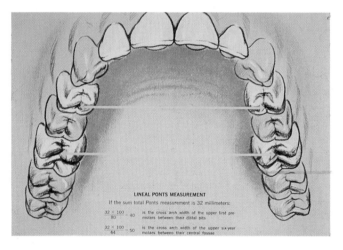

LINEAL PONTS MEASUREMENT
If the sum total Ponts measurement is 32 millimeters:

$$\frac{32 \times 100}{80} = 40$$ is the cross arch width of the upper first pre-molars between their distal pits

$$\frac{32 \times 100}{64} = 50$$ is the cross arch width of the upper six-year molars between their central fossae

(B)

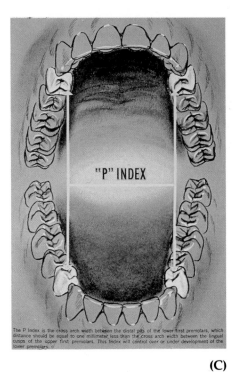

The P Index is the cross arch width between the distal pits of the lower first premolars, which distance should be equal to one millimeter less than the cross arch width between the lingual cusps of the upper first premolars. This Index will control over or under development of the lower premolars.

(C)

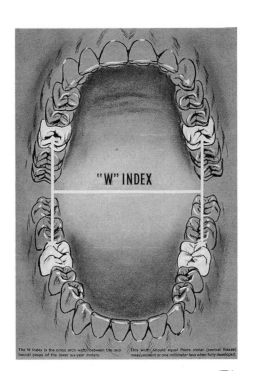

The W Index is the cross arch width between the mid-buccal cusps of the lower six-year molars. This width should equal Ponts molar (central fossae) measurement or one millimeter less when fully developed.

(D)

The ideal molar width for the upper arch is calculated in a similar manner with a slightly different ratio. The width transversely across the arch of the upper first molars is determined to be the linear distance from central pit to central pit and is calculated by the following formula:

$$\text{Pont's molar index} = \frac{SI \times 100}{64}$$

This gives the calculated ideal Pont's molar width for the maxilla relative to the measured value SI for a given case. Subtracting the patient's actual central pit to central pit linear distance, or width, taken from the study model from this calculated Pont's width, gives the development needed laterally in millimeters in the molar region.

As can be seen from the formulae above, they consist again of one variable and a constant ratio. Simple algebraic principles tell us that such a series of formulae with constant ratios such as logarithms, sines, cosines, etc, may be represented by precalculated tables of values, and in fact one exists for the Pont's index as listed below (see Table 5-1). This makes the determination of the Pont's premolar and molar indices a simple matter of obtaining SI from the study model and reading the appropriate values from the table.

Table 5-1
Average Length and Width of Upper Dental Arch

Sum of Incisal Widths.	Distance 4 : 4.		Distance 6 : 6.		Distance 1/1 : 4/4. Length of Dental Arch according to Korkhaus.
	Linder: Harth $\frac{SIW \times 100}{85}$	Pont $\frac{SIW \times 100}{80}$	Linder : Harth $\frac{SIW \times 100}{65}$	Pont $\frac{SIW \times 100}{64}$	
27	32	33·5	41·5	42·5	16
27·5	32·5	34	42·3	42·95	16·3
28	33	35	43	44	16·5
28·5	33·5	35·5	43·8	44·5	16·8
29	34	36	44·5	45·3	17
29·5	34·7	37	45·3	46	17·3
30	35·5	37·5	46	46·8	17·5
30·5	36	38	46·8	47·6	17·8
31	36·5	39	47·5	48·4	18
31·5	37	39·5	48·5	49·2	18·3
32	37·5	40	49	50	18·5
32·5	38·2	40·5	50	50·8	18·8
33	39	41	51	51·5	19
33·5	39·5	42	51·5	52·3	19·3
34	40	43	52·5	53	19·5
34·5	40·5	43·5	53	53·9	19·8
35	41·2	44	54	54·5	20
35·5	42	44·5	54·5	55·5	20·5
36	42·5	45	55·5	56·2	21

Determining the Pont's values for the lower arch form can be confusing if not approached in an orderly and clear-cut fashion. It is not difficult once the principles are understood. The determination is entirely dependent on the values obtained from the upper model and its calculated ideal Pont's indices.

We know the maxillary linear width from central point first bicuspid across to central point first bicuspid as measured from the model. We now measure the linear width from the tip of the lingual cusp of the first bicuspid to the tip of lingual cusp first bicuspid from the model. We subtract the latter width from the former, thus:

$$\text{Central points } 4/4 - \text{Li cusp tips } 4/4 = X$$

This value, X, represents the conversion factor or the linear *difference* between the widths of the central points and the tips of the lingual cusps. This difference remains *constant*. No matter how far out the teeth are spread from their original starting point, the *difference* in these two measurements remains the same. Since the cusps are attached to the same teeth as the cen-

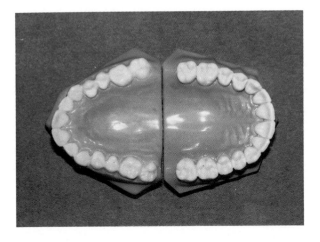

(A)

Figure 5-4 **(A)** Ideal arch form of right upper model exhibits Roman arch outline, well-rounded in cuspid area as opposed to left upper model which loses some of Roman-rounding in cuspid and bicuspid area due to slight narrowing. The compromised left arch outline is only slightly approaching the Gothic arch shape. **(B)** Comparing the two arches to a common chicken egg, one clearly sees the difference between the two arches is similar to the difference in outline of the two ends of the egg. **(C)** Outline of more correct arch form (Roman) corresponds to more rounded end of egg whereas outline of the compromised arch (Gothic) **(D)** with its narrower bicuspid area, corresponds to the more pointed end of the egg. This has possible far-reaching implications in treatment of orthopedically induced TMJ problems resulting from retruded mandibular arc of closure.

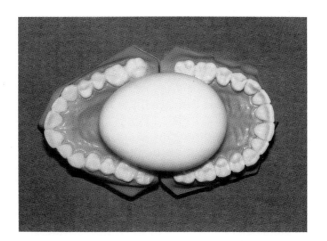

(B)

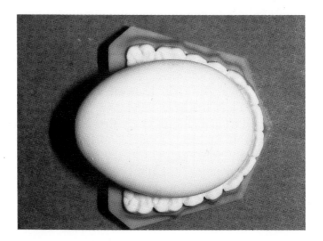

(C)

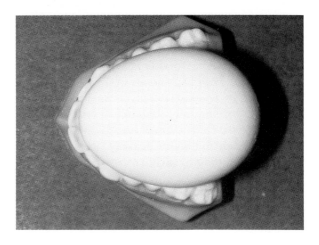

(D)

tral points are; as the points spread apart, the cusps follow by the exact same amount. As the points of the central fissures go, so go the lingual cusp tips. Hence the conversion factor X remains the same. We will use this value in calculating the patient's lower ideal width.

Understanding this calculation is dependent on realization of an identical anatomical relationship. The lingual cusp tip of the upper first bicuspid occludes with the *distal pit of the lower first bicuspid*. This means that if we know the ideal distance these upper first bicuspid lingual cusp tips will be at in an ideal calculated Pont's arch, we then automatically know the ideal transverse width of the lower first bicuspids across their distal pit width. Now the distance of the upper ideal Pont's central point to central point first bicuspids is determined from the table and SI. Then the upper ideal calculated lingual cusp tip to lingual cusp tip first bicuspid width may be determined by subtracting X, the constant difference or conversion factor, from the table-read Pont's index. Thus Pont's premolar index (ideal, calculated) − X = Li cusp width 4/4 (ideal, calculated).

This Li cusp 4/4 width is referred to as Pont's P. It represents, as seen from the abovementioned identical anatomical relationship, the distance of width distal pit lower first bicuspid to distal pit lower first bicuspid!

LI cusp tip 4/4 (ideal, calculated) = Pont's P = distal pits 4/4 (ideal, calculated)

So we now know the Pont's P, or ideal, calculated width for the lower bicuspid area of a given case. Now simply take the patient's actual measured P width from distal pit lower first bicuspid to distal pit lower first bicuspid taken from the study model, and subtract it from the ideal calculated Pont's P. The difference represents the lateral development necessary in the *lower* bicuspid region. Thus Pont's P (calculated from upper model) − Patient's P (measured from lower model) = development needed laterally in bicuspid region of mandible.

Fortunately, the calculation of the molar width for the lower is much easier. Another identical anatomical relationship exists here too. The upper Pont's ideal molar width central pit to central pit is read off the chart relative to the value SI. Now since the buccal (middle) cusp of the lower first molar articulates with the central pit of the upper first molar, the value of the ideal Pont's upper molar width gives the ideal Pont's lower molar width measured from tip of buccal (middle) cusp lower first molar across to tip of buccal (middle) cusp of opposite lower first molar. Well, almost! Since it is easy to continue on to develop laterally in the lower but a bother to have to bring molars back again lingually to avoid overdeveloping to a posterior crossbite, the values used for the lower are always a millimeter less than the upper. This gives a half millimeter leeway on each side to cushion the lower against overdeveloping to such a crossbite. The ideal calculated distance from buccal (middle) cusp to buccal (middle) cusp lower first molars is referred to as Pont's W. Now from the models we take the the actual buccal cusp to buccal cusp measured distance, patient W, and subtract it from Pont's W to get the amount of width needed in the molar region: Pont's W (calculated

Pont's molar index − 1) − Patient's W (measured from patient's lower model) = width needed in molar region mandible.

Thus our calculations for the amount of expansion needed in both maxillary and mandibular bicuspid and molar regions are complete. Well, almost, again! There is only one problem in turn with this detailed, beautiful, and refined system: It's not accurate! The arches defined by this method turn out to be a little too wide. But there is a reason.

When Dr Pont made his original measurements years ago, he studied the Basque people of the south of France. They are a hearty breed of people with generally meso- to euryprosopic tendencies as a physical trait. Other researchers such as Korkhaus, Linder, and Harth knew this and did studies of their own on the peoples of central Europe and found their arch width values to be, on the average, lower. Thus a "corrected Pont's" table was developed which utilizes these different figures. Table 5-1 shows the comparison between the original Pont's and the Linder-Harth corrected Pont's values. Each has its own value relative to the type of skull structure and facial type the patient may present. With the existence of the two tables, one for wide-faced euryprosopic-type individuals and one for more normal mesoprosopic-type individuals, the Pont's index along with the Linder-Harth corrections offers the clinician almost as much diagnostic versatility as the facially corrected Schwarz method. Both Pont's and Schwarz indices are used throughout the orthodontic community with the Schwarz possibly being the slight favorite due to its mathematical simplicity.

As stated previously, the original Pont's calculations were made using the *center of the central groove* of the upper first bicuspids for the maxilla and the *contact points* between the lower bicuspids for the mandible. Here in America, the *distal pits* are often used. The difference is slight and thought to reflect the Linder-Harth corrections somewhat. Whatever point you measure from, and they really are quite close, and whichever chart you use, these numbers are just that—numbers. They are only to act as a guide in helping the doctor decide what is best for the patient. The doctor is the one who assumes responsibility for determining when the case is correct, not some chart or mathematical formula. Diagnostic aids are the clinician's servants, not his masters.

THE "LOST C TRAP"

In the determination of arch width deficiencies using the Schwarz index that has been corrected and coordinated to facial type, one must be aware of a set of circumstances which may come about in the mixed dentition which would give a false indication of arch width deficiency and as a result may lead to improper treatment. It is a phenomenon known as the "lost C trap." In the old Palmer method of designating deciduous teeth, the teeth are assigned the letters of the alphabet in a manner such that the centrals are tooth A; laterals, tooth B; cuspids, tooth C; deciduous first molars, D; and deciduous second molars, E. Hence, with the qualifying terms of upper and

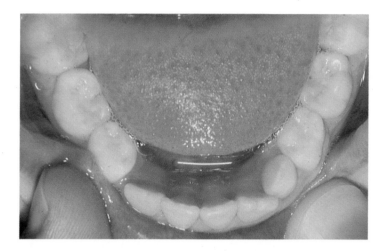

Figure 5-5 Lost "C" trap. Note how lower right quadrant has collapsed forward into space vacated by prematurely lost lower right deciduous cuspid. This places deciduous first and second molars and adult first molar farther forward on the arch than normal. This may lead to a false impression that the arch is narrower than it actually is due to the forward movement of the arch. This in turn could deceive the clinician into attempting to regain lost arch length by developing it primarily laterally instead of primarily anteroposteriorly, which would have been the original plane of arch collapse. This is all the more obvious in cases where both lower cuspids are prematurely lost and the anteroposterior collapse occurs bilaterally!

lower, right and left; a given deciduous tooth might be described as an upper right D, etc. In light of this naming system, the phenomenon of the lost C trap describes a process whereby the deciduous cuspids are lost prematurely either unilaterally or bilaterally in a given arch which allows the D's, E's, and first permanent molars behind the space created by the lost C to drift mesially en masse (which they often like doing). Left undetected and unprevented for a long enough period of time, the lost C space can become quite closed by the mesial drifting of the remaining teeth in the posterior quadrant. Realizing that the case will become crowded eventually once the permanent cuspids try to erupt, the treating clinician can perform both a Schwarz analysis *and* a mixed dentition arch length evaluation (as previously described) to determine the amount of crowding present and the direction his future treatment will take. Measuring the distal pits of the deciduous D's and adding 2 mm as a substitute for the first bicuspids which are developing right beneath them, he will invariably find the arch is short of width. Well, it may be, but then again in actuality it may not be! What happens that may deceive him with respect to interpreting the findings of the Schwarz analysis is that in drifting part of the way forward into the space vacated by the lost C, the D moves mesially to a naturally narrower portion of the young, growing, smaller dental arch. This deludes the diagnostician into surmising the case is narrower than it actually is. With one C gone, it is easier to detect such a phenomenon taking place because the other quadrant in the arch has the C present and its remaining teeth may be seen to reside by the resultant corresponding distance farther back on the dental arch as opposed to their comrades on the opposite, shortened side. It becomes truly deceptive to the eye and reflects an even greater apparent arch width loss when both C's of the same arch are lost simultaneously. Thus positioned forward on a naturally narrower portion of the arch (as the pediatric arch narrows rather abruptly in the cuspid area), a diminutive arch width measurement at that point may confuse the clinician into thinking the treatment of choice is to regain the arch width by lateral development with appliances designed for such, like the lower Schwarz or lower Jackson appliances, when in fact the true treatment of choice is to distalize the posterior quadrants, first molars and all, with common Sagittal I technique to regain the lost space given up by the premature loss of the C. Then the teeth will have been moved back to a wider point on the crest of the arch more distally and the arch width may be reassessed again at that position and any major gross arch width deficiencies still present can be corrected by lateral development techniques if need be. *Barring lingual incisor drift,* the mere fact that C's are lost and their spaces on the arch are closed in should be an adequate indication that the case is, in fact, crowded due to mesial posterior quadrant migration. Mixed dentition arch length analysis will confirm this, but it may also be analyzed cephalometrically according to what may be termed Ricketts' rule of permanent first molar positioning. From the 50-point computerized cephalometric analysis devised by Ricketts et al,[22] a handy relationship may be observed and proves to be practical here. Ricketts et al state that the distance from the pterygoid vertical to the distal of the upper first permanent molar should be equivalent to the age of the patient plus 3 mm! Tracing out these two components of this relationship and measuring the actual distance between the two on the tracing paper gives the clinician a quick and easy verification that a pair of upper first molars are, in fact, drifted mesially due to both upper C's being prematurely lost. Should only one C be lost in the arch, such cephalometric verification would not be necessary as the arch segment remaining intact with the C present would verify mesial drift of the opposing quadrant by simple model analysis and visual inspection. Should the upper arch be intact but the lower arch in turn exhibit this phenomenon, the case will reflect the common Class I dental relationship of the adult dentition. This is evidence enough that lower quadrants have drifted forward into the lost C space as the normal first permanent molar relationship for the mixed dentition stage is a *flush terminal plane,* not dental Class I molar interdigitation. The only way such a molar interdigitation would be possible would be if the uppers were back too far (nearly impossible), or if the lowers were forward too far (which they invariably are in a lost C space closure situation). When upper C's are gone, but lower deciduous cuspids are intact, the dental relationship of the upper and lower first permanent molars assumes the relationship of a dental Class II. Here molar distalization is required, not mandibular advancement, to correct the dental Class II which again is verifiable cephalometrically. Should, by some rare set of circumstances, all four C's be missing with resultant space closure, the mixed dentition analysis, application of Ricketts' rule, and common sense would indicate distalization techniques to be instituted *first* prior to the consideration of any sort of lateral arch development. The same may be said for the crowded-out deciduous cuspid. It is pushed labially and cannot provide its normal space-holding functions at the corner of the dental arch and invading posterior teeth will invariably migrate mesially wherever they can. Though arches may in fact be narrow laterally, if they also have missing C's or D's allowing arch length loss due to posterior quadrant mesial drift, they are also short anteroposteriorly, which only falsely accentuates the arch width discrepancies.

As previously stated, distalizing posterior quadrants is relatively easy in the early mixed dentition as the permanent second molars are so far down in the developing alveolar crest that they offer little or no resistance to the distalizing effects of the sagittal appliance.

Another factor to consider is the angulation of the anterior incisors. Extremely lingually verted anteriors may invade some of the space represented by the lost C. This is again verifiable by the use of cephalometrics and checking such values as those of the interincisal angle or the upper incisal angle or lower incisal angles of the Bimler analysis or the incisor-mandibular plane angle (IMPA) of the Tweed analyses to see if labial crown torque is required. Once the C space is opened by the amount required by the molar's mesial drift component of the space closing (determined cephalometrically and by interarch comparison of the flush terminal plane), fixed Straight Wire mechanics may be employed in the form of the Brem Utility arch to impart desired arch expansion and correct remaining labial crown torque as needed. The point being made is that the direction of development in these circumstances is primarily anteroposterior first, then only laterally if need be.

Yet even with these technical considerations aside, a clear understanding of the principles involved in mixed dentition arch length loss correction may be derived from a simple consideration of the basic tenets of arch-lengthening and arch-widening appliances. The arch-widening appliances, such as the Schwarz, Jackson, or other similar devices are designed to move posterior quadrants away from each other laterally across the arch. This may in fact provide first a generally wider arch but not necessarily a longer arch, at least not that much longer. It may prove useful to do so in order to provide an arch closer to the more accepted mean values of arch width relative to the size of the teeth involved and may provide more room to align crowded anteriors, including cuspids, across the *front* of the arch. This is essentially a function of increasing the purely lateral dimension component of the actual arch length which is a combination of both components of *width and length* (which means anteroposterior length). For the purposes of clearer understanding, we must accept that both the deciduous and permanent cuspids, which sit on the corner of the arch where the dimension of width laterally changes to a dimension of length anteroposteriorly, assume the role of posterior teeth and should be thought of as such rather than in terms of anterior teeth. This is especially true in lost C situations. When resultant mesial drift occurs into the space, it is by teeth that reside on the antero-posterior length component of the arch, the posterior quadrants, not on the lateral dimension component, as do the anteriors. Therefore, to correct such anteroposterior arch length deficiencies, appliances should be used that ad-dress *this* dimension directly in an *anteroposterior direction* as do the Sagittal appliances. To illustrate this more readily in mathematical and geometric terms, take the following example. If a permanent cuspid is crowded on each side by 2 mm of arch length loss in a given arch by virtue of sitting at the corner of the arch where lateral and anteroposterior dimensions meet, if the posterior quadrants are each distalized 2.4 mm, the arch may be rounded out and the cuspid crowding reduced. Yet if the case is developed in a purely *lateral* direction, it might take up to 8 mm per cuspid to relieve the potential crowding for a total of 16 mm across the width of the entire arch! It is also estimated that over 60% (5 mm) of the original 8 mm (10 of the 16 mm) is highly susceptible to the ravages of relapse. This places the posterior quadrants in an extremely unstable situation and all this instability is right in the future path of the gigantic forward thrust of the second molars that are lying in wait down in their developing embryonic buds in the developing alveolar processes. When posterior permanent deciduous teeth are lost prematurely, arch *length* is lost, not arch width. The concept of the deciduous cuspid being a posterior tooth makes it reasonable that distaliza-tion procedures should be employed first to regain the lost length prior to considerations of any possibly attending arch width discrepancies. This is why mixed dentition crowding, or potential crowding, often respond so well clinically to arch-lengthening procedures effected via the distalization of posterior segments with basic Sagittal appliance technique and relatively infrequently require arch-widening techniques. Distalization (to a more posterior, naturally wider point in the arch) has a certain modicum of arch widening inherent in the process. If initiated early enough, it is facilitated with ease. If initiated in the late mixed dentition stage with the benefits of second molar extraction, it is still facilitated with ease. This early mixed den-tition type of treatment represents one of the important exceptions (and there are others mentioned later) to the "develop laterally first" axiom, which is more applicable to the *early adult* dentition stage of development where the correction of true arch width lateral deficiency problems becomes a race against time.

DIRECTIONAL DECROWDING

On the heels of the phenomenon of the lost C trap follows what may be one of the singularly most important concepts regarding the solving of orthodontic treatment problems on a daily clinical basis, the notion of "direc-tional decrowding." Dental crowding is one of the major aspects of any type of malocclusion and is a result of the collapse of the dental arch in either an anteroposterior direction, a lateral direction, or the most common variety which is a combination, to varying degrees, of both. Since it is of such clinical importance to the practitioner, and its proper correction is so important to the successful outcome of the treatment plan, understanding of the principles of decrowding arches becomes critical. Since the type of arch that exhibits relatively equal amounts of both lateral and anteroposterior collapse appears at first to be the most difficult to decipher and treat successfully, we will first examine the problem at its extremes: (1) cases that are crowded as a result of nearly entirely lateral collapse, and (2) those of almost entirely anteroposterior collapse. Obtaining a categorized and clearer picture of the therapeutic approach used to handle these simpler types of single element crowding of the crowded arches makes for a more organized and methodical approach to dealing with cases that may at first *appear* more difficult and confusing by virtue of exhibiting a considerable amount of *both* elements of crowding simultaneously. One must first understand the extremes before one can understand the means. Previous to the changes in thinking concerning the relief of dental crowding by means of extracting teeth, the problem of gaining arch length in cases of the severe jumbling and crowding of teeth in the arch was "solved" by the extraction of bicuspids.[23] On the surface this seemed like an easy and expedient way out of the dental crowding problem, albeit seemingly this was done in complete disregard for any orthopedic considerations on a deeper level. And even though the bicuspid extraction technique offered the benefits of immediate space gain in the anterior half of the mouth with respect to arch length, ironically, in the long run it did not necessarily relieve the problem of crowding of certain other teeth in the posterior portion of the dental arch.[24] This phenomenon clearly expresses itself in the form of that age-old posttreatment nemesis of the early orthodontists — relapse! When cases relapsed, the teeth didn't drift farther apart, they drifted closer together resulting in rotations, especially in the anterior regions. And in the *anterior* regions, by geometric and stereoscopic necessity, rotations give up space, and that means shortened arch length! In retrospect, it may now be seen that this is often a result of the failure not of the patient to wear the retiners long enough, nor of the clinician's particular appliance technique, but rather of the failure of the treatment plan to remove one of the *major contributors* to anteroposterior crowding, the second molar! Not every individual actually possesses second molars that are capable of thrusting the entire dental arch forward to the point of causing collapse of the arch and dental crowding. Some individuals' second molars are much more "anterior-thrusting" than others. There is currently no way of determining *which type* a given patient might have other than the belated telltale signs of the status of the degree of rotations, or anteroposterior forward drift of permanent teeth in the dental arch as it is developing. Yet often that alone is enough of a clue.

Anteroposterior crowding of the dental arch can only result from an excessive expression of one of two (or a combination of the two) forces on the arch. The first is the force exerted on the anterior portion of the dental arch in primarily a posterior direction by the perioral musculature. As biological forces go, it can be quite formidable as is evidenced by the Class II, division 2, angulation to the upper anteriors seen in that type of malocclusion.[25] The second type of force is that of the thrust of the second molars (as well as the other posterior teeth in the quadrant actually) on the dental arch in an anterior direction. As biological forces go, this one can be enormous! When the forces from the perioral musculature in a posterior direction meet the forces from the second molars in an anterior direction, the teeth in the dental arch will bear the brunt of the "collision" at about the halfway point, the cuspid area. If the integrity of the arch is great enough to withstand these forces, everything stays put. If it is not, the anterior teeth and posterior teeth are forced just a little closer together with the result that the corner of the arch buckles and the cuspids become crowded out labiobuccally. This is the characteristic appearance of an arch suffering primarily from collapse in an anteroposterior direction. The four anterior teeth, be they uppers or lowers, are in reasonable lateral alignment across the front of the arch with their respective interproximal contacts in reasonably proper proximity to one another, relatively free of major rotations. The posterior teeth, bicuspids and molars, are also in a fairly "straight line," contacts all approximating properly. It is just that as a whole, the posterior quadrants are drifted bodily forward. Thus the cuspid is deprived of its normal amount of linear space on the corner of the arch (about 7 to 9 mm) and as a result forces its way past the distal contact of the lateral in an anteroposterior direction, the only way it can, and the resultant crowding of the arch becomes manifest. Only the slightest collapse laterally may be evident, but this is due primarily to the fact that the teeth in the posterior quadrants have drifted forward to a slightly narrower anterior portion of the dental arch.

Treatment for such classic anteroposterior collapse of the arch follows the simple reversal of the process by which the arch collapsed in the first place, that is, development of the arch in an anteroposterior direction once again, and that means Sagittal appliances. Correction may take the form of second molar extraction and distalization of the posterior quadrants until the crowded-out cuspid may be repositioned at its proper place on the arch once again. Or it also may take the form of first repositioning the anteriors to a more correct interincisal angle by imparting labial crown torque to them first, using second molars as anchorage in accordance with proper Sagittal II technique; then once that component is corrected, the second molars may be extracted and the remainder of the correction completed by distalizing the posterior quadrants as necessary, in accordance with proper Sagittal I technique. The selection of which method to use is determined cephalometrically, or by simple visual inspection if the Division 2 retroclination of the anteriors is great enough. The key to the fact that anteroposterior arch development is the treatment of choice is the spread of the four anteriors across the front of the arch. If the collapse is primarily in an anteroposterior direction, these anteriors, upper or lower, will remain intact and uncrowded, or nearly so. The arch will be near Schwarz or Pont's corrected indices for width and the cuspids will also be blocked out labiobuccally, evidence of the anteroposterior collapse.

On the contrary, if collapse of either arch is primarily in a lateral direction the four anteriors will most likely be jumbled, exhibiting various forms of crowding and/or rotation. The contact between the distal of the permanent cuspid and the mesial of the first bicuspid will usually be disrupted to some extent, or if not that, then the disruption occurs between the mesial of the cuspid and its adjacent lateral. The anteriors may also be excessively "bowed" out labially causing a very pointed appearance to the outline of the anterior part of the arch. If by some miracle the four anteriors retain their integrity of lateral spread across the front of the arch, remaining free of rotations, jumbling, or other forms of crowding, and lateral collapse is still present, it will at once be obvious to the eye as the arch form would be quite distorted with the extremely lingually positioned bicuspids and molars. Treatment here is obviously a matter of lateral development. The permanent cuspids must be far enough from each other across the front of the arch to allow the proper alignment of the four anterior teeth that must be positioned between them, an alignment free of rotations or any other form of crowding. The key to seeing that this type of arch is crowded due to *lateral* collapse of the arch form is the loss of the integrity of the spread of the four anteriors in conjunction with moderate to severe deficiencies in Schwarz or Pont's indexed values for width.

Now that we have seen how to "decrowd" an arch that has collapsed either laterally or anteroposteriorly, it may be more clearly understood as to how to view the slightly more complex problem of decrowding an arch that is collapsed both laterally and anteroposteriorly.

If narrowness of the arches exists, it is due to a specific reason. That reason is believed to be an imbalance in muscle function. The shape of a dental arch may be simplistically thought of as the line of demarcation be-

---

Figure 5-6 Directional decrowding. **(A)** Being on a curve and due to its trapezoid or nearly triangular shape, upper cuspid crowded out and 2 mm short of arch length results from posterior segments drifting forward approximately 2.4 mm. **(B)** To regain 1 mm of space for cuspid, posterior segments would have to be distalized 1.2 mm along crest of ridge, and to gain 2 mm for cuspid, posterior segments would have to be distalized 2.4 mm. **(C)** However, to gain 1 mm of arch space for each cuspid by means of lateral development, each arch would have to be moved 4 mm laterally for an increase of total arch width of 8 mm (5 mm of which is quite likely to relapse back); to gain 2 mm of arch space for each cuspid, each would have to be moved 8 mm laterally per side for a total of 16 mm (10 mm of which would be suspect with respect to stability). The reason stability is a problem here is that teeth are being forced into an area where they do not naturally belong. Lateral collapse was not the problem to begin with, but rather the crowding was initially of an anteroposterior nature. **(D)** Directional decrowding of arch implies choosing correct method that most nearly reverses how arch came to be crowded in the first place.

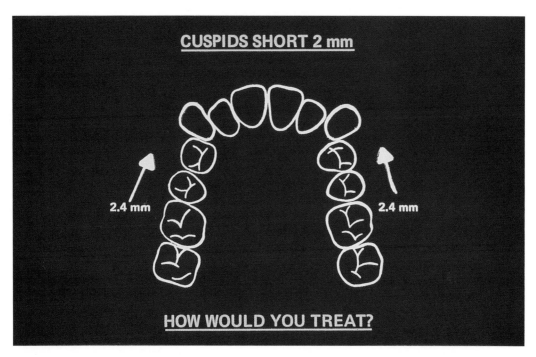

(A)

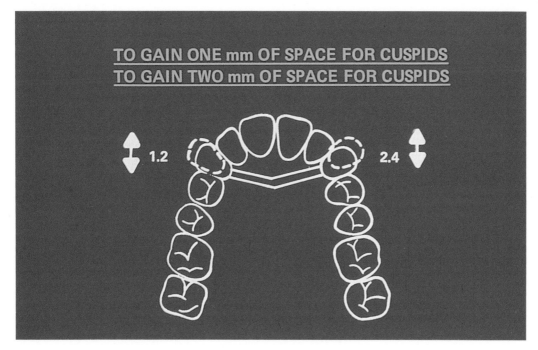

(B)

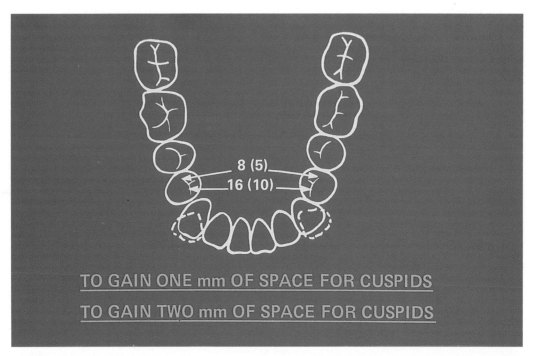

TO GAIN ONE mm OF SPACE FOR CUSPIDS

TO GAIN TWO mm OF SPACE FOR CUSPIDS

(C)

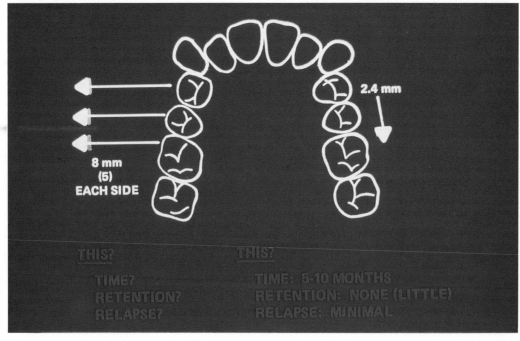

(D)

tween the forces pushing out and the forces pushing in, with the teeth and even the alveolar processes occupying the neutral zone between these two opposing forces. Improper arch form may be thought of as an expression of an imbalance in either direction of these two counteracting forces. If that imbalance is great enough and is shifted in favor of the external force in primarily the lateral plane, it will cause a substantial collapse in the arch and its aberrant state must be addressed directly by means of active lateral development appliances that not only restore the outline of the dentition to a more acceptable level of arch form, but also can "hold their own" against the persistent intentions of the muscles to return to their old ways. Not only arch form correction, but also muscle retaining and rehabilitation are implied in all cases of lateral development. This muscle retaining and rehabilitation may often take the form of overcorrection and/or prolonged retention of active plates so common to efforts at lateral development or occur as the result of having enlisted the services of the muscle-oriented functional appliances that often follow active plate arch preparation.

However, in cases where lateral development is not critical, the decrowding of dental arches may often be best accomplished by combining the slight lateral and slight anteroposterior arch collapse correction efforts into just the anteroposterior lengthening of the arch alone! This is a concept that proves especially useful in the late mixed and early adult dentition stages and in those individuals of the *narrow* frontal facial type. It must be remembered that lateral development of dental arches has always been a venture plagued with the problems of relapse.[26-28] It must also be remembered that the facially corrected Schwarz and Pont's indices are only mathematical mean values. This means that though certain individuals' arch widths may fall on or beyond the mean values, an equally important number of cases will be found to be less than these values. It is difficult to predict prior to treatment the limits of tolerance to lateral development a particular case may exhibit. Therefore, it is often wise to "make peace" with the "external" muscles as soon as possible and avoid any forms of lateral expansion of the arches wherever practicable. Thus it may be seen that in certain cases a compromise might readily be struck between Nature and the treating clinician concerning the correction of the crowded, anteroposterior foreshortened but only *slightly* narrow arch in the form of relieving the crowding exclusively in an anteroposterior direction when only small amounts of extra development in that direction would be needed to completely correct and decrowd the case. This process, where applicable, accepts the arch width at the levels Nature has already preselected for the individual, provided it is also compatible with the demands of functional balance and harmony for that given individual. Very pointed arches are of course also very narrow, but seldom crowded. Lateral development is more associated with correction of arch form, less so with crowding, with the aforementioned four anteriors being a possible exception. Lateral development is a price that must justifiably be paid by the treating clinician, but only upon formidable demand. Serious consideration must be given to its circumvention wherever possible, resorting to more naturally stable forms of arch crowding correction such as *sagittal* development which may be on proper occasion truly substituted with impunity. In the posterior quadrants, sagittal development is always more stable than lateral development. Stability is often aided by listening to the arch width suggestions Nature has already made and trying, wherever possible, to comply with Her demands. Each patient is unique, never ordinary, never the same. The patients are separate and distinct individuals, not walking tables of statistical norms. Unnecessary or excessive amounts of lateral development may not be what is actually on their list of needs. Where decrowding is concerned, an enormous amount of arch length can be gained by development in the highly stable anteroposterior direction, *especially* when second molars are removed.

Directional decrowding is a matter of utilizing various model analysis methods to determine just how the arches became crowded initially. Also efforts should be made to determine as to what degree each component of total arch length, anteroposterior and lateral, has been compromised in the collapse of the arch. Though serious lateral width discrepancies *should be directly addressed,* one must remember that it is not to be thought of as being on an equal par as anteroposterior development. Its use must be governed with temperance and respect for the desire to "get away with anteroposterior development only" wherever the arch crowding-arch form-arch width situation permits. A decrowded, nicely rounded, very stable, but only slightly narrower than normal arch is a very sound and acceptable treatment result. There is a steadily growing contingency of modern-day clinicians, especially in Europe, who feel the strict adherence to Pont's tables represents, for a certain formidable percentage of patients, a slightly unrealistic treatment goal.

The key to correct use of model analysis systems, the Carey, Schwarz, Pont, etc, is in their *coordinated* use as a team to give the clinician direction in his treatment planning. Using only a Carey, for instance could lead to a false impression as to how to approach a case. Checking only the width of an arch and not its length or symmetry is also an unbalanced approach. Full knowledge of the meaning of the shape of the arches the patient presents before orthodontic therapy is begun is mandatory to correctly diagnose the individual case and select appliances for treatment. The more complete and thorough the gathering of information beforehand, the better the resultant delivery of care.

"The great end of life is not knowledge,
but action."

Thomas Henry Huxley

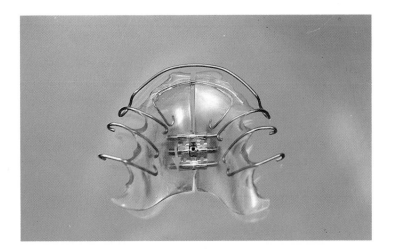

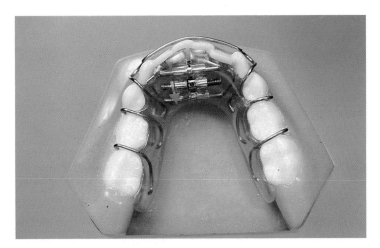

(B)

(C)

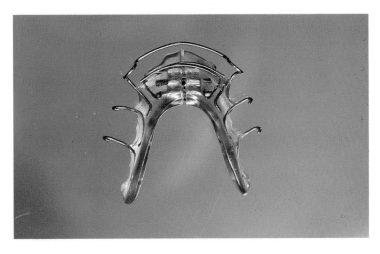

(D)

of these teeth will tip in lingually. This is possible *only* if the lingual acrylic in the palatal portion of the appliance behind the cingula of these teeth is reduced to give them room to move lingually. Remember the old adage, "Teeth move through bone, but not through acrylic." Therefore, as the appliance expands, the position labiolingually of the anterior teeth can be controlled. Once the position of the anteriors is satisfactory, and if more lateral expansion is necessary posteriorly, the action of the bow may be stopped by periodic relief of its tension on the teeth by opening it at the cuspid loop portion with a small three-prong pliers. This of course raises as well as advances the labial bow. Compensatory bends at the right-angle bend where the wire turns horizontally across the facial surfaces of the teeth bring the bow into correct position once again after being expanded at the cuspid loops.

Another point to remember is that the interproximal acrylic in the palatal area just lingual to the inner surfaces of the anterior teeth, on both upper and lower appliances, acts as an active orthodontic force during appliance expansion. Simply inspecting the position of these acrylic projections prior to expansion, and envisioning where they will rest after future expansion laterally, will divulge the effect they will have on the adjacent teeth. If the results of this process would be undesirable, reduce the acrylic lingually so that as the appliance expands laterally, it will not interfere with the pretreatment position of the teeth. By proper adjustment of the labial bow and judicious grinding of the lingual acrylic, crowded anteriors may be "expanded" apart and allowed to reposition themselves by means of "controlled relapse" from the expanded position on the arch, a function of wire and acrylic adjustment.

The same principles apply to activation and adjustment of the lower appliance. Selective grinding coordinated with controlled expansion allows individual teeth in the arch that are particularly out of place to receive specific attention. A small amount of ingenuity and a lot of common sense, after careful observation and deliberation, usually solves most cases of lateral development. Plus, the clinician always has the various model analysis systems to serve as an approximate goal and guide.

Another adjustment to be performed as the plate expands laterally is to relieve the acrylic adjacent to the tissues in the palatal vault area. Excessive reduction is not necessary but merely sufficient amounts of removal to allow the vault of the palate to "drop down in" a little as the two alveolar processes separate from one another. A millimeter per 2 months or so usually proves adequate. This allows a better fit of the appliance over the long term. As the posterior alveolar processes move laterally apart from one another, the edge of the palatal vault may have a tendency to lower itself at the junction of the horizontal and vertical sections. Simple checking with pressure indicator paste, similar to the technique used for checking for sore spots in a denture, will indicate any areas on the roof of the appliance that would benefit from slight reduction. Of course, the acrylic adjacent to the alveolar processes need not be reduced. That is where the orthodontic and orthopedic forces are delivered to the arch.

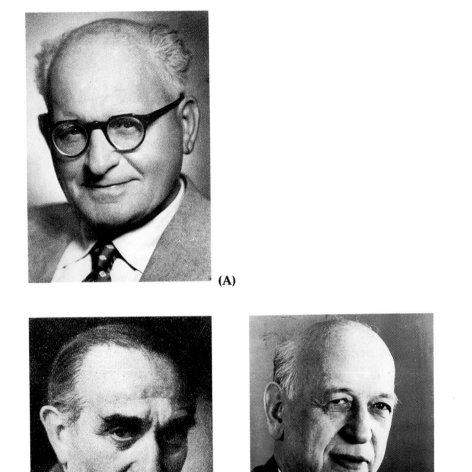

Figure 5-8 **(A)** A.M. Schwarz **(B)** A. Kantorowicz **(C)** Gustav Korkhaus

The frequency of opening the expansion screws is usually a function of patient age, arch development needs, patient cooperation, and various other physiological and logistic factors. Usually one-quarter turn of the expansion screw representing 0.25 mm every four to seven days is the rule; with shorter intervals in younger patients, slightly longer intervals in adolescents or adult patients. As the case expands laterally, periodic tightening of ball and Adams clasps is required. Adams clasps often must be "rolled upward" as the plate expands. The length of time required to attain ideal indexed width can be calculated by multiplying the number of millimeters short of Pont's or Schwarz the case is at the start by four times the number of days the patient waits between turns of the screw. Always leave a little more time for delays and as always, with all forms of orthodontic movement, overexpand a little, usually 5% to 10%, and retain 3 to 6 months in the mixed dentition, longer in the adult dentition.

If expansion takes place too fast, as in a young and very cooperative patient turning the screws every two to three days, the teeth will have a tendency to tip out buccally ahead of their apices. If this happens, longer periods of retention are required to allow function (or sometimes more active forces) to upright the teeth to a more vertical inclination buccolingually. But if expansion stays in the four- to seven-day range of screw activation, the function of the inclined plane action of the teeth keeps the roots, and bone, developing in the correct manner as the arch is developed laterally. *Function* is what prevents stripping of the subcoronal portion of the roots through the alveolus with resultant loss of gingival attachment and gingival crest.

The other critical factor to remember concerning the importance of function is that the acrylic not only pushes against the teeth as the appliance

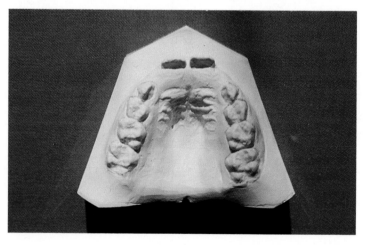

(A)

Figure 5-9 **(A) (B)** Pretreatment model and appliance for typical maxillary arch widening in mixed dentition. **(C) (D)** Posttreatment model and expanded appliance—note improvement of arch form to more rounded Roman arch shape.

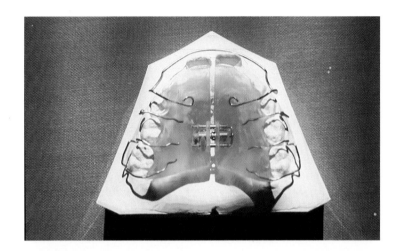

(B)

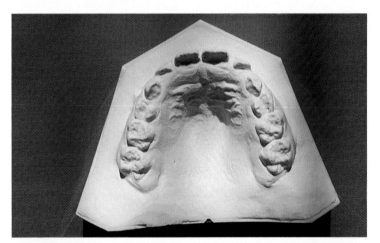

(C)

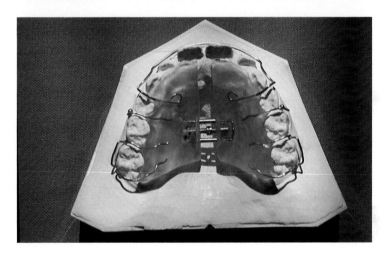

(D)

expands but also against the alveolar bone. This orthopedic/orthodontic combination is capable of moving the tooth and its alveolar process together as a single unit by separating the midpalatine suture in a process of "slow disjunction."[30,31] Function during this movement is always a goal.

THE TRANSVERSE PLATE—A SPECIALIZED APPLIANCE FOR UPPERS ONLY

The Transverse active plate is nothing more than an upper Schwarz plate with acrylic covering the occlusal surfaces of the teeth to act as a bite plate. This is handy as a palliative effect in patients who would benefit from immediate bite opening due to TMJ involvement. It also acts as an aid in "freeing up" the occlusion in cases where the movement of the upper teeth in a lateral direction might be inhibited by the inclined plane action of the lower teeth.

The Transverse is activated and adjusted in a similar manner to the Schwarz plate. It may or may not possess a labial bow, depending on needs. However, the use of the bow is quite common. As it expands laterally, each half of the plate requires the conventional adjustments of the acrylic just lingual to the maxillary anterior teeth to obtain the desired control, movement, or nonmovement of these teeth. This is usually done in conjunction with the use of the labial bow. Also, the palatal acrylic adjacent to the tissues of the palatal vault should be monitored and adjusted by slight reduction where necessary as the plate expands. The occlusion of the lowers against the upper acrylic bite planes is also periodically adjusted so as to remain balanced on both sides of the arch.

Figure 5-10   (A) Pretreatment status of maxillary arch with simple Schwarz plate in place shows pointed or gothic outline of maxillary teeth. Also note blocked-in maxillary right lateral incisor. **(B)** After period of treatment, note how arch form is both developed laterally and shortened anteroposteriorly to more acceptable outline. This is a combined product of widening of the appliance, contraction or flattening of labial bow, and "judicious" adjustment (reduction) of palatal acrylic adjacent to lingual surfaces of upper incisors. Note how acrylic lingual to upper right central was reduced to permit its retraction lingually by steadily flattening labial bow, but also note how the acrylic lingual to lateral was judiciously left intact to force tooth both laterally and labially as the two halves of the appliance were gradually expanded during treatment. Remember, in order to retract upper anteriors during treatment with Schwarz plate, labial bow must be kept in contact with labial surfaces of teeth and palatal acrylic of appliance must be reduced sufficiently so as not to act as its own interference to desired retraction. **(C)** Reduce palatal portion of acrylic slightly as appliance expands laterally to avoid sore spots and to allow palate to "drop in" slightly as it is developed laterally.

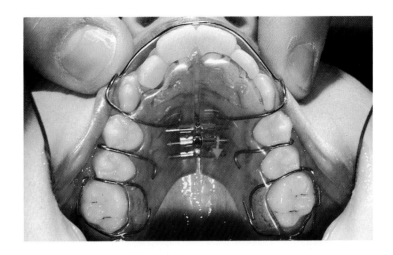

(A)

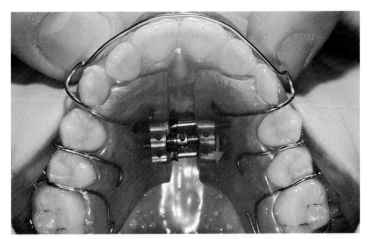

(B)

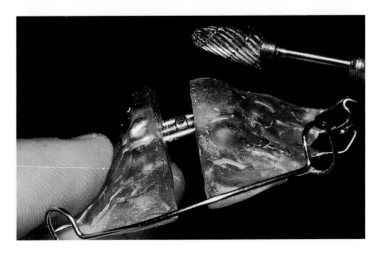

(C)

The Transverse appliance is constructed on a model of the upper arch with a wax bite registration of approximately 2 mm thickness between the posterior teeth to relate the lower model to the upper in such a way that comfortable and proper functioning interocclusal acrylic pads may be processed onto the plate. Actual measurement of the wax bite registration may prove handy in saving the clinician much tedious acrylic reduction.

The acrylic occlusal covering pads need only be 2 to 3 mm thick. Commonly, the construction bites for this appliance (as well as for the Sagittal) are incorrectly taken at too great a thickness of wax between the posteriors or with wax that is not adequately heated so as to be soft enough. Too great a thickness of a construction bite will result in an appliance with pads that are correspondingly too thick. And if the wax is not heated to the correct degree of softness, the appliance may not only be too thick in the pads but the bite will tend to be open in the anterior region of the plate as well. Pads that are too thick are more difficult for the patient to accommodate to and more difficult for the clinician to adjust. Two millimeters is all that is needed.

In the mixed dentition, if a Schwarz plate is used to treat a maxillary bilateral posterior crossbite, the use of acrylic coverage of the upper occlusals becomes important. If the "bare" Schwarz is used, as it expands it has a tendency to "drag the lowers" with it. The action of the inclined planes of the uppers against the lowers during function tends, in some cases, to cause the lowers to be forced laterally also. If the lower anterior area exhibits any degree of crowding, the occlusals of the uppers may be left exposed to possibly help with relief of same as the upper is expanded. If the lowers are in reasonably correct arch arrangement, coverage is often considered mandatory to prevent any further widening on the bottom. Of course, the most positive form of orthodontic control for the mandible during upper arch-widening cases such as described is with an appliance designed specifically for that purpose.

The Molar–Inclined Plane Action Debate

Quite a good deal of debate takes place among some clinicians as to the question of occlusal coverage of the upper posterior teeth with acrylic pads in the treatment of posterior bilateral crossbites in the mixed dentition. Those in favor of it say that it is useful because it prevents the inclined plane action of the lowers from interfering with the movement of the upper

---

Figure 5-11   (A) (B) (C) Maxillary Transverse Appliance. The Maxillary Transverse Appliance for adult dentition usually is constructed with two expansion screws and acrylic occlusal coverings approximately 2 mm thick. This allows appliance to serve as intraoral splint in TMJ patients and also helps free occlusion in bilateral posterior crossbite situations so bite may be corrected laterally without cuspal interference from lowers.

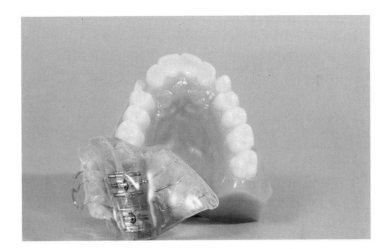

(A)

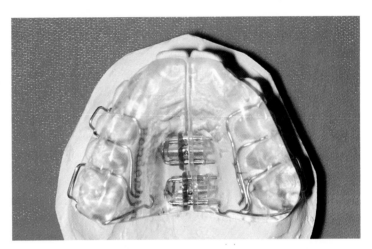

(B)

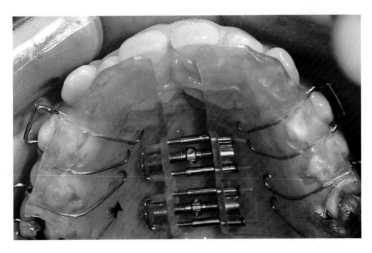

(C)

posterior teeth. This camp also feels the function of the pads on the upper teeth themselves act to keep the teeth upright and prevent tipping. They feel the force of the lowers on the acrylic bite surface of the appliance acts to stimulate the tooth in the proper manner and help "lock it in" to the appliance so that lateral development of the upper arch proceeds smoothly and correctly. They will also acknowledge that this process implies that the acrylic surfaces must be adjusted at the periodic checking appointments, about monthly, to keep the appliance balanced in a manner similar to a splint. This means keeping the occlusion of the lowers against the acrylic quite even and reasonably symmetrical so the stimulation is universal throughout most parts of the moving arch. After the appliance has completed the orthodontic movement on the upper, one is also left with the problem of rearticulating the teeth arch-to-arch once the problem of lateral development has been corrected. Careful observation of the patient on a timely basis will usually divulge the best time to withdraw the appliance and allow the case to start "settling in." Immediate and total withdrawal of the appliance would result in a high risk of some degree of relapse. Using the appliance as a nighttime retainer is advantageous at this point. Using a second appliance that is "next up" in the treatment plan, such as a Bionator, also acts as a form of retention for the newly obtained, increased arch width while completing the case. But when the Transverse is the last appliance in the treatment sequence, meaning the *only* removable appliance, the combination of function *without* the plate during the day and function of the plate in the form of retention during the night usually acts as an effective combination for settling a case in to correct occlusion. It may take a while, possibly as long or longer than it took to accomplish the arch widening in the first place, but it's an easy time for the patient. However, one must not expect miracles from this technique. If the arches are not reasonably close when the expansion is complete, further work with fixed or removable appliances on both upper and lower arches may be needed to bring about correct alignment buccolingually.

The opposing camp disdains the use of acrylic covering pads for the occlusals of the upper arch, saying that the inclined plane action of tooth against tooth is necessary to bring about the proper development of the arch. They feel "expanding" an upper arch with a Schwarz plate will also bring about some naturally occurring development of the lower. As the teeth on the maxillary arch widen farther and farther apart, the function of the inclined planes of their cusps on the inclined planes of the cusps of the lowers acts to drive the lowers buccally. If this is desirable and the desired action is completed on a given case, fine. If not, a lower appliance may always be called upon to help the case along. But this is true only in cases of mild to moderate bilateral posterior crossbite with some crowding of the lowers. It is not a technique indicated when both arches are articulating properly posteriorly and are free of any crossbite, yet still mutually collapsed and both in need of lateral development. But this "occlusally bare" or uncovered-appliance theory leaves the followers of this technique with the problem of expanding the upper arch in a crossbite situation when the lower arch is free of any anterior crowding or lateral collapse. In such cases one would want to be sure no inclined plane action would spoil the lower arch. Some say use retention of some sort or another on the lowers during treatment of the uppers with the Schwarz plate. It is simpler to use the Transverse and protect the lower arch form with acrylic pads.

So the choice is up to the practitioner. Use the acrylic pads to cover the occlusals of the upper and "destroy" the functional occlusion, or leave them off and run the risk of inclined cusp plane interference or expansion of the lower arch where undesirable. Individual diagnosis of each case will usually dictate the better choice. The point to remember is that it is not the appliance that is the key but the doctor's ability to simply look in the mouth, observe the present condition, and use his skill and clinical experience to determine what is needed, and what is the best way to get it. When confronted with such situations, most clinicians after careful deliberation will do what works best for them in their own hands.

The construction bite for the Transverse appliance is the same as for a Sagittal. Schwarz appliances need no construction bite.

THE JACKSON APPLIANCE—A SPECIALIZED APPLIANCE FOR LOWERS ONLY

The Jackson appliance is used exclusively for arch development in the mandible. Though an upper Jackson appliance was developed, it was so inefficient that it has become obsolete and is seldom, if ever, used. The Jackson appliance is one of the oldest in the "body-wire energized" active plate repertoire. It dates back to 1887![32] It was in that year Victor Hugo Jackson published an article on an appliance he had developed for the purposes of lateral expansion of the dental arches. It was composed of German silver, spring gold, and piano wire! It also utilized a clasping device known as a "crib." These prototype cribs were inefficient but would be vastly improved by George Crozat a generation later. Like all the great founding fathers of orthodontics in America of that era, Jackson also published a book in 1904 entitled *Orthodontia and Orthopedia of the Face*. Even back then the distinction between these two aspects of the science was recognized.

The lower Jackson appliance is primarily indicated for the use in mixed dentition. It operates on the same principle as the lower Schwarz, that is, pressure is applied to the lingual surfaces of the lower teeth and lower alveolar crest by means of acrylic plates that fit snugly against them but do not cover the occlusal surfaces. The appliance does not usually possess a labial bow but does have the capability of having lap springs bilaterally on the lingual. The appliance has paddle springs resting against the cuspids and is held in place with finger or ball clasps only. This is due to the fact that slight vertical or "pumping" actions of the appliance are desirable.

Though the action of the appliance on the mandible is similar to that of the Schwarz, its source of active force for expansion comes not from an expansion screw but rather from a lingual body wire. The appliance is open across the lingual of the anterior region and the two acrylic halves are held together by a large lingual wire running the entire length of the lingual arch. This lingual arch body wire exits the acrylic on each side of the appliance just distal to the last molar. The wire comes out (not down) here and travels the entire distance of the lingual surface of the lower arch to the same place on the opposite side of the appliance. It is this wire that gives the appliance its springiness and provides the source of power for lateral development.

Adjustments

To expand a lower Jackson appliance, two Boley gauges and a three-prong pliers are needed. First, measure the appliance with a Boley gauge from right angle bend to right angle bend on the body wire where the wire exits the acrylic at the distal end of the appliance. Add 3 mm to this measurement. Measure the anterior part of the appliance from paddle spring to paddle spring with the second Boley gauge. Add 3 mm to *this* measurement. Now take the three-prong pliers and with the single beak on the tissue side and the double beaks on the tongue side, crimp the lingual body wire slightly at the midpoint of the wire just behind the lower centrals. It is desirable to expand the appliance in the preceding manner such that the distal ends separate by 3 mm, checked by the first Boley gauge. This expansion at the center of the lingual body wire opens up the appliance at the distal end, but by virtue of the design of the appliance and the geometry involved, this action brings the anterior parts of the two halves of the appliance closer together. Now taking the appliance in hand, bend the two acrylic halves buccally with firm but gentle pressure to the point where the distance across the paddle springs (or any other landmark spot on the anterior parts of the appliance that is consistently used) corresponds to the distance of the sec-

---

Figure 5-12   The Jackson appliance. **(A)** Maxillary Jackson appliance. **(B)** Mandibular Jackson appliance. **(C)** Lower Jackson appliance off model, viewed from above. **(D)** Close-up view of how finger clasps positively engage interproximal spaces, a clasping system far more practical for retaining springing action of appliance. **(E)** V.H. Jackson.
Figure 5-13   Adjustment of mandibular Jackson appliance. **(A)** Measuring distal extensions of Jackson appliance. **(B)** Expansion of distal ends of appliance laterally by crimping body wire with three-prong pliers in anterior lingual area—single beak on outside of arc, double beaks on inside of arc. **(C)** Measurement of anterior portion of appliance (prior to expansion of body wire which brings anterior arm tips in lingually as posterior extensions expand out laterally). **(D)** Holding body wire with pliers as vise, the acrylic arm is bent laterally. This is done on both sides of appliance equally to place appropriate load on appliance. Once this is accomplished, lap springs (crossover wires) may be adjusted with finger pressure or three-prong pliers to place appropriate forces on lower four anteriors as desired.

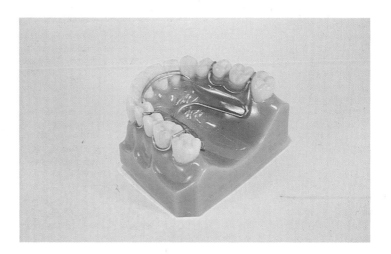

(A)

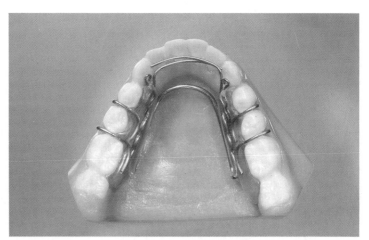

(B)

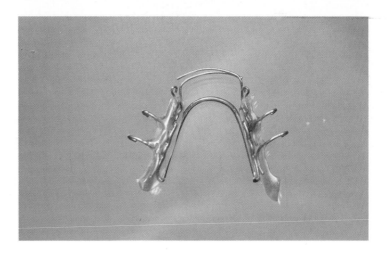

(C)

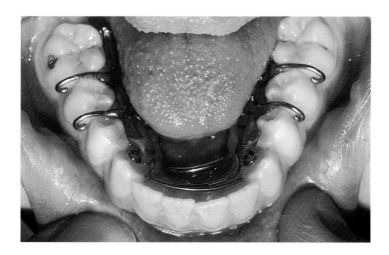

(D)

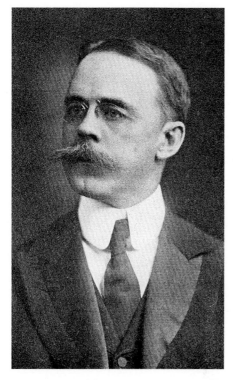

(E)

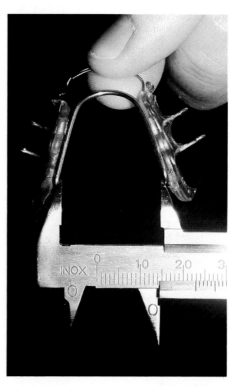

Figure 5-13A

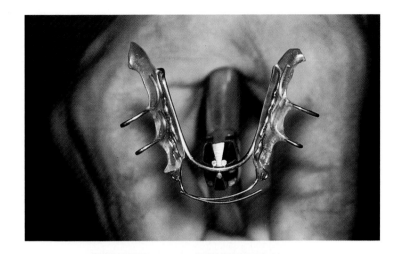

(B)

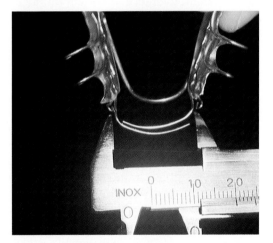

(C)

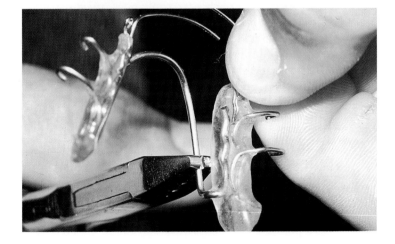

(D)

ond Boley gauge, the original distance plus 3 mm. This causes the appliance to be expanded equally by 3 mm in both the anterior and posterior area. This will give the patient the impression that the appliance "feels springy" while worn in the mouth. This is normal and a different sensation than that derived from wearing a Schwarz plate. As may be surmised from the preceding description of adjustments, this appliance requires a deft technique and adroit hands to adjust properly. Clinicians with Crozat appliance experience find this appliance easy to use, as the two appliances are adjusted in somewhat a similar manner. Finesse is required.

The lap springs (crossover wires) may be adjusted to apply labial pressure to the lower anteriors either singly or as a group. Again, fine adjustment, about the thickness of the diameter of the wire, in a labial direction is all that is indicated. This process may be repeated at routine checking appointments to keep tension on the wires constant. The same three-prong pliers is used here for these adjustments.

Certain problems are associated with the use of this fine appliance. First is patient tolerance. A certain number of patients are unable to tolerate the presence of the lingual body wire or the springy feel of the appliance as it is worn in the mouth. In these cases substitution of the Jackson with a Schwarz is indicated. Secondly, the lingual plates of acrylic must be constructed and adjusted properly so as to avoid engaging the lingual undercut of the myohyoid ridge. Since the appliance springs up and down slightly during wear, any impingement of acrylic into this undercut area would result in ulceration of the lingual mucosa at the crest of the myohyoid ridge.

Another problem to take into consideration is that which some clinicians refer to as "whiplash." This is the process whereby too much buccal flare is applied to the premolar area over too long a period of time during treatment resulting in the premolars being expanded out beyond the crest of the alveolus and being tipped out of the path of the arch. This may happen either bilaterally or unilaterally. Careful observations over more frequent office visits at the time when the premolar area is nearing the outer limits of its required development usually prevents this problem.

As with the Schwarz appliances, no construction bite is necessary for the Jackson appliance.

If a labial bow is desired for specific purposes in lower incisor movements or if intercanine development is imperative, the use of a Jackson appliance is usually abrogated in favor of a Schwarz plate, as the labial bow would all but eliminate the springing action of the Jackson. The one advantage of the Jackson over the Schwarz is that the Jackson may be expanded eccentrically in the anterior region only.

THE NORD CROSSBITE APPLIANCE—A SPECIALIZED APPLIANCE FOR ONE SIDE ONLY

The Nord crossbite appliance is a one-side-only lateral expansion active plate. It is designed for correcting *unilateral* posterior crossbites. It is similar in design and appearance to the Transverse active plate except that it has an acrylic bladelike projection running the length of the posterior segment along the palatal lingual line angle. This blade drops down to abut against the lingual surfaces of the lower posterior teeth on the side that has the normal bite.

Dr C. F. L. Nord presented his first paper on removable active plates utilizing expansion screws to the European Orthodontic Society meeting in Heidelberg, Germany, in 1929.[29] This marked the rebirth of popularity of active removable plates. Their primitive use dates back to the late nineteenth century, but as previously alluded to, their popularity was diminished with the rise of the fixed appliances of E. H. Angle. Though Nord's reintroduction of the removable active plate was at first met with only mediocre acceptance in Europe, it initiated a movement that was to be carried on by others such as Tischler, Von Thiel, and Schwarz. So many excellent modifications have been made to active plates over the decades by so many different practitioners, especially A. M. Schwarz, that none of the prototype appliances of Nord survive to this day except for the crossbite appliance.

Oddly, it is quite likely the single most incorrectly used appliance of the active plate family, not because of improper adjustment but because of improper diagnosis!

In cases of true unilateral posterior crossbite requiring one posterior segment to be moved laterally, the Nord appliance is indicated. The plate, as stated previously, is a Transverse appliance with occlusal pads covering the upper posterior segments and an acrylic blade extending from the occlusal lingual edge of the correct side down to abut against the lingual surfaces of the lowers. Thus when the expansion screw is activated, the plate tries to expand bilaterally, but the constant closure of the lingual surfaces of the lower molars against the blade of acrylic on the correct side acts as a form of anchorage to prevent that side from moving laterally. Then the only direction remaining in which the expansion may take place is laterally, the direction of the deficient quadrant. This results in eventual correction of the crossbite without moving the upper and lower arches apart on the correct side. Patients do quite well with this appliance, and many can even eat with it about as well as with the standard Transverse!

Once the expansion is complete, the blade may be trimmed off (which the patient greatly appreciates), and the appliance may be used as its own retainer. Retention should extend for a considerable period and be phased out gradually. Should slight relapse be evident, the plate may be closed slightly by turning the screw backward and reinstituting treatment once the trimmed stabilization blade is replaced in the form of quick-cure acrylic.

The problem facing clinicians is not in how to use the Nord crossbite appliance but rather *when* to use it. Cases of true unilateral crossbite are not quite as frequent as might be thought. When examining a patient suspected of this condition, check the midlines of the arches: either the frenums or the interdental spaces between the upper and lower centrals. If they align vertically and the case is still in unilateral crossbite, then the case is probably a "pure" unilateral crossbite. But if the midlines of the upper and lower arches are off slightly, the direction of shift is almost always in the direction of the deficient maxillary quadrant. As the mandible closes on the upper, it simply finds a more stable final resting place in an occlusion in which it is shifted to the side of the deficient maxillary quadrant to allow more complete intercuspation, even if the path of closure must be more deviated.

However, this is not as serious a problem as it may at first seem. The appliance is inserted and the treatment carried out until a portion of the unilateral expansion is complete to a point where, when the bite is closed and the appliance is out, the midlines align with an equal amount of deficiency exhibited by both posterior maxillary quadrants. Many cases of one-sided crossbite are actually bilateral in nature with one side more deficient than the other, and it is the shift of the mandible that disguises the case into appearing as if it is of a unilateral nature. Sometimes the collapse of the upper arch is symmetrical, not enough to cause a full-fledged maxillary bilateral crossbite but merely enough to cause the posterior cusp tips to align vertically over the lowers in a tip to tip arrangement. This causes the mandible to shift to one side or the other for more stable interdigitation. Having the patient close so the mid lines of the arches align vertically easily divulges this situation. A Schwarz or Transverse plate is the appliance of choice here as the collapse of the upper arch is symmetrical and not a true unilateral type. The shift of the mandible only makes it appear that way. Therefore, once the case is expanded unilaterally for a time, the acrylic anchor blade may be removed and the case continued on as if treated with a standard Transverse appliance. This circumstance occurs more frequently in the mixed dentition where it is easiest to correct. Adult unilateral crossbites often require finishing with fixed Straight Wire–type appliances. As with all forms of lateral development, the sooner the case is diagnosed and treated, the better.

> *"Ay, he does it well enough if he be disposed, and so do I, too. He does it with a better grace, but I do it more natural."*
>
> William Shakespeare
> Twelfth Night

Figure 5-15 Nord crossbite appliance on model; note unilateral deviation of midline cut to side that is to be unilaterally pushed laterally.
Figure 5-16 Anchorage side of appliance sports acrylic wing that drops down to engage lower posterior quadrant on anchorage side.

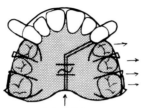

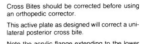

Cross Bites should be corrected before using an orthopedic corrector.

This active plate as designed will correct a unilateral posterior cross bite.

Note the acrylic flange extending to the lower arch.

The acrylic cut can extend the full length of the mid-palatine suture or it can angle to one side as shown here.

Use one screw in the appliance in the mixed dentition, and two screws in the permanent dentition.

WAX BITE FOR A CROSS BITE APPLIANCE

Place the warm Modern Materials Mfg. Co. Shur Wax (Pink Base Plate Wax) on the upper posterior teeth leaving the anterior teeth free of wax. Have the child close slowly in his natural centric bite until there is about 1½ mm of space between the upper and lower posterior teeth.

Chill in cool water.

FORESTADENT SCREW
#150-1322 (6mm Expansion) or
SCHEU SCREW #714 (8mm Expansion)

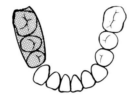

Figure 5-14

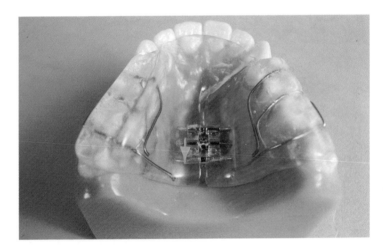

Figure 5-15

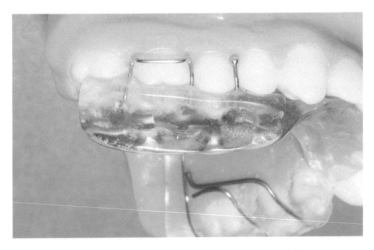

Figure 5-16

What we have discussed so far are a few basic methods of lateral arch development. As stated previously, various other techniques have been developed over the decades which may be utilized to combat this particular problem. However, an in-depth discussion of all possible methods would not only be impractical at this point but also beyond the scope of this text. Lateral development with active plates represents one of the most basic and commonly used techniques which is capable of handling the greatest percentage of cases of that type that present to the clinician on a daily basis.

Some areas of endeavor to consider beyond this basic level are two appliances which represent disciplines on *opposite ends* of the spectrum relative to the approach to lateral development problems. Each appliance has its place in the total picture of treatment methods, and the clinician may wish to advance his knowledge and skill in these areas as individual needs and preferences dictate. One appliance relies on the gentle tension of wrought wires while the other relies on the brute force of an expansion screw. They are the Crozat appliance and the Rapid Palatal Expander.

THE CROZAT APPLIANCE

The Crozat appliance may be reasonably likened to an active plate stripped of all its acrylic leaving only the metal skeleton behind. The all-metal removable wire appliance relies on the tension produced by sprung body wires to produce the light and intermittent active forces that combine with the natural forces of occlusion to produce bodily tooth movement. It may be used for lateral development at any age except the late mixed dentition, where the lack of deciduous root structure obviates orthodontic-type force application to primary teeth.

History and Development

The first prototype of this appliance dates back to the turn of the century when Dr Ernest Walker of New Orleans developed an early forerunner of the modern appliance which he constructed out of gold and platinum wires.[33] Unfortunately, he died in 1914 before being able to meet Crozat, who graduated from the Dewey School of Orthodontia in 1916. The problems Walker had with his appliance were in the area of retention. The clasping mechanisms simply were not efficient enough. Dr George B. Crozat had been made aware of Walker's work from one of his instructors who also trained him in the use of the early appliances of V. H. Jackson. Jackson's appliances of that time made use of a special clasp design referred to as a "crib." But the cribs of that time were made of soft wires and retention was poor. As a result the early Jackson appliances met with poor acceptance.

When Crozat settled in New Orleans, he started seeing some of the patients Dr Walker had treated. Inspired by what he saw, he advanced the design of the appliance and improved the clasping mechanism of the cribs.

He drew on his experience and knowledge of the Jackson appliances to design a cribbing mechanism made from a harder solder and added a Roach-type clasp to improve retention. This design proved so successful and improved retention so much that the appliance took on the mechanical resemblance almost rivaling the fixed appliances.

He presented the "new" appliance to the orthodontic community in 1919 and began teaching its use to a small band of devoted followers. He was asked to speak before the American Association of Orthodontists in 1920.[34] But he was met there with only polite indifference. He addressed the same body again 20 years later with the same result. In the years between 1919 and 1964, a mere four or five articles appear in the literature concerning the appliance[35,36]: two by Dr Crozat and one by the eminent Martin Dewey himself![37] This lack of exposure in the literature plus the singularity of the methodology in the utilization of the appliance originally led to the development of a following of zealous practitioners that may be viewed by those unfamiliar with the technique as something approaching that of a cult, especially since clinicians of a gnathological persuasion have "homed in" on the appliance and the philosophy behind its use. However, in more modern times most operators take advantage of the speed and efficiency of fixed appliances to finish cases they treat primarily with Crozat appliances.

Dr Crozat did not believe in moving teeth by sheer force alone but rather by more natural methods using light and intermittent forces allowing function to have its way. The philosophy he generated also called for taking advantage of periods of rest. As a result it is not uncommon for treatment to easily extend over a period of years. By virtue of the tight clasping mechanism, the appliance allowed Dr Crozat to rotate molars. This relieves anterior crowding somewhat and also increases the vertical slightly. He could also distalize molars which moved them to a wider spot on the arch and this also increases vertical. But he was not an advocate of lateral expansion or development with the appliance! That was to remain for one of his students to bring to the forefront. He believed his appliance merely helped Nature bring about growth and development that was being hindered or misdirected. Natural function played a critical role in accomplishing the orthodontic objectives. Molar rotation was also one of the key objectives.

Dr Crozat died on October 2, 1966, essentially spurned by the majority of the fixed appliance–oriented American orthodontic community. But his philosophy and technique had other champions to carry on after him: Dr Wendell Taylor of Birmingham, Alabama, and Dr Albert T. Wiebrecht of Milwaukee.[38]

Dr Wiebrecht studied with Dr Crozat every year at his office in New Orleans for a period of over 40 years. He was also knowledgeable of the efforts of Dr Pont of France and his work with the indexing of values of lateral arch width measurements for ideal arch form. Wiebrecht used the Crozat technique to expand the arches actively out to the Pont's values.[39] This produced a great improvement in the problem of relief of anterior crowding as with wider arches and the distalizing techniques already developed by Crozat, the movement of anterior teeth became more readily correctable. He also advanced the design of the appliance to where now there are a few devotees of the system that use the appliance exclusively for the treatment of almost every form of malocclusion.

Dr Wiebrecht also taught the use of the appliance and advanced its capabilities to the point where mandibular orthopedic repositioning may be resultant to treatment. One way in which this happens is in the widening of the upper arches in Class II cases. As the maxillary arch is widened, it "unlocks" the arch occlusion which prior to treatment has been held distally by the occlusion in order to interlock lower mandibular cusps with the narrow upper arch but only back on a more distal, wider part of the upper arch. This results in the Class II condition. But as the upper arch is widened out, the mandible is free, via intercuspation guiding plane influences, to travel forward to its most natural position, thus effecting a change from Class II to Class I and relieving the compression of the temporomandibular joint. Like Crozat, Wiebrecht's philosophy was oriented toward the use of gentle pressures and reliance on function to develop the natural growth potential of the maxillofacial system rather than the active forceful movement of teeth to a predetermined place. They are in good company as similar views form the basic tenets of the "therapeutic matrix" concepts behind the treatment philosophies of one of the great German orthodontists, Hans Peter Bimler.

Appliance Design

The maxillary Crozat appliance is composed of omega-shaped palatal body wire usually made of 16-gauge tempered Nichrome, or formerly gold, with the bow of the omega across the roof of the vault of the palate facing the premaxilla (the opposite direction of the Coffin spring in the Bionator). The base of the omega loop descends from the roof of the palate on each side to the lingual surface of the maxillary first molars where it attaches to the crib or clasping mechanism. Occasionally, this palatal body loop may be reversed and run posteriorly for special cases. The body wire is bent in such a way as to come as close to the palatal tissues as possible without impingement.

The cribs, which almost always are attached to the first molars, must fit precisely in order to provide the formidable retention necessary to carry out the desired orthodontic movements without dislodging the appliance. Accurate stone models must be trimmed slightly at the gingival area to accentuate the anatomy to allow the crib to fit properly. Stone representing the gingival tissue is trimmed, not the teeth. Crib wires were traditionally made of 21-gauge gold; 0.7-mm tempered Nichrome is now used almost exclusively. The crib design, essentially circular, encompasses the entire tooth

---

Figure 5-17 (A) (B) (C) Basic maxillary and mandibular Crozat appliances. (Figures B and C *courtesy of Dr Jerry Barnes, St Paul, MN.*)

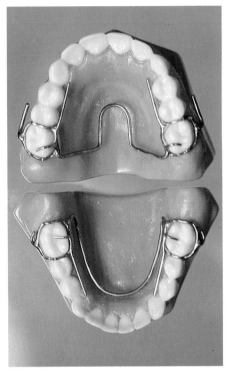

(A)

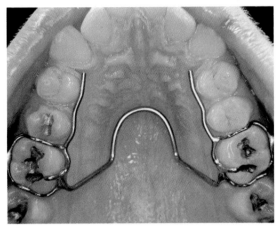

(B)

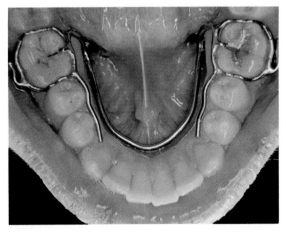

(C)

and by virtue of its horizontal and vertical components, which are usually parallel to each other, takes on the appearance somewhat of two Adams clasps soldered together buccal to lingual. The crib is made on a surveyed cast to reveal the height of contour on the molars they encompass. The horizontal components of the crib should rest just on the survey line and be parallel not only to each other but to the buccal cusps as well. To increase retention, Roach-like clasps called "crescents" are added on the buccal or labial of the crib just below the height of contour and are extended into the mesial and distal undercut areas. Small holes are drilled into the cast at these areas by the laboratory technician to facilitate construction of the appliance. This is why the crescents must be shortened by cutting them so they just clear the contact area on the path of origin and insertion. After they are retrieved from the casts on which they have been made, this may be done

---

Figure 5-18 Maxillary Crozat appliance. The basic appliance is composed of the following standard components: (1) The body wire, which is omega-shaped in maxillary appliance and is adjusted in a manner identical to body wire of Jackson appliance in mandible. (2) Both upper and lower appliances are held in place by circular clasping components called cribs. These cribs always possess (3) occlusal stops to prevent overseating of appliance and (4) crescents (shown here adjusted out and away from embrasure area for better visualization), which are small buccal clasps soldered to buccal surface of crib wire. They are made a little too long by drilling small holes into buccal interproximal spaces of construction model. Therefore they must be ground and adjusted by hand to exactly proper length to allow proper seating and retention in mouth. They are ground back to proper length with common green stones or heatless stones and set with small oculist pliers by crimping them in toward interproximal undercuts. (5) Lingual arms (which may be bent according to contours of bicuspids or left straight) extend from lingual portion of crib and are used to flare bicuspids buccally. (6) Extensions from buccal portion of crib (sometimes used for Class II elastics) on maxillary appliance are referred to as 1/2-high labials. Auxiliary springs are often placed on lower (similar to lap springs or criss-cross wires) to control lower anteriors.

Figure 5-19 Crozat appliance adjustments. **(A)** Holding the three-prong pliers in this fashion on omega loop of body wire of this maxillary Crozat will expand molar cribs outward but bring tips of lingual arms inward. **(B)** Holding the three-prong pliers in opposite fashion on body wire of this mandibular Crozat will contract molar cribs inward but bring tips of lingual arms outward. **(C)** To rotate molar cribs (usually counterrotation buccally after expansion of body wire), place three prongs of pliers around junction of body wire and crib and using pliers as a vice **(D)** gently but firmly rotate the body wire away from the crib in a level manner in appropriate direction. **(E)** Lingual arms may be adjusted as needed for management of bicuspid teeth.

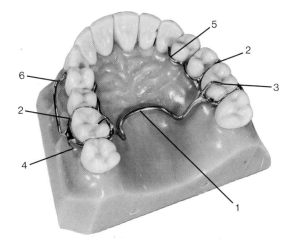

Figure 5-18

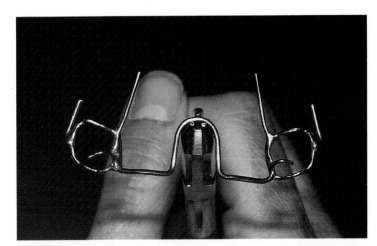

Figure 5-19A

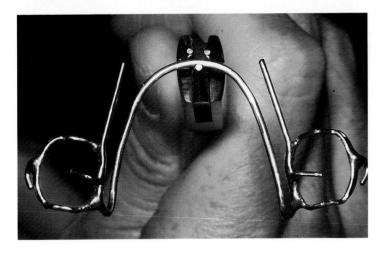

(B)

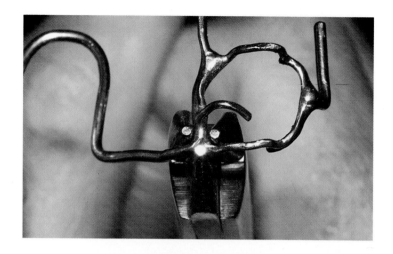

(C)

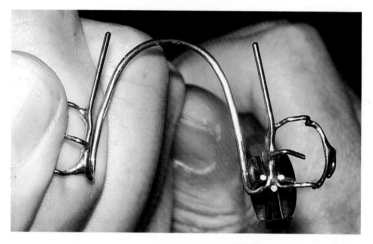

(D)

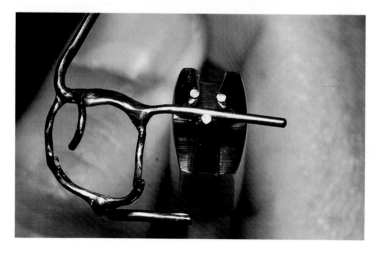

(E)

with the benefit of the presence of the patient to "try in" the appliances to determine where to place the cut. This may also be done ahead of time in the laboratory. After the crescents are cut, the cut edge is flattened by grinding with a green stone to improve contact with the tooth surface. Then the tip of the crescent may be "set," that is, adjusted so it engages the undercut area gingival to the interproximal contact. Back when primarily gold wires were used, they could be flattened by simply squeezing with a flat-on-flat pliers. Again 0.7 mm or 0.28-inch wire is most popular.

The crib usually has an occlusal wire rest running up into the lingual groove to prevent displacement of the wire gingivally.

Lingual arms, usually of 18 gauge or .036-inch Nichrome, are extended from the lingual surface of the crib forward to the first bicuspid area. They may be adjusted to apply pressure on the lingual surface of the bicuspids. Occasionally, an auxiliary buccal arm known as a half-high labial may be added.

The mandibular appliance is constructed in a similar manner with the lingual body wire running from lingual first molar to lingual first molar complete with cribs, crescents, lingual arms, occlusal rests, and auxiliary springs.

What these represent are the most basic of appliances. Additions may consist of short "pins" added to the body wire and sharpened at the tip to a point, or major arm wires or springs for the purposes of individual tooth movement. A certain form of pin with a 90-degree bend in it that was flattened on the end instead was referred to in the early literature as a "golf stick" because of its resemblance to that device. Now they are referred to as "pin-putters," a further allusion to "a more specific club!" (I wonder what their nickname would have been if Dr Crozat had come from Montreal where the major pastime is hockey?!)

By combining these basic elements with every conceivable type of loop, bend, hook, and wire, the variations of the Crozat appliance are limited only by the type of case presented and the skill and imagination of the treating doctor. Elaborate designs are possible which enable the treating clinician to deal with almost every type of malocclusion.[40] But with complexity of design also comes difficulty of adjustment and length of treatment time. However, in its basic form the Crozat is an excellent and efficient appliance for lateral arch development. It is inefficient only in its ability to produce finishing positioning and final alignment.

Adjustments

Since the appliance is composed of metal wires that constitute a single unit, adjustment of *one part* of the appliance affects *all parts* of the appliance. It is that principle that requires that the appliance be adjusted with extreme care and with very precise and knowledgeable technique. In the initial phases of Crozat therapy, the appliance is used to expand or laterally develop the arches. This consists of expanding or opening and flattening out the omega loop of the body wire on the upper, or the lingual arch of body wire on the lower, and counterrotating the cribs and lingual arms. To accomplish this requires a three-prong pliers, a flat-on-flat, an oculist pliers, and two Boley gauges.

After setting and adjusting the crescents, the new appliance should fit snugly in the mouth and be ready for activation. First measure the distance from the innermost lingual side of one crib to the same area on the opposite crib on the other side of the arch. With the second Boley gauge, measure from the tip of the right lingual arm to the tip of the left lingual arm and set aside. Now with a flat-on-flat pliers, gently compress the centermost point of the main body wire so that the arch is expanded so that the cribs have separated by 3 mm over their initial distance from each other represented by the first Boley gauge. This will also cause the lingual arm tips to come in closer to one another. Since the axis of rotation of the expanding arch wire is in the midline of the curve, as the cribs move out, the tips of the lingual arms move in.

Now the cribs must be counterrotated at their junction with the main body wire to bring the lingual arms into their proper position. With the three-pronged pliers, place the middle prong inside the loop of the crib and allow the body wire to pass between the two opposing prongs so a tripodization or bracing effect is realized. Now while firmly holding the crib to prevent slippage, use the pliers as a vice against which you rotate the entire rest of the appliance by hand so as to rotate the crib gently in a buccal direction. Do this slightly on both cribs so that the tips of the lingual arms are 3 mm farther apart than their initial distance represented by the second Boley gauge. Obviously, an adroit technique is mandatory. The appliance now has what is referred to as a "3-mm load" to it. When reinserted into the mouth, the "spring" of the appliance will offer a slight-to-moderate resistance to insertion. Once it is snapped into place, it immediately starts tipping teeth buccally, but the *constant functioning* of the teeth during swallowing, mastication, etc, keeps the molars upright and allows for proper bone deposition as the teeth move bucally. Upper bicuspids are limited by the apical base.

At approximately 4-week intervals this procedure is repeated, first measuring the appliance inside, then outside the mouth to determine how much expansion must be added to maintain the 3-mm load.

Crozat appliance methodology represents one of the most natural and logical of the disciplines of orthodontics. It is a form of treatment requiring the utmost in manual skills and creativity on the part of the clinician and produces results of which its proponents may be justly proud. But for all its elegant and erudite treatment procedures and philosophies, the technique is not without its problems. The greatest of these concerns both the patient and the doctor, and revolves around the issue of practicality.

Figure 5-20   (A) Auxiliary springs (similar to lap springs or crossover wires in active plates) are often added to Crozats, especially in lower anterior area, to manage incisor teeth. **(B)** After development anteriorly.

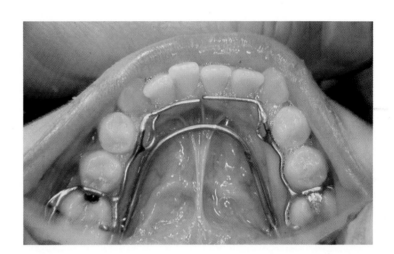

(A)

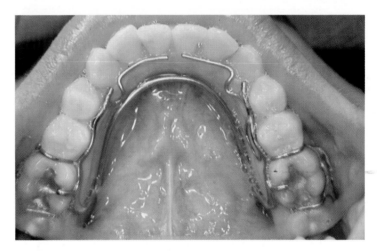

(B)

The cardinal feature concerning the patient relative to being treated exclusively with Crozat appliances is that of time. It is not uncommon for treatment in such cases to extend over 3 or 4 years; and since the appliance acts as its own retainer, this time period may easily extend longer. Patient cooperation becomes a problem over such periods of time. In an age oriented toward instant gratification and expediency in all aspects of life, the chances of patient "burnout" are high in a technique involving the volatile combination of both a long period of time and a removable appliance. As the case improves, patients weary of wearing the appliance are apt to leave it out, feeling the teeth look "good enough," and thereby fail to avail themselves of the final perfections capable with the technique. By virtue of being removable, the appliance is also subject to being damaged by the patient, especially in appliance designs of a more complicated nature. The slightest distortion could have far-reaching effects.

As far as the doctor is concerned, the problems associated with exclusive use of the appliance for the complete treatment of the malocclusion

Figure 5-21 Crozat technique is capable of true orthopedic development of dental arch as is depicted by these before and after cross-section views of maxillary arch. **(A)** Pretreatment condition of arch—note inclination of molars and level of their respective occlusal tables. **(B)** Posttreatment view—note entire maxillary arch is wider and molars retain their original inclination and level occlusal surfaces, showing that no tipping buccally has occurred.

Figure 5-22 Crozat appliance study case: early expansion in a 7-year-old. **(A)** Pretreatment study model of maxillary arch. **(B)** Initial appliance inserted with cribs on maxillary deciduous second molars and simple lingual arms extending to deciduous cuspids. This basic form of appliance was used for lateral arch development. Later as first molars erupted and anterior permanent incisors started to appear, **(C)** auxiliary springs were added to lingual arms in cuspid area to assist in controlling erupting anterior incisors, and distal extensions were soldered to body wire to engage first permanent molars. Note also how omega shape of palatal body wire has been flattened due to expansion of the appliance. A total of 12 mm of total arch width across the deciduous second molars was gained by this treatment. **(D)** Pretreatment study model of mandibular arch. Note there is no room for lower permanent lateral incisors to erupt. **(E)** Initial basic appliance inserted in mandible with similar construction, ie, cribs on mandibular deciduous second molars and lingual arms extending to deciduous cuspids. **(F)** As case progresses and permanent first molars erupt and permanent incisors appear, distal extensions and auxiliary springs are added to basic appliance to complete development of arch form. Note that not only is lower arch "decrowded," but an actual surplus of arch length exists as evidenced by diastemas present. A total of 6 mm across width of mandibular deciduous second molars was gained in this case. (*Courtesy of Dr Jack Hockel, Walnut Creek, CA.*)

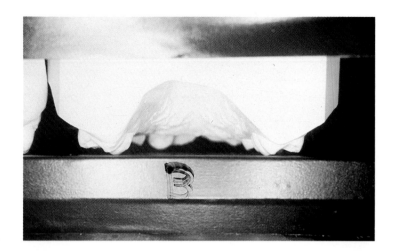

Figure 5-21A

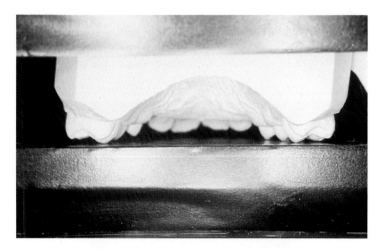

(B)

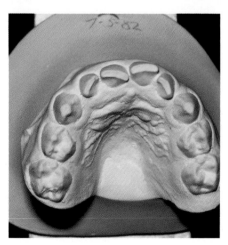

Figure 5-22A

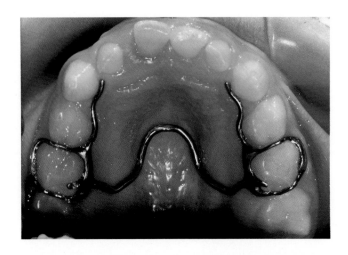

(B)

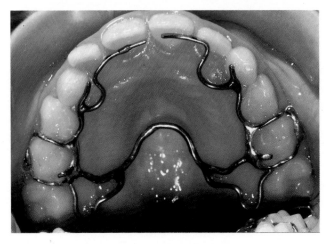

(C)

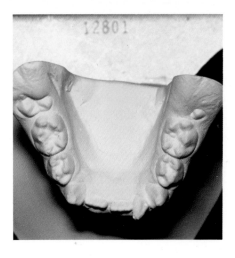

(D)

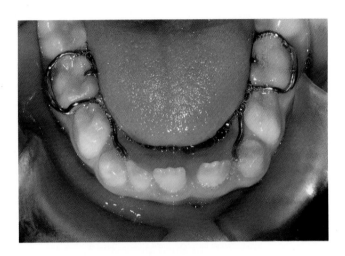

(E)

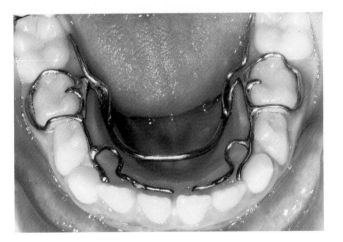

(F)

are far greater in number. The first is that of the skills and discipline necessary for proper adjustments. The seeming simplicity of the design of the appliance can be deceptive. When cribs are counterrotated, extreme care must be exercised to keep them at the original occlusal plane level so as to prevent vertical torque of the crib.

When breakage occurs, repairs are recommended to be done by the doctor himself to save the time loss of sending the appliance to a laboratory. But this in turn demands more of the doctor's time and requires extra training and materials. There was even a period in the early development of the use of the appliances that was dominated by the philosophy that "If a doctor can't make one, he shouldn't use one!" Thankfully, times have changed.

Another fact is that severe rotations of teeth other than the first molars are difficult to correct, as they are with any removable appliance. Torque of the roots also obviously presents problems. And though some mandibular orthopedic repositioning changes may be initiated by means of the use of intra-arch Class II–type elastics running from half-high labial hooks on the upper to buccal elastic hooks on the cribs of the lowers, far easier and quicker methods exist for this purpose.

Yet, in spite of some of the problems Crozat appliance technique presents, there are those practitioners whose skill and interest are of such levels that the future of the appliance seems assured. The Crozat appliance truly represents a valued alternative to certain lateral development problems in adult cases. The appliance will no doubt keep its rightful place in the armamentarium of the orthodontic community among the other great appliances and techniques that have been developed over the years.

Figure 5-23 Crozat appliance study case: late mixed dentition. In this case, use of lap springs is illustrated. **(A)** Maxillary arch with appliance inserted which is modified by means of extending would-be lingual arms to form lap springs to develop anterior incisors as well as usual lateral development in bicuspid area. **(B)** Completed development. **(C)** Mandibular appliance upon insertion with lap springs. **(D)** Completed development. (*Courtesy of Dr Jack Hockel, Walnut Creek, CA.*)
Figure 5-24 Crozat appliance study case: adult dentition. **(A)** Basic maxillary appliance, cribs on first molars, lingual arms extended to first bicuspids. **(B)** Developed case. **(C)** Basic mandibular appliance. Note small auxiliary spring added to tip of left lingual arm to aid in movement of left mandibular cuspid. Also, right lingual arm was initially shorter than normal until room was made for first bicuspid, which was originally completely blocked out to lingual. Later additional auxiliaries were employed to complete the development. **(D)** Note also how central grooves of lower first molars indicate molar rotation that was accomplished. (*Courtesy of Dr Jack Hockel, Walnut Creek, CA.*)
Figure 5-25 **(A)** The basic rapid palatal expanding appliance: a century-old concept. Its inherent relapse must be planned for, and compensation takes the form of overcorrection.

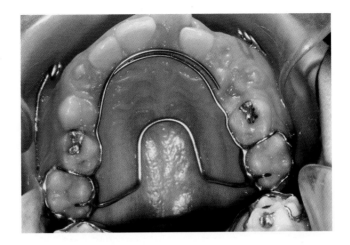

Figure 5-23A

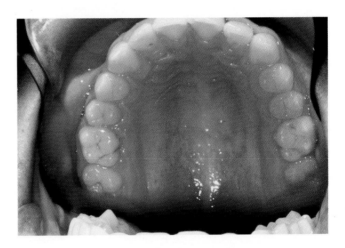

(B)

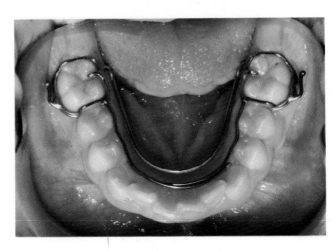

(C)

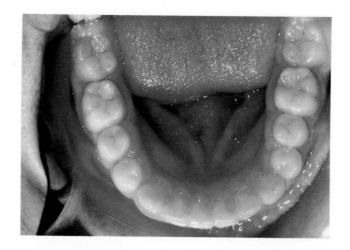

Figure 5-23D

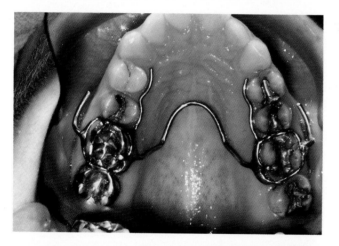

Figure 5-24A

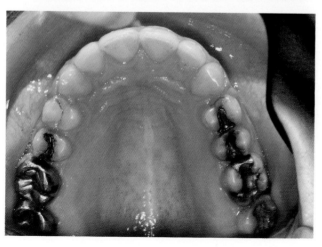

(B)

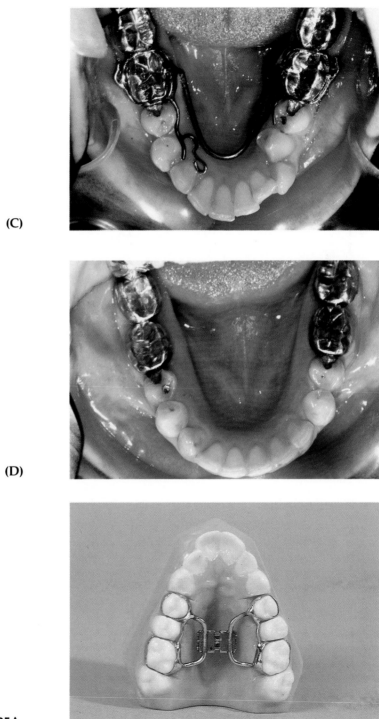

(C)

(D)

Figure 5-25A

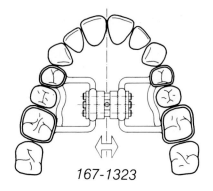

167-1323

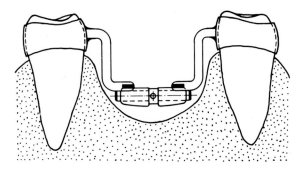

Figure 5-25 (B) Variation of basic Rapid Palatal Expander screw designs in Forestadent screw 167-1323. Its smaller body design allows it to be placed closer to surface of palate due to offset design of appliance arms. It opens to a full 10 mm, providing an extra 2 mm expansion over more conventional variety screws.

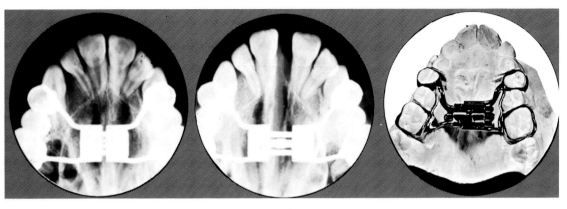

(A)   (B)   (C)

Figure 5-26 **(A)** Pretreatment x-ray of Rapid Palatal Expander in place in maxillary arch. **(B)** After activation (a period of time spanning about 2 weeks), note separation of midpalatal suture and diastema formation between centrals. This closes back together again spontaneously due to elastic memory of transseptal fibers. **(C)** Clinical appearance of appliance in mouth. (*Courtesy of OIS/Orthodontics, Wilmington, DE.*)

> *"Nothing great was ever achieved*
> *without enthusiasm."*
>
> *Ralph Waldo Emerson*

THE RAPID PALATAL EXPANDER

The Rapid Palatal Expander is a fixed appliance that is usually attached by means of orthodontic bands and/or stainless steel crowns to the maxillary first permanent molars and maxillary first bicuspids, or deciduous teeth, in the younger patient. Rapid expansion, by means of a fixed jackscrew, is obtained over a 2- to 3-week period by means of turning the screw twice a day and thereby creating pressures great enough to separate the palate orthopedically at the midpalatine suture. The appliance is stabilized and retained for a period of 3 to 4 months to allow the separated sutural edges to reapproximate by means of osseous healing. It is the most purely orthopedic appliance in the repertoire, with the possible exception of the Bionator. It is also one of the oldest. Its first appearances date back to 1860, the year of the first pony express, the election of Abraham Lincoln, and the secession of the state of South Carolina from the Union!

Controversial times indeed, and no less so for dentistry, for in that year a far-sighted genius of a man named E. C. Angell published an article entitled "Treatment of Irregularities of Permanent or Adult Teeth."[41] In it the author claimed he widened the palate by splitting it at the midpalatine suture by means of a metal appliance which obtained its force from a jackscrew. Since this was in the days before the advent of radiology, the evidence Angell cited was strictly empirical. As might be imagined, he met with extreme resistance as his ideas were considered by the bulk of the professional men of the time as being utterly absurd![42-46] What is incredible is that even after the development of x-rays, soon after their discovery in 1895 by Wilhelm Roentgen, the resistance to suture separation techniques remained adamant *in spite* of the indisputable proof provided by the radiographs. For nearly a century the Rapid Palatal Expansion appliance languished in a limbo of rejection and apathy.[47-50] Its resurgence to the forefront of modern-day orthodontic procedures may be chiefly credited to the crossing of two paths: that of the teacher Professor Gustav Korkhaus[51] and the clinician Dr Andrew Haas. They met at the University of Illinois in 1956 where Haas was a graduate student. The rest is history.[52,53] As the new champion of rapid maxillary expansion devices, Dr Haas has, through numerous research projects and lectures, made the old appliance "new" again but this time with a far more favorable level of acceptance. Indeed, "self trust is the essence of heroism." Finally, after 100 years, this technique is given its full recognition.[54-64]

Appliance Design and Adjustment

The Rapid Palatal Expander may be an all-metal device or may have acrylic additions to it. The first principle of its action is that it is fixed and not removable. Orthodontic bands are fitted to the maxillary first permanent molars and either maxillary first bicuspids or, if they have not erupted yet, deciduous first molars. In the case of the deciduous first molars, stainless steel crowns may be used. An impression is made with these elements in place. When the impression is removed, the bands usually stick to the teeth and must be accurately replaced in the impression and "sticky waxed" into position so the model can be poured. This also creates a void in the model to facilitate soldering. Once this is completed, if acrylic palatal portions are to be added, a .045 round stainless steel wire is made to engage the bands on the lingual surface and travel palatally so as to also engage the acrylic pad area. The expansion screw is then mounted and soldered into place along with the wires. The entire metal unit is now one piece. The acrylic is then added in two sections, one for each side of the appliance. It covers only the midpalatal vault area. The acrylic should be free and clear of the midline palatal screw area and also be polished to remove any irritating rough edges. Such appliances with the acrylic additions are considered more original and are definitely preferred by Dr Haas. Some clinicians, however, omit the acrylic entirely, feeling it only acts to irritate palatal tissues and fails to add an appreciable degree of extra stability to the appliance in the retention phase of treatment. Also, some practitioners will omit the bicuspid band or deciduous stainless steel crown in early mixed dentition stages and simply solder only the lingual arm, running it anteriorly from the lingual of the first permanent banded molar. The appliance is cemented in the mouth with standard fixed appliance cementation methods. Coventional methods of separation, ie, elastic separators, brass wires, loop separators, etc, may also be needed prior to cementation.

Once the appliance is securely cemented into place, the operator initiates expansion for the patient in the office at the initial appointment. The wire key or lever is inserted in the holes of the central cylinder of the expansion screw and rotated one quarter turn by pushing the key from anterior to posterior. A long piece of dental floss is tied to the loop handle of the key to prevent aspiration of the key by the patient should the key slip loose from the hands while turning the screw. Be sure to have plenty of length to the floss, at least 2 or 3 ft, for should the rare event take place that one is aspirated, there will be plenty of floss left to retrieve it. The first two turns are effected by the operator about ten or 15 minutes apart; then another one or two turns are also performed at the same intervals of time, but this time the parent or other adult responsible for the patient performs them under the supervision of the clinician. The person who will be performing the turning of the screw for the patient must be fully confident of his or her abilities to carry out these actions once the patient is dismissed. It is not difficult. The patients and parents are then instructed to turn the screw once in the morning and once in the evening every day until the procedure is complete. The patient is seen approximately twice a week in the office so that the clinician may maintain careful supervision of the progress. Expansion takes place rapidly as the suture is opened in the first week and necessary expansion is usually complete in 2 weeks or so. The first noticeable sign that suture opening is taking place is when a diastema starts to appear between the two maxillary centrals. The split in the palate occurs in a V-shaped pattern with the widest part of the separation taking place in the anterior premaxillary area and the more narrow portion of separation taking place in the posterior. The fulcrum of rotation for the inverted V-shaped space created between the two halves of the palate is in the area of the fronto-maxillary suture. Some alveolar bending and orthodontic tooth movement does occur also. Therefore, overcorrect almost to the point of developing a buccal crossbite before initiating retention. But since there are maximum forces being applied somewhere in the vicinity of 20 lb, this type of orthodontic movement or bending in the alveolus is minimal. Actual suture splitting is the major effect of the heavy forces used. What tipping of teeth buccally that does occur is another reason for the overexpansion. During the 3-month retentive phase of treatment, the functioning of the lower teeth on the slightly tipped uppers causes the uppers to upright themselves to a more favorable vertical position. But in so doing, they will also rotate on a horizontal axis which brings them back in again lingually. This, in combination with a certain amount of natural anticipated relapse, will bring the case into correct occlusion with the lowers.

Retention consists of simply tying the central cylinder of the expansion screw with brass ligature wire and allowing the appliance to remain in place for 3 to 5 months. This allows time for the bone to fill in the open suture area and for any uprighting that might be needed to take place as a result of function. The separated centrals usually close themselves at this time also due to the elastic transeptal fibers of the periodontal tissues of that area.

Skeletal Effects

The shape of the space opened between the two halves of the palate is always an inverted V type due to the resistance of the zygomas in the posterior area of the palate. Since the source of applied force is inferior to the zygomas and their bracing effect against sideways displacement, and since resistance in the anterior premaxillary area is minimal, absolute parallel opening of the suture, anterior to posterior, is impossible. The expansion will always be slightly greater in the anterior part of the suture. This is a beneficial effect also; if true parallel opening occurred all along the entire length of the palatal suture, the frontal processes of the maxillary bones would be forcibly moved laterally into the orbital cavities. Thus this pyramid effect to the opening causes greater width to be realized at the occlusal level than at the palatal level and so forth through the nasal cavity as one ascends superiorly through the maxillofacial complex. Generally the separation stops at the resistant point of nasion. Since some separation is effected in the nasal area inasmuch as the roof of the palate forms the floor of the nasal cavities, improved air flow is observed also. Early authors noted this effect and many, including Korkhaus, reported that the lowering of the vault of the palate contributed to the straightening of the deviate nasal septum. This technique brought favorable acclaim from many of the rhinologists around the turn of the century who were impressed with the improved respiratory abilities this technique brought.[65-72]

Though it has been generally accepted that palatal widening techniques improve air flow through the nose as an aid to mouth breathers and that the technique lowers the palatal vault and may straighten deviant nasal septa, there has been some controversy as to what happens to A-point. (A-point: junction of maxillary alveolar bone and maxillary basal bone taken at the innermost curvature from anterior nasal spine (ANS) to crest of the maxillary alveolar process.) Haas, Davis, Kronmann, and others have reported that A-point moves down and forward after treatment. Others contest this. It may, but if it does, it does not move much. Wertz reported an advancement of 1.5 mm; Haas reported increased Sella-Nasion–A-point (SNA) angles of 2.5 degrees, a slight increase at best. Haas also reported that in half of his cases A-point not only moved forward on the horizontal plane but downward on the vertical plane. The theory behind the forward and downward movement of A-point is founded in the mechanics of the movement and resistance of the bones during expansion. First, as for the forward movement, as the palatal halves are split, with the greater increase in the anterior region due to the resistance of the buttressing zygomas, the posterior tuberosities would be rotating about an axis in the posterior nasal spine area into the pterygoid plate area. This area is well fortified and were the tuberosities and their adjacent osseous structures to be rotated into them from a buccal direction, it would imply either bony resorption, an unlikely event in just 2 weeks, or the movement of the entire body of the palatal halves forward away from this area against which they abut. This would account for the advancement of the apical base of the denture in a forward direction if such should occur at all. The same is true for the downward movement of the A-point on a vertical plane. This is also felt to be the effect of the way the bones are disarticulated and rotated apart. But not every case demonstrates this phenomenon and when it does appear, it usually is slight.

Very little discomfort is experienced by the patient during expansion therapy. At the initial appointment when the appliance is "primed" with the first four turns, the patient will obviously experience a sensation of pressure or tightness in the maxillary arch. But this is usually well tolerated by the patient. The technique is best suited for mixed or early adult dentitions. In the late teen or young adult patient, the degree of calcification of the suture may necessitate less frequent turning of the expansion screw to a frequency of once per day. Sometimes headaches, dizziness, blurred vision, or facial pain are a consequence of attempts to split the palate too rapidly in the adult patient. Again, this is rare if the appliance is used at the correct time in the patient's growth and development, ie, the mixed or early adult dentition. Adult treatment past 20 to 23 years of age often requires modified techniques employing surgical osteotomies prior to insertion of the appliance.

Indications for Use

The most obvious choice for employment of the Rapid Palatal Expander is the case in the mixed or early adult dentition that exhibits a bilateral maxillary posterior crossbite as a result of deficiency of the maxillary apical base. As the deficiency may be rapidly regained, this appliance is an excellent choice and will give consistently good results. But certain factors come into consideration even for the ideal Rapid Palatal Expander case. The first is that as the vault is lowered, the bite also opens the vertical slightly as there is a certain amount of extrusion of the crowns of the posterior teeth due to the forces of expansion. This is due to the quite common event observed of downward movements of the maxilla. It averages about 1 to 2 mm of downward development. This then would lower the point of initial closing contact of the posterior teeth also and thus open the vertical. This would tend to cause the mandibular plane angle to open also and cause a slight distalization of B point on the mandible as it rotates back due to its arc of closure on the lower maxillary occlusal plane. Similar effects are noticed when denture patients suffering from lost vertical have what appears to be worn Class III-looking dentures replaced with new ones at more correct open vertical; the mandible appears to retrude back to normal Class I facial appearance. Less consistent is the observance of the downward and forward advancement of A-point.

This overall effect of lowering of the maxilla and possible advancement of A-point with concomitant slight distal rotation of the mandible due to the steepened mandibular plane lends this technique to the treatment of certain Class III malocclusions also. If the case is not too severe, the anterior as well as posterior crossbite may be corrected by rapid expansion as a result of the accumulative effects of the above. Biederman has demonstrated this conclusively.[73] The nonsurgical Class III and pseudoskeletal Class III patients are likely candidates for rapid palatal expansion when their condition is compounded by posterior bilateral crossbite.

The appliance is *contra*indicated in cases of Class II, Division I, malocclusion or prognathic maxillas as rapid expansion techniques would only intensify these effects. The same is true for patients with an already steep mandibular plane. This also is intensified by rapid expansion.

Another important effect to consider is the difference between a true unilateral posterior crossbite and a bilateral posterior crossbite with a concomitant mandibular shift to make it appear unilateral. In the latter situation the case would respond well to rapid expansion and allow the mandible to correct itself relative to its midline shift, resulting in a correct occlusion and balanced and correct condyle-fossa relationship.

Like many techniques of orthodontics before it, the Rapid Palatal Expander is associated with various controversies as to appliance design. Some clinicians insist on cementing two bands on each side (or stainless steel crowns [SSCs] in mixed dentition if first bicuspids are unerupted); others claim that first molar banding and soldered lingual bars are sufficient in the mixed dentition. One school of thought championed by Haas mandates that acrylic pads must be used in the vault of the palate as an aid in dissipating expansion pressures and as an increased buttressing effect during stabilization. The opposing school says these are not necessary and only cause hygiene and tissue irritation problems. Some say you need buccal bars soldered on; others claim they are redundant. One might traverse the spec-

---

Figure 5-27 Correction of maxillary arch form with rapid palatal expansion and fixed appliances. **(A)** Pretreatment intraoral view of maxillary arch form. **(B)** Pretreatment maxillary palatal x-ray. **(C)** Rapid Palatal Expander cemented to place. **(D)–(N)** As appliance is activated over a period of only weeks, note how palate sequentially separates along midpalatal suture as is evidenced by separation of right and left central incisors, and radiographic evidence of separation of right and left halves of maxilla. Often fixed appliances such as the straight wire-type appliances are called upon after the 3- to 4-month retention phase of treatment with the Rapid Palatal Expander is complete in order to obtain more individualized tooth movements in the production of proper final dental arch form. (*Courtesy of Dr Jay Gerber, St Mary's, WV.*)

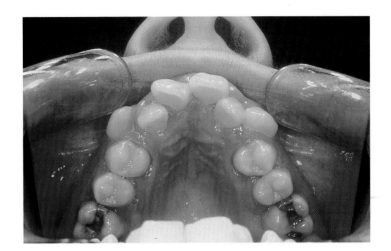

(A)

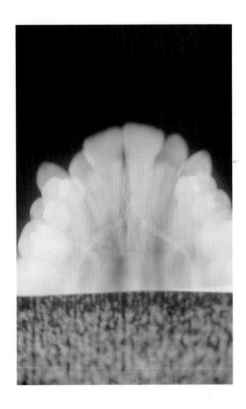

(B)

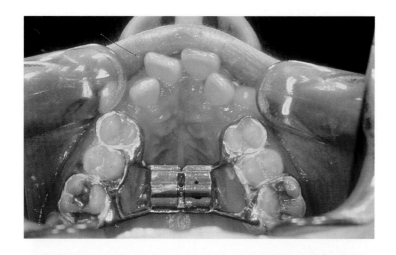

(C)

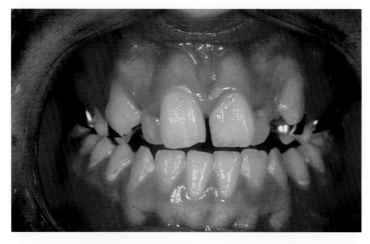

(D)

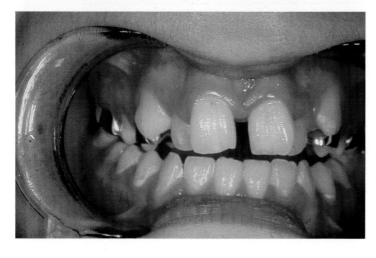

(E)

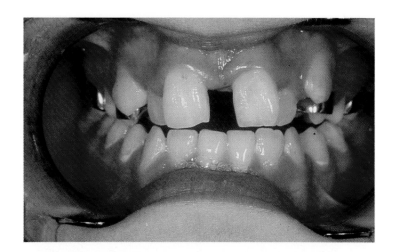

(F)

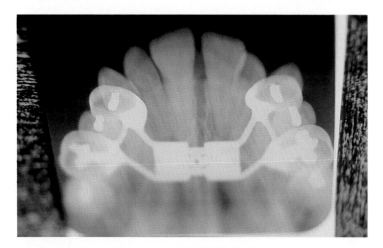

(G)

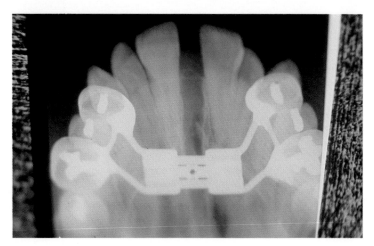

(H)

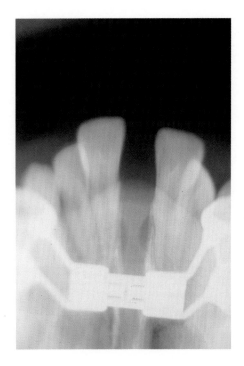

(I)

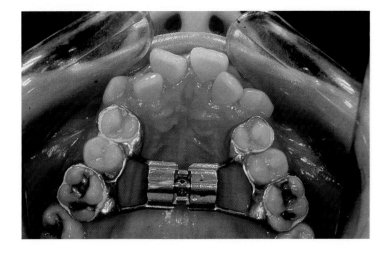

(J)

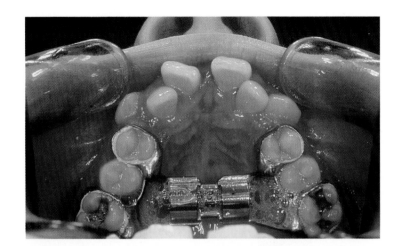

(K)

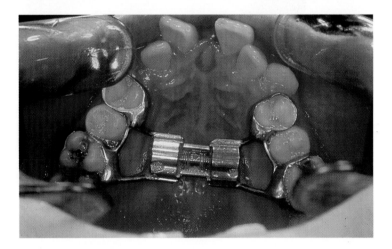

(L)

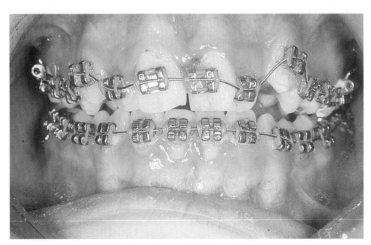

(M)

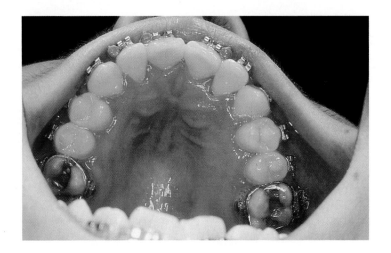

(N)

trum of appliance designs from the simple Hyrax, an all-metal appliance, to an Isaacson or Haas appliance with the full complement of options. They all work.[74]

But likewise there are several facts that are quite indisputable. The maxillary palatal suture does separate and the entire case can be expanded out in 2 weeks or so. Retention must be maintained by the appliance itself for at least 3 months. Less, even by 1 month, will result in almost total relapse. Following appliance removal, acrylic Hawley-type retainers may be inserted if needed. The technique is surprisingly painless, though some patients report tenderness in the nasal area to touch. Properly retained, the cases can be reasonably stable. They are easy to make, especially if one relies on professional laboratories. (All that is needed is an accurate stone model!)

Expansion screws may be used that range from 8 to 16 mm expansibility, though cases seldom, if ever, require more than 15 mm expansion. They work best in the mixed or early adult dentition. Adults that undergo this type of treatment exhibit more alveolar bending and orthodontic tooth movement due to increased ossification and rigidity of the facial skeleton.

THE STEINHAUSER-LINES PROCEDURE— MAXILLARY BILATERAL CORTICOTOMY

Older patients such as late teens and early adults are more resistant to rapid expansion of the palate due to the rigidity of the facial skeleton, chiefly the zygomaticomaxillary, zygomaticotemporal, zygomaticofrontal, and frontomaxillary sutures. When the technique is instituted in these individuals, the pressures generated by the expansion screw are absorbed by the periodontal membranes of the teeth and the cortical plate rather than effecting separation of the midpalatal suture. This also can lead to improper axial tilting of the banded teeth and dehiscence of the roots, through the buccal alveolar plate. Tenderness or soreness of the cheekbone area is also an observation often reported.

In an effort to reduce these side effects and assist the action of the rapid expansion appliance in the mature patient, Steinhauser developed a simple yet ingenious technique to surgically correct palatal width insufficiency. The LeForte I-type osteotomy was refined slightly by Lines several years later and consists of the following. Incisions are made high in the maxillary buccal vestibules running from the distal of the second molars, or third molars if present, and extended horizontally to the maxillary cuspids where they drop perpendicularly to the gingival crests. A periosteal flap is reflected exposing the cortical plate of the upper maxilla. Using a straight bone bur of a fissure type, a cut is made through the surface of cortical plate from the distal of the last molar or the area of the pterygoid fissure, horizontally about 3 mm above the apices of the roots of the maxillary teeth to the cuspid root area where it drops vertically between the cuspid and first bicuspid roots to the crest of the alveolar ridge. This is done bilaterally and the flaps sutured shut.

In the palate, a full palatal flap is reflected and bur cuts are made parallel to either side of the midpalatal suture and vomer bone in the posterior nasal spine area forward to the area in line with the apex of the cuspid root tip where again the cut drops to the alveolar crest between the cuspid and first bicuspid roots. The flap is then repositioned and sutured into place by running the sutures interdentally with the fixed buccal mucosa. Some surgeons prefer to suture a petrolatum gauze pressure pack into the palatal vault for 24 hours after surgery. Patients do surprisingly well and the procedure may be done in the surgeon's office using only local anesthesia.

A short period of time is required before cementing the appliance to place after surgery. About 2 weeks.

Activation in the standard manner may begin immediately with little or no pain or discomfort to the patient since the only resistance to lateral expansion now that the dense, brittle cortical plate has been sectioned are the lateral nasal walls, the pterygopalatine sutures and the cancellous spongy pliable bone of the alveolar interdental spaces between the cuspids and first bicuspids. As expansion takes place, there is still enough residual rigidity in the bone to transmit enough orthopedic pressure to cause separation of the central incisors as usual. And, as usual, the amount of elastic resistance in the periodontium and transeptal fibers is sufficient to cause this space to close itself as the centrals relapse back to their original position and the case proceeds normally. However, in a given number of lateral expansion cases augmented surgically by the above procedure, certain problems persisted.

THE EPKER-WOLFORD PROCEDURE—THE EXTENDED MAXILLARY CORTICOTOMY

Although lateral maxillary and palatal osteotomies greatly aided maxillary expansion techniques in adult treatment, a certain number of cases were still bothered with age-old problems of both instability and relapse. As a result of empirical observation of these posttreatment problems, it was theorized that the three main buttressing sutures, the midpalatine, the zygomaticomaxillary, and pterygomaxillary, should all be sectioned to effect better results. Subsequently, more intrepid surgeons developed a highly advanced technique to move the two halves of the maxilla away from each other more completely at their natural sutures. The technique as described by Epker and Wolford[75] is comprised of the following.

A circumvestibular incision is made high in the buccal and labial vestibule from the region of one upper first molar completely around the

Figure 5-28 The Epker-Wolford procedure: advanced maxillary bilateral corticotomy. Pretreatment condition of 20-year-old adult female with severe maxillary bilateral crossbite. **(A)** Narrow maxillary arch with anterior crowding, lingually locked laterals. **(B)** Final arch perfection obtained with fixed appliances.

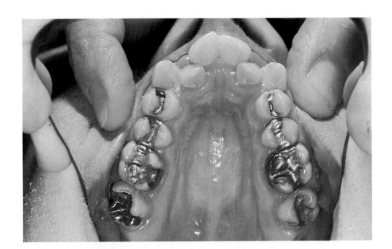

(A)

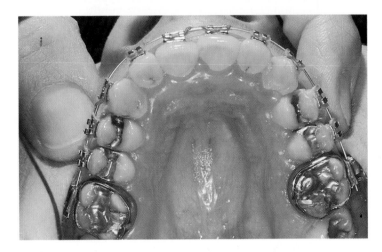

(B)

arch to the region of the opposite first molar. Collateral circulation is adequate to supply the attached gingivae below the incision. A periosteal flap is reflected superiorly opposing the maxilla and piriform apertures bilaterally. Even the mucoperiosteum of the lateral and inferior border of the nasal opening is reflected slightly. At the lateral aspect of the maxilla, the flap is undermined clear back to the pterygomaxillary junction even though the incision is not made that far back, as it would allow the herniation of the buccal fat pad to interfere with the operative area. Retraction is provided prior to the osteotomy with conventional retractors such as the Minnesota retractor or large periosteal elevators. Under water irrigation, the osteotomy is made with common straight handpiece bone burs about 4 mm apical to the root tips of the maxillary teeth to insure vitality from the piriform aperture to the pterygoid plates. Using a periosteal elevator to act as a shield to protect the nasal mucosa from laceration from the bone bur, the anterior portion of the osteotomy is made through the anterior portion of the lateral nasal wall. Posteriorly, the osteotomy runs to the level of the second or third molar if present, and once distal to these teeth it drops off gradually toward the most inferior portion of the pterygomaxillary junction. This entire procedure is repeated on the other side also.

After the horizontal sections are made bilaterally, a vertical one is made at the anterior maxillary midline suture below the anterior nasal spine. After an osteotomy is cut midline between the maxillary central incisors, a fine osteotome is inserted and tapped gently to aid in completing the section. It is first directed directly between the roots of the centrals with a finger placed in the palatal area to detect and guard against penetration through to the inner lingual surface of palatal bone. Then the osteotome is redirected straight posteriorly to split the entire midpalatal suture! As the osteotome is tapped posteriorly through the midpalatal suture, it may be torqued to aid in completing the split posteriorly.

Lastly, the lateral nasal walls are cut with an osteotome from the edge of the piriform rim to a level of about 30 mm posteriorly, while using the aforementioned periosteal elevator to again protect the nasal mucosa. The only major bony attachment now left is the perpendicular plate of the palatine bone. Mobility of the two halves of the maxilla is checked and if inadequate, the pterygomaxilla areas are also sectioned with small curved osteotomes designed for such purposes.

Carefully, the maxilla may be tested for mobility with finger pressure making sure not to "down-fracture" it, which would then disadvantageously require vertical stabilization with suspension wires. Osteotomes may be used to mobilize the two halves of the maxilla. They are inserted into the lateral maxillary and midline osteotomy sites and gently torqued to test for adequate mobility. Of course both right and left halves must be equally mobile, or unequal unilateral expansion will occur once the appliance is activated.

The appliance is inserted prior to surgery so that it may be activated immediately upon completion of the osteotomies, even before closure! It is usually activated to 2 to 3 mm to insure expansion is bilaterally symmetrical. The incision is then preferably closed with a running suture of common resorbable gut. The remainder of the expansion is then carried out over the next week or so depending on the amount of expansion needed. Two to four turns of the appliance expansion screw per day may be used, and once activation is complete the appliance is left in place the usual 90 days to insure proper healing of bone. If greater distances are achieved in the 10 to 12 mm area, longer periods of appliance wear followed by several months of retainer usage are indicated to insure proper bone healing of a sufficient degree to prevent relapse.

"Never was born!" persisted Topsy;
"Never had no father, nor mother,
nor nothin'. I was raised by a
speculator" . . . ;
"Do you know who made you?" asked
Miss Ophelia.
"Nobody as I knows on," said the
child with a short laugh . . . "I s'pect I
grow'd."

Dialogue between Miss Ophelia Sinclare
and the black slave child, Topsy
Uncle Tom's Cabin
Harriet Beecher Stowe 1811–1896

Case Study Illustrations—Following Pages

Figure 5-29 Case study. In this case, combined techniques of initial rapid disjunction of midpalatal suture with Rapid Palatal Expander, continued slow disjunction of midpalatal suture with transverse appliance, molar distalization with Sagittal appliance, and autocorrection of slight crowding combined with second molar extraction principles are demonstrated in same case. At 12 years, 4 months of age this case of Class II, Division 1 bilateral maxillary posterior crossbite is described cephalometrically as a "high angle" case and exhibits 10.9 mm shortage of arch width across bicuspid area and 13.7 mm shortage across first molar area. **(A) (B)** Pretreatment views of severely collapsed maxillary arch with right maxillary posterior quadrant crowded slightly farther forward than maxillary left posterior quadrant. **(C)** RPE inserted to initiate initial sutural disjunction as soon as possible in treatment plan. **(D)** Original pretreatment mandibular arch form—slightly crowded. **(E)** After 6 mm of original deficiency of arch width was regained by the RPE following adequate periods of retention, appliance was withdrawn. **(F)** Arch-widening principles were temporarily suspended in this case in favor of securing the erupting cuspids into more favorable positions via the principles of directional decrowding theories. Maxillary left cuspid may be seen to have adequate space in which to be correctly repositioned; however, the maxillary right cuspid has its proper position on arch impinged upon by forward-drifting maxillary right posterior quadrant. Therefore, maxillary Sagittal I appliance is now seemingly preemptively employed to distalize upper right quadrant to make room for blocked-out cuspid. Second molars have been removed in all four quadrants at beginning of treatment. The Sagittal acting as back-up retention device for maxillary width already gained by previous appliance is used not only to make room for right cuspid, but also to tease both cuspids down and back into their proper positions on palatal arch. **(G)** With right cuspid arriving in correct position (cuspid on rugae) slightly ahead of left, remaining arch width discrepancy (slightly less than half the original amount) is gained by use of the **(H)** standard transverse appliance (no labial bow was used in this case). With insertion of transverse appliance, note how remaining crowding represented by overlapped four maxillary upper anterior teeth is expressed horizontally across front of arch and is due not almost solely to a deficiency in lateral arch dimension (note that Sagittal appliance has been used to correct anteroposterior crowding and forward crowded cuspids in that particular plane). **(I)** As appliance is activated, old "acrylic drop" technique is also called upon to aid in proper positioning of anteriors as plate expands. Once expansion is complete to desired widths, the space in appliance may be filled in with quick-curing acrylic to act as its own retainer. Now that major maxillary arch orthopedic portions of treatment plan have been accomplished, all that remains is correction in both arches of problems mostly of an orthodontic nature. **(J)** However, due to slight decrowding of mandibular arch resulting from extraction of second molars alone without benefit of any form of appliance therapy, the decision was made not to place any appliances on the lower but rather to simply "wait and see" if remaining crowding self-corrects spontaneously. However, the same does not hold true for upper arch, where more active forces will be required to level, align, and rotate individual teeth to obtain proper arch form. **(K)–(N)** Fixed appliances, which are best suited for such, may now be called upon to correct remaining tooth position discrepancies in upper arch. Once fixed appliance portion of treatment is complete, all appliances are removed. A maxillary Hawley-type retainer was employed in this case, and final results **(O) (P)** are evident. Completed case of proper arch form and occlusion now evident. **(Q) (R)** Pre- and posttreatment facial views. Though no Bionator was used in this case, note how original pretreatment retrognathic lateral profile is improved in posttreatment view. This is product of unlocking and balancing occlusion to allow mandible its natural opportunity to develop itself down and forward, as it would normally do in absence of any posteriorly locking form of malocclusion.

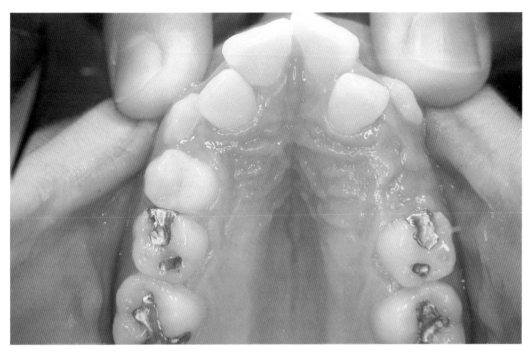

(A)

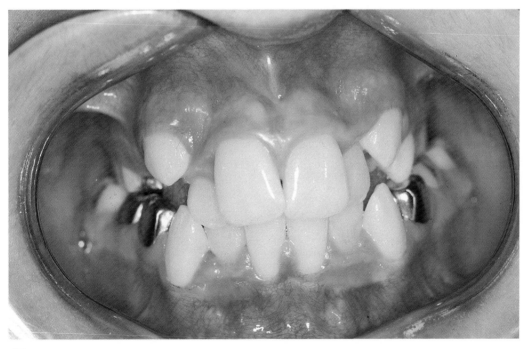

(B)

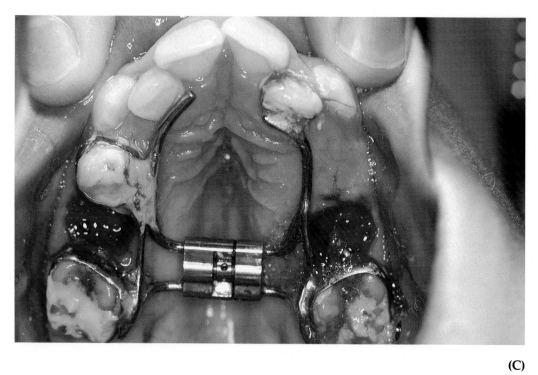

(C)

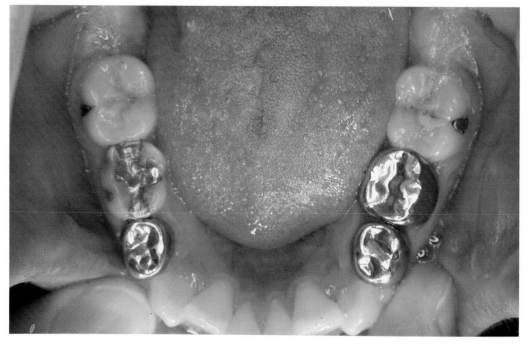

(D)

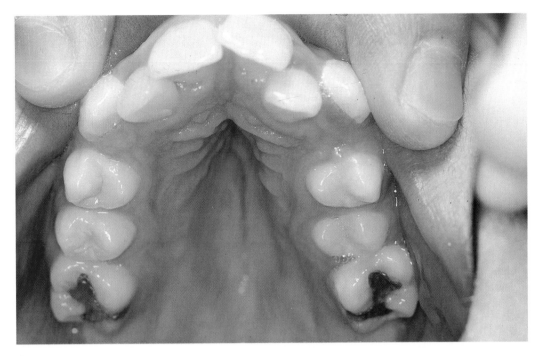

(E)

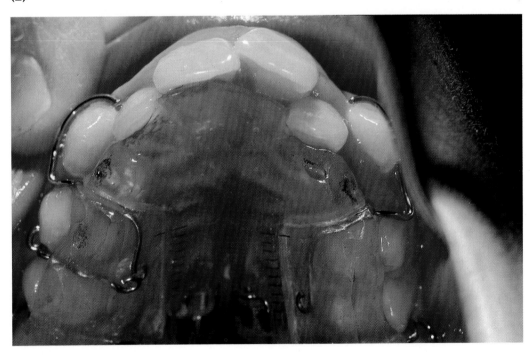

(F)

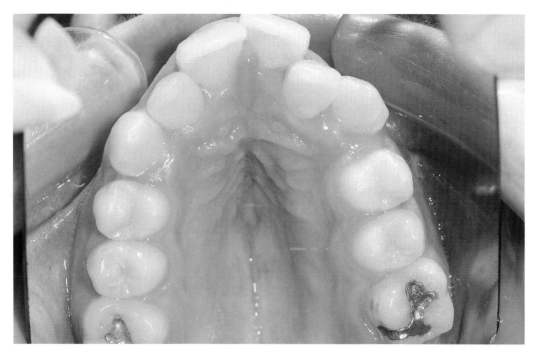

(G)

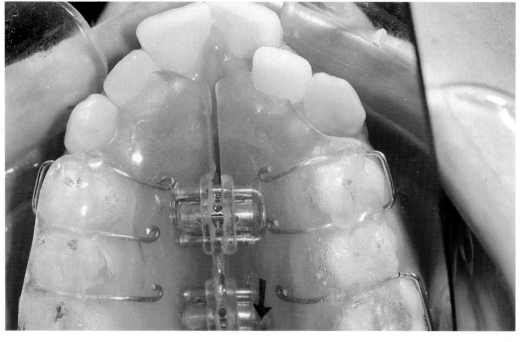

(H)

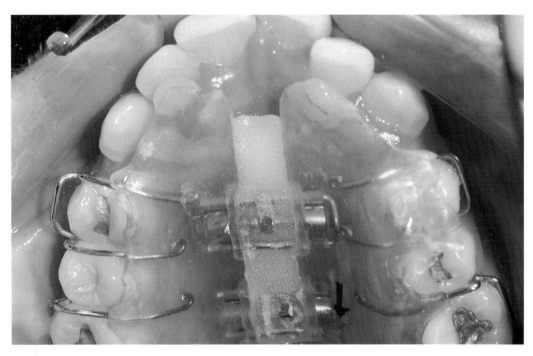

(I)

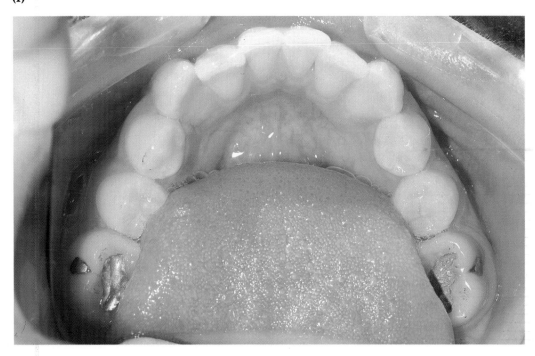

(J)

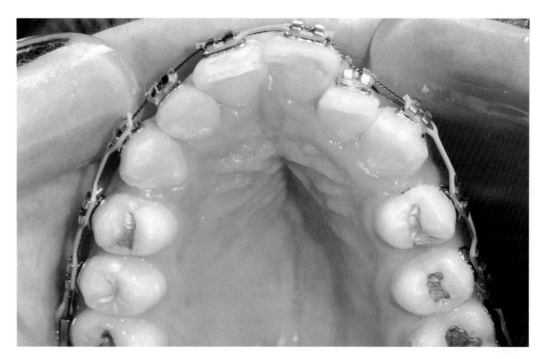

(K)

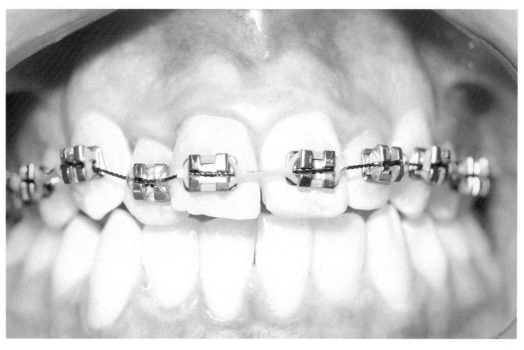

(L)

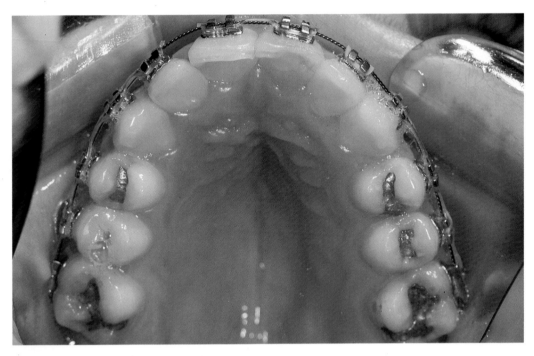

(M)

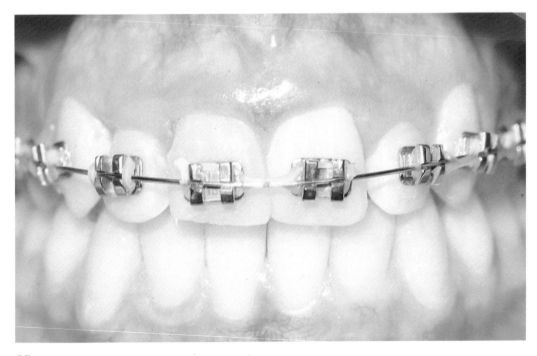

(N)

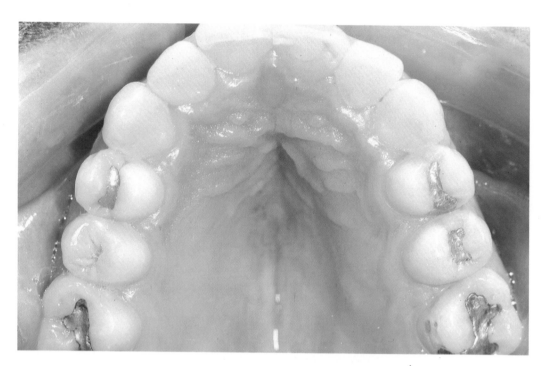

(O)

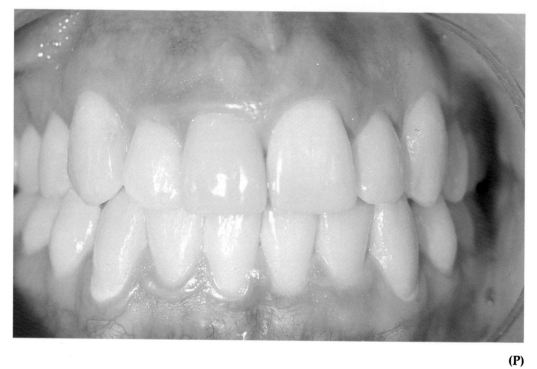

(P)

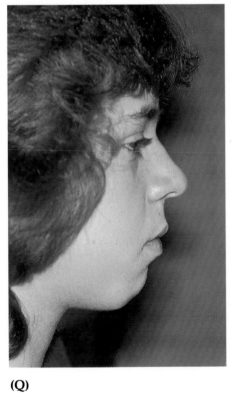

(Q)

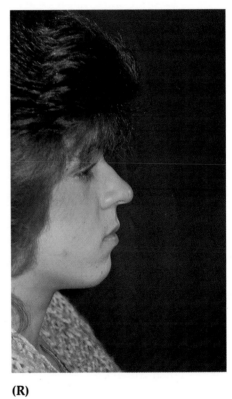

(R)

THE FAN APPLIANCE

The fan-type pivot screw active plate is an anterior maxillary arch-widening appliance. It is completely neutral as far as maxillary posterior cross-arch width is concerned. It is similar in appearance to the Schwarz plates, split down the middle with an expansion screw of a special type in the anterior palatal half, but in the posterior section, near the most distal limit of the appliance, it is held together by a nonexpanding pivoting flat horizontal hinge. When the expansion screw is opened, this posterior pivoting hinge allows the appliance to expand in the front half only. Actually, it opens in a V-shaped arc that has the posterior palatine midline area as the axis of rotation for "fanning" of the two halves of the appliance away from each other, hence the name. The primary purpose of these types of appliances is to expand a very pointed type arch, which requires the anterior segment be widened or developed more laterally than the posterior segments which themselves may have the molars already positioned in the correct or near-correct width relationships for that particular arch. When activated, they move the cuspids and bicuspids out laterally, retract protruding maxillary central and lateral incisors by virtue of the action of the labial bow, and either move upper first molars out sideways to a slight degree or leave them entirely alone to remain in their pretreatment position. To refer to the concept represented by the aforementioned Leghorn analyzer relative to the shapes of maxillary arches, they turn pointed ones into rounded ones.

Appliance Design and Function

The origins of the fanwise active plate are obscure and its lineage is difficult to trace.[76] But it, no doubt, arose during the heyday of active plate design and development in the 1930s and 1940s in Germany when men like Nord, Tischler, and Schwarz were bringing active plate usage to the forefront in orthodontics throughout Europe. It has gone through several changes over the years.

The appliance has been modified and specialized for various types of asymmetrical or eccentric expansion over the years by means of various types of screws designed for this purpose. Originally, expansion screws of the simpler type were placed in the anterior part of the appliance while the posterior parts were held together by means of a wire. As the anterior half of the appliance expanded, the posterior sections were held together by the wire allowing the fanlike expansion to take place in the bicuspid region. However, this allowed for only about 4 mm lateral development anteriorly. But then special screws came along that had their ends mounted in small flat drumlike fittings that could pivot around the two respective ends of the

Figure 5-30 **(A) (B)** Basic maxillary fan appliance. **(C)** Mandibular appliance. (*Courtesy of Ohlendorf Co, St Louis, MO.*)

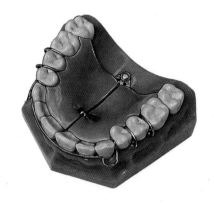

(A)

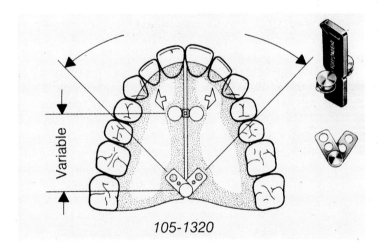

105-1320

(B)

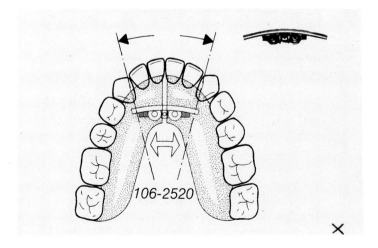

106-2520

(C)

expansion screw shaft as its central cylinder was rotated during activation. These modified screws allowed for up to 8 mm of anterior expansion. In conjunction with these screws there was also used a flat, pivoting-type hinge that was placed in the posterior border of the appliance that held the two halves stationary relative to lateral motion but allowed rotation of the adjacent edges away from each other angularly.

Another screw developed was a one-piece unit known as a Wipla screw. It consists of two flat parallel bars joined at the distal end by a freely rotating rivet and anteriorly by a jackscrew threaded through each end of the two bars. It also has two metal bars projecting out of the sides of each bar laterally which serve to engage the body of acrylic in the palatal vault. The entire appearance of this little device can't but be reminiscent of some sort of small crustacean that one would find under a flat rock in a tidal pool by the seashore. Wipla screws come in various sizes and are quite strong once processed into the acrylic of the appliance. Their only disadvantage is that the placement of the screw from the pivot point is always fixed and the angle of opening is always a function of the screw size used. On the other hand, the aforementioned two-piece units previously described allow the freedom to place the expansion screw as far away from the hinge as the operator may desire for a particular case. The farther away the expansion screw is placed anteriorly from the pivoting point in the posterior part of the appliance, the more nearly parallel, or less eccentric, will be the resultant expansion. Both work well in situations for which they are indicated.

For two-way eccentric expansion another type of screw is needed. Some cases need both anterior and posterior development laterally with the anterior region needing the greater development. The screws designed for this process are square-looking devices with, again, two parallel bars, one to be imbedded in each side of the appliance. But two jackscrews are incorporated, one anteriorly and one posteriorly. They are threaded through the two bars at right angles and engage the bars through fittings that allow both expansion at a given screw site and pivotal motion at the same time. Thus the screws may both be turned at the same time producing parallel disjunction of the two halves of the appliance to the point where the molars have been developed laterally to the desired width at which time the activation of the posterior screw is stopped and held while the anterior may be continually turned producing the fanlike expansion of the plate at that point and continued lateral development in the anterior region.

However, these early model double-bar–type screw designs were bulky and somewhat primitive in design and action. Something more streamlined and efficient was needed, and with "necessity being the mother of invention," a more practical design was evolved. Taking a cue from original Wipla-type designs, a two-way eccentric palatal expansion screw has been developed, the Nardella. Its initial appearance is that of a near cousin to the crustaceanlike Wipla. However, this eccentric two-way–type screw has two activating screws that run transverse to the midpalatal suture, one anteriorly and one posteriorly. This makes the Nardella the ideal choice for cases requiring more expansion in either the bicuspid or molar region due to the eccentricity of arch outline. Since both activating screws pivot equally, it may be used to widen the transarch bicuspid dimension only, the transarch molar dimension only, both dimensions in varying degrees, or both equally, by simply activating both screws.

A screw has been developed to produce eccentric, or anterior-oriented, expansion in the mandible. It has a curved bar that fits behind the lower incisor area and as the screw is opened, the appliance separates at the midline along the line of arc of the guiding bar, which is fine if that is the exact way the movement of the teeth in that area is desired. But there is also, due to the geometry of the movement of the two halves of the lower appliance away from each other, an inherent sagittal component of force in a distal direction delivered to the posterior segments in these cases. This may or may not be desired and has a tendency to cause the appliance to "pop up" off the posterior teeth. Extra added retention by means of more wire clasps is indicated as a result. Because of the problems associated with the design of this appliance, it is subject to limited use.

The maxillary fan appliances also have a labial bow identical to those used on the conventional Schwarz plates and it is used in the same manner. Usually the maxillary anteriors are protruding and exhibit excessive labial crown inclination in severely pointed arches and as the anterior segment of the appliance is expanded, the labial bow will flatten and aid in drawing the upper central and laterals back into their normal position. Also, like the Schwarz plates, the fan appliances are held in place with the usual Adams and ball clasps and the acrylic does not extend over the occlusal surfaces of the teeth.

As with all forms of retraction of protruding upper anterior teeth, the acrylic directly adjacent to the lingual surfaces of the upper anterior teeth must be adjusted as the plate is expanded to allow uninhibited movement of these teeth lingually as pressure is applied by the flattening labial bow. By proper adjustment of the bow coming in from the labial and the presence of acrylic abutting from the lingual, various individual movements and incidental 'decrowding' of individual teeth may be accomplished during treatment. These movements aid in the preparing of the teeth to assume their correct positions in the more normal, rounded arch form desired.

The appliance may be used as its own retainer or a more streamlined Hawley-type retainer may be constructed once the case is returned to normal arch form. However, these cases are almost always associated with Class II-type malocclusions since the narrowness of the upper arch anteriorly is often accompanied by a retrograde development of the mandible since the lower posterior molars tend to seek out the more stable occlusion on the wider more posterior part of the upper arch, thus producing the Class II condition. If the lower arch were of normal size and shape and were in its correct anterior-posterior cephalometric position against an upper arch that was V-shaped and narrow anteriorly, it would imply a bilateral crossbite. Either way the fan appliance usually serves as a preparatory stage of treatment getting the upper arch ready for the next battery of appliances that will be called upon to treat the remaining problems associated with the case.

Commonly, this means a Bionator and this appliance serves well as giving double duty in acting as not only an orthopedically corrective functional appliance but also as a retainer for the preservation of the development produced by the fan-type predecessor.

These fan-type active plates are not used as frequently as the other types of active plates, but they have a definite place in the repertoire of the clinician using removable appliances and they serve as extremely valuable tools for the cases in which they are indicated. To be deprived of their use would seriously hamper the clinician's ability to deal with the varied types of malocclusions with which he will be confronted.

"Yet how different the artists and their workmanship."

Epictetus AD *c60–c120*

MISCELLANEOUS TRANSVERSE APPLIANCES

It has been estimated by some experts in the field that there are in excess of 30 different varieties of arch-widening appliances of one sort or another with new ones being introduced steadily. Though they all develop arches laterally, some are more efficient than others. Some enjoy a relatively reasonable popularity while others remain more obscure. Usually the less frequently seen appliances are pet devices of certain clinicians or groups who have a special preference for them for various personal reasons and as a result develop extraordinary skills in their manipulation and use. However, their employment is not generally enlisted by the rank and file of most practitioners to the degree of more popular appliances previously mentioned.

One such appliance that enjoys a certain degree of popularity among certain clinicians is the Arnold expander. It is used for maxillary arch development only, and is a relatively simple device. It is made entirely of metal and is shaped like an open-ended box. Metal bands are placed on the first molars (or second molars if present) to which either .036 or .040 stainless steel wire arms are soldered. These arms extend anteriorly to the cuspids. In this area

---

Figure 5-31 **(A)** Wipla-type Forestadent screws 105-1310. **(B)** Bar-type two-way expansion screw (Dentarum Co FRG). (*Courtesy of Graber TM, Neumann B:* Removable Orthodontic Appliances, *ed 1. Philadelphia, WB Saunders Co, 1977, p 34.*)
Figure 5-32 The Nardella eccentric expansion screw. (*Courtesy of OIS/Orthodontics, Wilmington, DE.*)

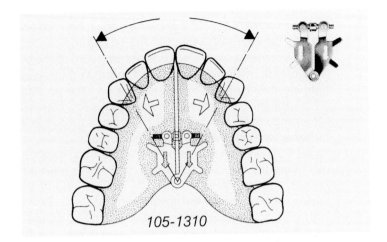

(A)

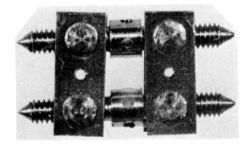

(B)

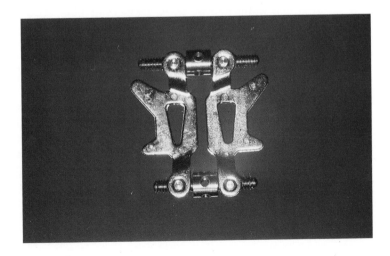

Figure 5-32

another similarly gauged wire is soldered at approximately a 90-degree angle to the lingual bars across the palatal ruga area. This transverse bar fits into a sleeve soldered to the opposing lingual bar. An open coil spring is placed on the bar that slides into the sleeve and the bar is inserted into the sleeve prior to cementation. The constant pressure of the open coil spring pushing against the male wire bar solder joint on the one side and the end of the female sleeve on the other side delivers the pressure necessary to expand the appliance and move the teeth laterally. This, of course, brings to bear the problem of the spring losing some of its power and getting weaker and weaker as the appliance expands. A modification was soon added that put a set screw on the male wire bar which had the ability to be loosened, moved along the bar, and tightened again. This placed the open coil spring between the set screw on one side and the end of the female sleeve on the other, against which the spring abutted flush. This modification allows the clinician to advance the set screw down the threaded male bar to keep the spring compressed as the appliance expands. By thus picking up the slack in the spring brought about by expansion of the appliance, the spring is kept at its near-maximum state of compression for the entire course of treatment. The adjustment of the set screw by rotating it with a small, special Allen-type wrench which allows its relocation down the male bar to maintain compression of the spring is usually done about every 3 to 5 weeks.

THE PORTER DERIVATIVES

Another old-timer in the all-metal lateral expansion appliance field is what is commonly referred to as the Porter lingual arch. Actually the term "Porter" may be a bit of a misnomer and may have to have been drafted, out of necessity. It was a name believed to have been applied to these appliances at St Louis University over a half century ago. The man who actually developed these appliances was Dr H. C. Pollock.[77] He was himself a St Louisan and his father Dr S. H. Pollock owned one of the original books that was published by V. H. Jackson in 1886. As a young man he met the aging Dr Jackson at an American Association of Orthodontists meeting in

---

Figure 5-33 **(A)** Maxillary fan appliance at beginning of treatment. This particular fan appliance design incorporates use of two-piece screw—pivoting hinge arrangement. This particular appliance does not make use of labial bow commonly used on fan-type appliances. Action of labial bow on maxillary anteriors as appliance is activated is similar in effect to that of labial bow of common Schwarz plate and requires similar wire and lingual acrylic adjustment technique. **(B)** Beginning of appliance activation. **(C)** Appliance completely activated.
Figure 5-34 The Arnold Expander. This simple device takes advantage of sliding set screw and open coil spring to provide gentle forces for lateral development of maxillary arch.

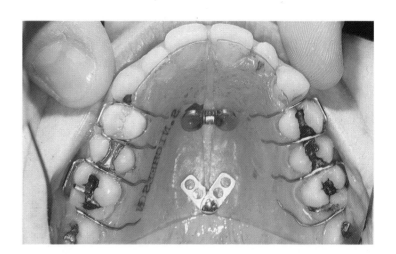

(A)

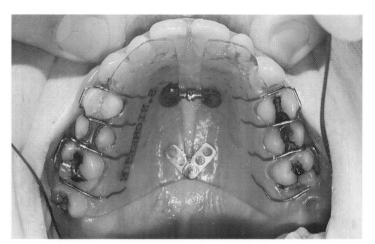

(B)

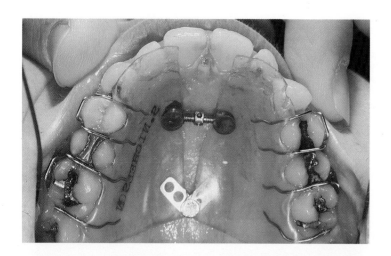

(C)

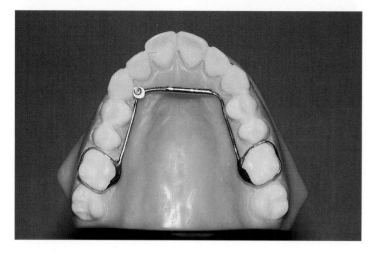

Figure 5-34

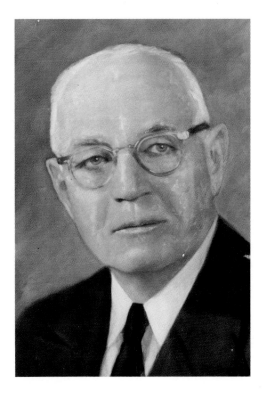

Figure 5-35 H.C. Pollock

Toronto, Canada.[78] But Pollock was also a contemporary of another individual who was also to become famous for the development of a removable
appliance, George Crozat. Like Crozat, Pollock also took additional training at the Dewey School of Orthodontia; but unlike Crozat who went to
New Orleans, Pollock spent his entire professional career in St Louis.
However, with respect to promoting his appliance designs, Pollock preferred
to remain relatively obscure. Possibly the cold indifference that was vested
upon his friend, Dr Crozat, by the fixed appliance–oriented orthodontic community of that day had some influence on him. Description of his appliances
surfaced around 1924,[79] but generally remained out of the literature of that
era. This no doubt accounts for the failure of his name to follow his basic
appliance designs. But after one look at these appliances, there can be no
doubt as to the influences both Jackson and Crozat had on him. These appliances are nothing more than Crozats with soldered molar bands as a
means of attachment instead of custom-soldered wire cribs. They are adjusted in the same manner as the Crozats; but being held in place with
soldered first molar bands usually requires that the entire appliance be
removed for adjustments, then recemented to place again. The relatively
light 20-gauge body wire of the appliance allows for a 2- to 4-mm load to
be placed prior to cementation. The "Crozat purists" claim that the cemented

bands fail to give the identical action as the free-moving crib for gnathologic effects. These appliances may also be used for either upper or lower arches[80-82] in conjunction with labial arch wires for anterior control. These labial wires may be attached to banded anteriors and inserted posteriorly into free-sliding buccal tubes on the molar bands.

Though these older-style soldered Porter-Pollock–type fixed appliances see little service in these modern times, they serve as an important prototype to appliances that would bring this type of mechanics to far more advanced levels of sophistication. The two men most intimately associated with the refinement of this technique are each in their own right men of true orthodontic genius. The first is Dr Robert Ricketts who developed, among other things, the original Ricketts-type fixed Quad-Helix appliance. The second is Dr William L. Wilson who brought the technique to its present state of the art with his concepts of combined fixed-removable modular orthodontic principles which find their chief expression in the 3D series of all-wire removable appliances that are held in place by means of friction locks to cemented molar bands. More than just a means of lateral development, the Wilson 3D series is an entire orthodontic system in its own right.

The first of the Porter-progeny for lateral palatal development is the Ricketts version of the Quad-Helix appliance.[83] This all-wire "uppers-only" appliance appears to be an offshoot of the Crozat philosophy upon initial inspection. It derives its name from the four helical coil loops which give it its active forces. It is usually constructed of .038 Blue Elgiloy wire and may be fabricated directly by the operator or at the laboratory from plaster casts. It is a "running W"-shaped piece of wire that comes preshaped in five sizes. After selecting the best size that corresponds to the arch being treated, the two lingual arms are soldered to preformed molar bands such that the posterior helical loops are about 4 to 5 mm distal to the point where the lingual arm is soldered to the molar band. From the posterior loop the wire runs forward to the anterior palatal area where it crosses over behind the maxillary anteriors with helical loops at each corner. The appliance is adjusted with appropriate wire-bending pliers so that it is as passive and close-fitting to the cast as possible before soldering. The lingual arms are cut and adapted to the lingual surfaces of the maxillary cuspids at the gum line and may be adjusted if needed in a Crozat fashion.

Figure 5-36 **(A)** Maxillary Porter appliance, the first prototypes of which were devised by H.C. Pollock. **(B)** Porter lingual arch mandibular appliance. **(C)** W appliance showing strong Crozat-Jackson influences and another link in the chain of steadily evolving all-wire appliances. (*Courtesy of DynaFlex Laboratories, St Louis, MO.*)

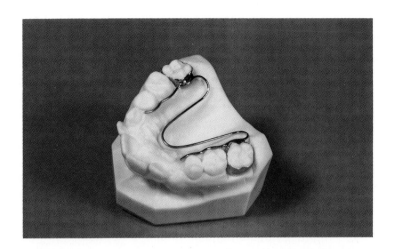

(A)

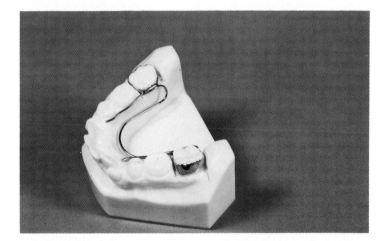

(B)

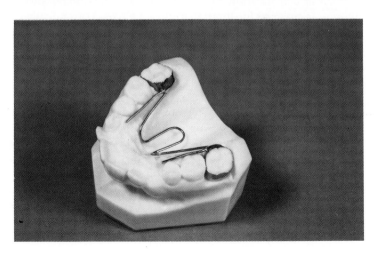

(C)

Adjustments

The appropriate-sized appliance is selected relative to a study model of the case and the wire is shaped with the fingers and a three-pronged pliers to adapt to the model as closely and as passively as possible prior to placement. The appliance is activated prior to cementation by any one, or a combination of, several different methods. Like the Crozat appliance, the Quad-Helix may be used to widen the overall arch as well as rotate, torque, or upright molars. Torquing molars buccally is a key adjustment to this appliance. Without doing so, the arch tends to suffer from buccally tipped molars as the case widens laterally. Discrete adjustments of the bands at their junction to the body wire to impart buccal molar root torque to the molars helps keep them upright during their migration laterally. Distal rotation at the molar band/body wire junction is also helpful in gaining arch space for what may be crowded arches anteriorly. In fact, distal rotation of mesially rotated molars is such a key element in the relief of crowding of anterior portions of the arch that Ricketts recommends it as the first form of activation to be performed when indicated (hints of the concept of directional decrowding). Molars may be widened by crimping the anterior bridge portion of the appliance between the two anterior helical loops with a three-pronged pliers placing the single prong against the anterior side of the wire and crimping until the desired separation of the posterior portion of the appliance is gained. Ricketts recommends 500 g of force for orthopedic disjunction of the midpalatal suture when needed. In the original Ricketts version of the appliance which is cemented into place, periodic checking of the appliance occurs approximately every 6 weeks. At that time activation is accomplished intraorally by placing the three-pronged pliers directly anterior to the posterior helical loop on the palatal bridge portion of the body wire. The pliers is placed such that the crimp would increase the force buccally, ie, the single prong on the medial portion, the double prongs on the lateral portion of the body wire (or palatal bridge). Slight crimping in such fashion at this location rotates the molar more distal and flares the anterior arms (similar to the lingual arms of a Crozat) out bucally (expansion adjustment). Reversing the pliers would expand the molars only while pulling the anterior arms in lingually (reverse adjustment). The anterior arms of the appliance (lingual arms) may be adjusted independently of the molar activation. They

---

Figure 5-37   (A) Fixed maxillary Quad-Helix (Ricketts). Original design of this appliance was introduced by Dr Robert Ricketts and represents essentially fixed appliance since body wire was soldered to bands that required entire appliance to be cemented to place at once. **(B)** Removable maxillary RM Quad-Helix. Variation of Ricketts appliance was subsequently developed by Rocky Mountain/Orthodontics and consists of appliance with male wire pins that fit horizontally into female RM lingual sheaths A-186. This version is available in stainless steel. (*Courtesy of Rocky Mountain/Orthodontics.*)

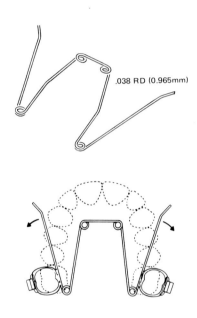

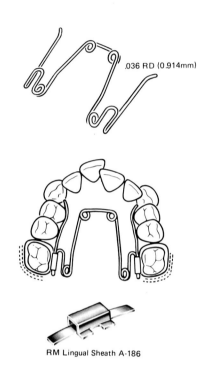

.038 RD (0.965mm)

.036 RD (0.914mm)

RM Lingual Sheath A-186

(A)   **(B)**

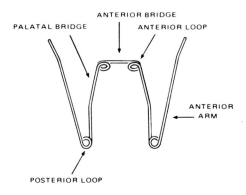

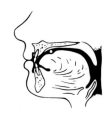

Figure 5-38A

ACTIVATION (INTRA-ORAL)

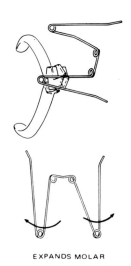

EXPANDS MOLAR

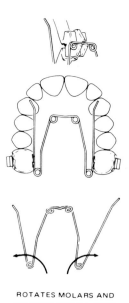

ROTATES MOLARS AND
EXPANDS BUCCAL ARMS

Figure 5-38B

may be activated as needed prior to the insertion and once the appliance is cemented in place, they may be adjusted intraorally to increase pressures buccally on the bicuspids and cuspid as needed by placing the pliers anterior to the molar. Augmentation of lateral forces of expansion may also be carried out intraorally by additional crimping of the anterior bridge portion of the body wire. Ricketts prefers to give the anterior arms (lingual arms) only slight activation or none at all at first, keeping them out of contact with the more anterior teeth entirely until any necessary molar rotation is complete. The problems with these adjustments of course is that they require a certain "feel" on the part of the operator as the activations are being performed on an appliance that is already cemented to place and is nonremovable. It is theorized that once activated and cemented to place, the appliance provides for the more stable slow type of disjunction of the midpalatal suture similar to that obtained by Schwarz and transverse active plates.

THE WILSON SERIES

Advancing one step further, the Wilson series[84] of all wire 3D appliances show not only a strong Porter-Crozat–type heritage but also reflect certain Mershon influences as well.[85-87] Unlike more traditional heavy wire lingual arches, the Wilson-type lingual arches are of a lighter, more resilient wire. Marketed in a variable-sized prefabricated nature under the trademark "3D," these devices are not meant to replace other orthodontic techniques but rather may be incorporated into existing systems to supplement the clinician's versatility in an overall coordinated fashion. The Wilson series of appliances, which may be used in upper or lower arches, or even in sectional forms for single tooth movement within a particular quadrant, take advantage of minute adjustments of the activating portions of the pentagonal wire "loops" (or activators) incorporated into the mandibular appliance or helical loops in the palatal version of the appliance to gain a steady, active force as a result of the elastic memory of the activated (spring) wire. What makes this system extremely practical is that the wire portion of the appliance is held in place in the mouth bilaterally by two friction locks which consist of two loops bent into the wire and flattened to form small posts which fit into two specially designed matching vertical 3D tubes on the lingual surfaces of first molar bands. Therefore they may easily be removed; activated by bending, expanding, or crimping the wire in the appropriate manner in various places on the appliance; and then reinserted by "plugging in" the friction lock posts into their matching double vertical lingual tubes on the 3D first molar bands that are used in this technique.

One slightly simpler appliance of this sort used in the palate is the 3D multiaction palatal appliance. It is the one most similar to the Crozat in both appearance and action and has only a Crozat-like body wire with no helical loops at all. Fittings soldered to the molar area portion of the appliance allow the appliance to be easily inserted into the two vertical tubes of the lingual portion of the 3D upper first molar bands. The diamond-shaped activating loop in the midpalate, which mimics the omega loop of the Crozat, is of .036 wire, while the lingual arm areas are of .025 diameter wire. Used primarily for lateral-type development of the maxillary arch, the appliance is adjusted similar to the Crozat appliance with the incorporation of similar 3-mm loads of tension.

Another more advanced appliance of this series for the palate is the 3D Quad-Helix appliance of Wilson. It also has the advantages of modular components making it easily removable, which obviously facilitates adjustments. It is adjusted similarly to the Ricketts version of the Quad-Helix, with the advantage that it may be done so without removing the entire appliance, as the Wilson version removes only the body wire portion. The Wilson appliance is also made of the .036 wire in the body portion tapering to .025 in the lingual arms. These lingual arms are contoured around the inside of the entire anterior upper arch, unlike the Ricketts versions which stop short at the cuspids and are flared slightly labially at that point. However, the lingual arms on any of these appliances may be custom-shaped by the operator with various favorite wire-bending pliers to suit the individual needs of various types of labial or lateral tooth movement during full arch lateral development.

Adjustments

All of the palatal "quad" appliances may be adjusted in a similar fashion to the original Ricketts version, which has been previously described. Another adjustment technique which some clinicians use consists of using a Jarabak pliers inserted into the appropriate helical loop acting as the vice and applying finger pressure to the arms and/or body wire. Adjusting the appliance at all four helical loops in such fashion, a 4-mm load of overexpansion is placed on the appliance prior to insertion, 2 mm at each posterior loop, 2 mm at each anterior loop. Due to the removable aspects of the appliance, this is easily maintained. Adjusting the anterior arms at the two posterior loops only will obviously produce an eccentric, fanlike development in the bicuspid area along with corresponding molar rotation. The appliance may also be adjusted as needed for eccentric lateral force in the anterior portion of the palate by flaring the wire arms out slightly in the bicuspid area. The expansion adjustments of the anterior bridge and reverse

---

Figure 5-39 **(A)** 3D multiaction palatal appliance. **(B)** Multiaction palatal appliance fitted to model.

Figure 5-40 **(A)** **(B)** Arch development with 3D multiaction palatal appliance.

Figure 5-41 **(A)** **(B)** 3D Quad-Helix palatal appliance (Wilson).

Figure 5-42 **(A)** **(B)** Arch development with 3D Quad-Helix palatal appliance (Wilson).

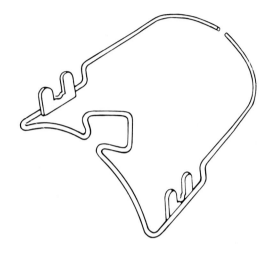

(A)

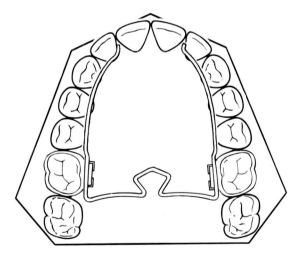

(B)

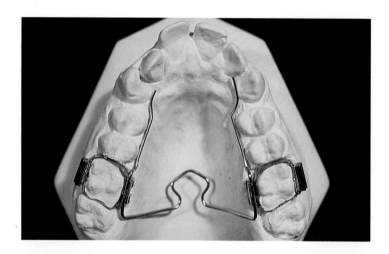

Figure 5-40A

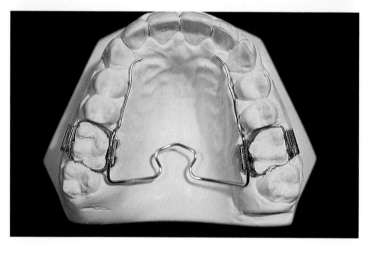

(B)

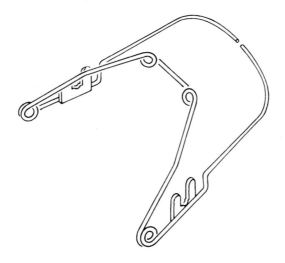

Figure 5-41A

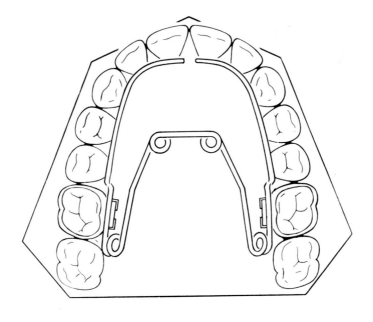

(B)

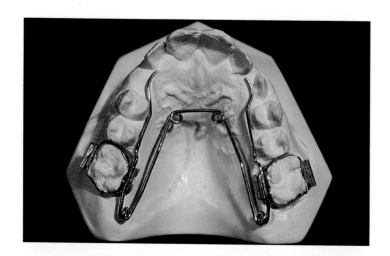

Figure 5-42A

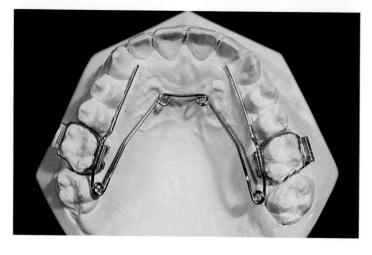

(B)

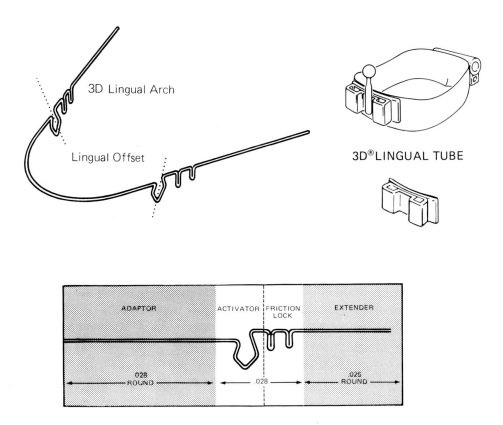

Figure 5-43   Wilson 3D lingual arch.

adjustments of the palatal bridge portions of the body wire tend to widen molar areas only. The load must be augmented "Crozat fashion" about every 4 to 8 weeks as the palatal arch spreads out laterally and the resultant tension of the appliance becomes less as it expresses itself. Thus depending on the type and combination of adjustments used—anterior arm (lingual arm) and posterior loop only for fan-type development, palatal bridge reverse adjustment for molar widening as in some crossbite cases, or combinations of both for overall arch development—a great variety of arch development, molar rotation and arch decrowding situations may be addressed in the maxillary dentition.

The counterpart to the Quad-Helix palatal appliance for the mandibular arch is the Wilson 3D Quad-Action mandibular appliance. It is the most recent descendent of the older original Wilson 3D lingual arch, which was actually the first of the entire series to be developed. The original Wilson lingual arch was a modification and an advancement over other more heavily wired lingual arches that were in use up to that time. It had the two friction grip interlocking posts processed on it that were made of bent and flattened arch wire loops that fit into vertical lingual tubes of the custom 3D molar bands. It also had bilateral pentagonal activating loops formed in the wire which were situated just ahead of the friction locks. In spite of its seeming simplicity of design, the original Wilson lingual arch was developed to serve a variety of functions. There are several basic components to the original lingual arch:

The Adaptor. The Adaptor portion of the arch rests against the cingulae of the anterior mandibular teeth. This provides a source of applied pressure for certain anterior tooth movements and the main source of anchorage for other functions that the lingual arch may be used to carry out such as Class II mechanics, etc. It is of .028 "round wire" and may be readily soldered to accept finger springs, etc, for additional treatment functions.

Activator. Part of the genius of design of the Wilson lingual arch is reflected in the Activator portion of the device. It is a pentagonal loop with five separate internal angles to it, each of which is numbered as such and identified for instructional purposes accordingly as 1 through 5. The first bend, going from distal to mesial is 1, the second, 2, etc. It also is of .028 diameter wire. The unique geometric design of the Activator loop allows for three-dimensional active force mechanics to be instituted with a vast variety of movements possible. Slight adjustment of the various angles of the Activator loop at any one, or various combinations of the internal or external angles, by a small round-on-flat pliers provides the force for active movements. These adjustments are kept to 1.0 mm or less as the force dissipation is 100%, due to the resilience of the wire; therefore movements are both rapid and controlled. The Activator loop is offset lingually slightly to avoid gingival impingement.

Friction lock. The removable aspect of these appliances is accomplished via the twin posts engineered into the arch wire in what would be the first molar area. Of the two posts that make up one attachment mechanism, the mesial post is longer than the distal post to facilitate insertion into the matching 3D vertical lingual tubes of the molar band. The locking posts are inserted initially, mesial post first, into the lingual tubes by means of a How pliers and seated completely to place with any of a variety of common amalgam pluggers, a i-67 band director, or similar instrument. Removal is easily accomplished by inserting the tip of an ordinary heavy-duty scaler under the horizontal wire portion of the lock and, bracing the tip of the scaler against the lingual occlusal surface of the band, rotating the instrument occlusally. This levers the posts vertically free of the lingual tubes.

Figure 5-44 3D Quad-Action mandibular appliance (Wilson). **(A)** This removable all-wire mandibular appliance is advanced form of simpler Wilson 3D lingual arch. **(B)** Appliance inserted. **(C)** Occlusal view.
Figure 5-45 Adaptor portion of 3D lingual arch of Wilson may be used to advance or hold mandibular incisors, depending on how activator loop of appliance is adjusted.

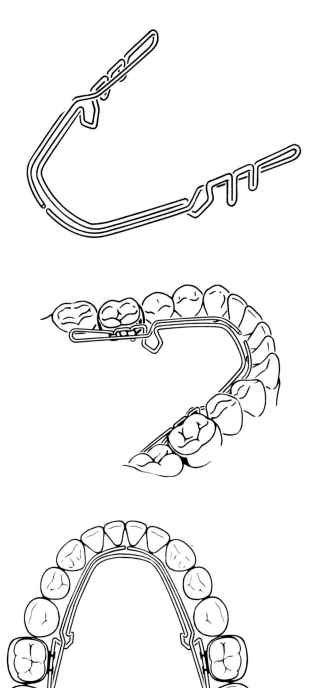

(A)

(B)

(C)

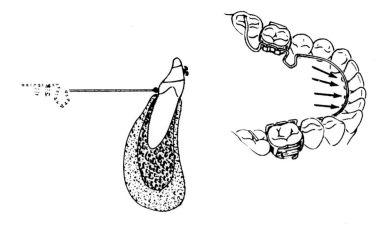

Figure 5-45

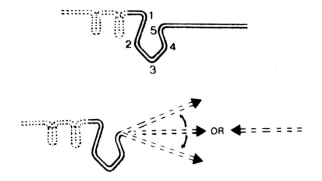

Figure 5-46A

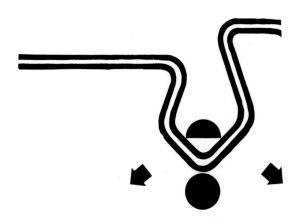

(B)

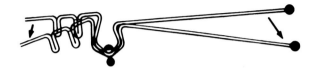

(C)

ACTIVATOR

PLIER TIP POSITIONING	SLIGHT ADJUSTMENTS ──→ ACTIVATE ──→ 1.0mm OR LESS	

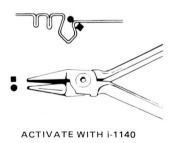

ACTIVATE WITH i-1140

(D)

FITTING 3D LINGUAL ARCH INTO THE 3D LINGUAL TUBE

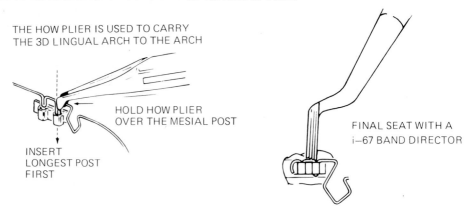

THE HOW PLIER IS USED TO CARRY
THE 3D LINGUAL ARCH TO THE ARCH

HOLD HOW PLIER
OVER THE MESIAL POST

INSERT
LONGEST POST
FIRST

FINAL SEAT WITH A
i—67 BAND DIRECTOR

REMOVING THE 3D LINGUAL ARCH

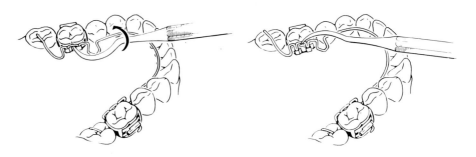

Figure 5-47   Friction lock.

Extender.   The portion of the lingual arch extending distally from the friction lock is of .025 diameter wire and is referred to as the extender. It may be modified in the original version of the lingual arch to perform a variety of tooth movement or anchorage functions. It is used in its shorter version for such purposes. However, if it is lengthened and bent forward, one from each side meeting anteriorly to form a second lingual arch lying over the first, split in the midline to allow for a variety of adjustments which facilitate various situations of lateral and anterior arch development, what we now have is the most recent of Wilson's developments, the 3D Quad-Action mandibular appliance. It serves as a counterpart to the Wilson Quad-Helix of the maxillary arch and provides for a variety of functions including lower incisor advancement, molar distalizing or uprighting, bilateral expansion, molar rotation, and asymmetrical lateral expansion such as fan-type expansion in the mandibular bicuspid area. Like its maxillary counterpart, its multipurpose nature also provides a handy alternative for the patient whose compliance with removable appliance treatments is less than satisfactory.

3D lingual arch adjustments. The Wilson 3D Quad-Action mandibular appliance comes prefabricated in four sizes. A size most closely corresponding to a model of the mandibular arch is selected. Prior to activation for treatment purposes, the appliance is adjusted to fit the model as closely and passively as possible. Its width may be altered by means of gentle finger pressure. The base wire (body wire or Adaptor) should rest just free of the cingula of the lower incisors. Adjustments of the Activator loop portions of the appliance with a round-on-flat pliers will bring the Adaptor wire into exact position. During the process of adapting the wires of the appliance to the model, the extenders (lingual arms) are temporarily raised out of the way.

The appliance is first leveled by placing the friction lock into one side of the molar band. The other side should correspond; but if it needs to be raised or lowered, it may be done by removing the appliance and holding the friction post that was inserted with a How pliers and raising or lowering the opposite side by the appropriate amount with finger pressure. When accomplished, the two friction locks should rest passively adjacent to their respective lingual tubes. Rotation and/or torquing of the friction locks is always accomplished by holding the *mesial* post of the lock in the pliers and adjusting as needed.

In activating the appliance for treatment, the two extenders (lingual arms) and the two body-wire Activators allow for both sagittal and transverse development of the arch along with other types of selective movements as well.

For sagittal development of the arch in an anterior direction the Activators may be adjusted to advance the Adaptor wire anteriorly against the incisors. They are adjusted bilaterally with the customary 1.0-mm activations in sequential adjustings until the desired amount of movement is effected. The extenders may also be enlisted to aid in this action. One problem, however, in this type of action is in preventing the activated wire, especially the extenders, from merely riding up the lingual surfaces of the anteriors instead of moving them bodily forward. This problem is solved simply by the placement of lingual buttons on the cuspids by common acid etch direct-bonding techniques. This provides control of the wires, keeping their action at the gingival areas of the teeth where they belong, thus assuring proper bodily movement of the teeth.

Lateral development is accomplished by widening the body wire and enlisting of the extenders to apply pressure in the bicuspid area. The use of lingual buttons on the bicuspids proves a handy way of keeping the extender wires under control in that region when forces are exerted laterally.

Molar distalization is accomplished by adapting an extender wire on the side of the molar that is to be moved so that the extender wire braces against the distal of the first bicuspid. This in conjunction with close adaptation of the base wire (Adaptor) to the cingula of the anteriors engages cross-arch anchorage principles to provide the anchorage for distalizing the molar by means of activation of the Activator loop. Activator adjustments again should be kept in the 1.0-mm range and molars should be distalized one at a time.

Fan-type expansion in the bicuspid region may be accomplished by use of extenders alone (most likely aided with the use of lingual buttons) with or without molar rotation as is needed. Molar rotation, accomplished by means of holding the mesial post in a How pliers and bending the rest of the appliance either buccally or lingually depending on the type of molar rotation desired, is best carried out through a series of minimal adjustments over a period of several visits. However, it must be remembered that when the friction lock mechanism is adjusted to effect a distal molar rotation, the corresponding extender on that side will produce an active force on the bicuspids due to its displacement buccally. If this is not desired, it must be adjusted back lingually to its original preadjustment passive position.

The multiple uses of these appliances make them practical enough in their own right, but it must be remembered that the Wilson series, especially the mandibular lingual arch and sectional arch, were originally designed to be used in conjunction with other treatment modalities as well. For instance, the buccal surfaces of the first molar bands may be fitted with edgewise or Straight Wire molar brackets. Thus fixed appliance mechanics may be employed simultaneously with the actions provided by the removable aspects of the system. This results in efficiency of operation and greatly reduced treatment time.

Many other more individualized movements and actions are also possible with the Wilson series of appliances. However, it is not within the scope of this text to discuss them all here. Dr Wilson has made a major contribution to the profession by means of the series of removable wire appliances he has devised. They will definitely occupy a permanent position in the standard armamentarium of practicing clinicians in the years to come. Doctors Jackson, Crozat, and Pollack must surely be smiling, wherever they are!

Figure 5-48 Extender. **(A)** Distal extension, referred to as extender, may be used for a variety of purposes. **(B)** One purpose may be to upright tilted molars, as when erupting third molar occasionally "sticks" behind a first in second-molar replacement technique.

Figure 5-49 **(A)–(F)** Wilson 3D lingual arch adjustment series.

Figure 5-50 Arch development with Wilson 3D lingual arch. **(A)** Pretreatment. **(B)** Posttreatment. (*Figures 5-38 to 5-50 courtesy of Rocky Mountain/Orthodontics.*)

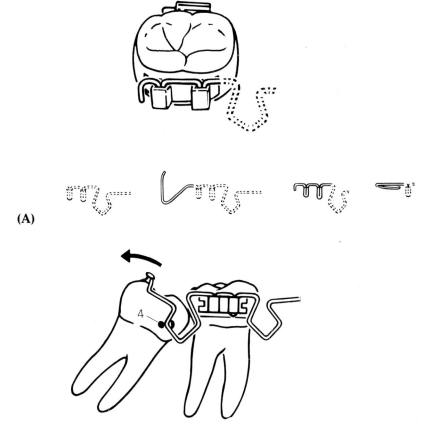

(A)

(B)

STEP **1**

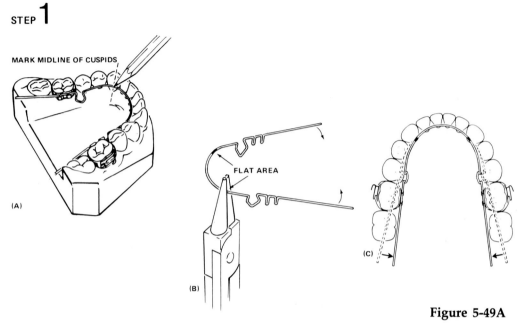

(A)

FLAT AREA

(B)

(C)

Figure 5-49A

STEP **2**

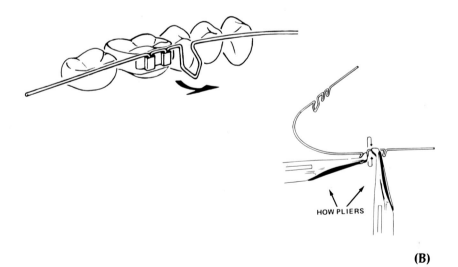

HOW PLIERS

(B)

STEP 3

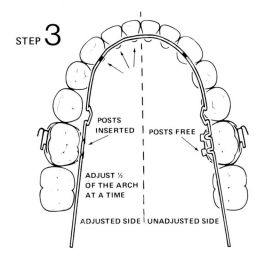

POSTS
INSERTED | POSTS FREE

ADJUST ½
OF THE ARCH
AT A TIME

ADJUSTED SIDE | UNADJUSTED SIDE

(C)

STEP 4

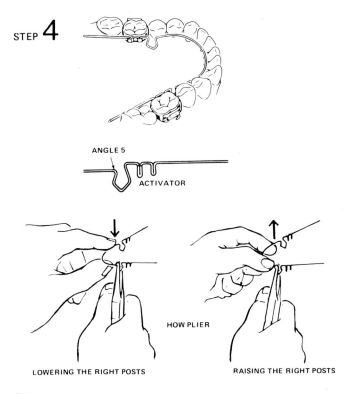

ANGLE 5

ACTIVATOR

HOW PLIER

LOWERING THE RIGHT POSTS   RAISING THE RIGHT POSTS

(D)

STEP **5**

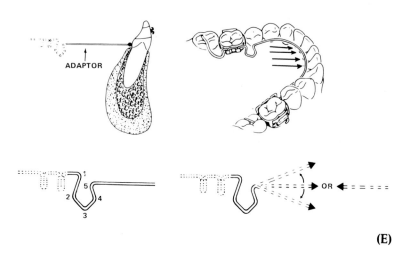

(E)

Arch Size Selection

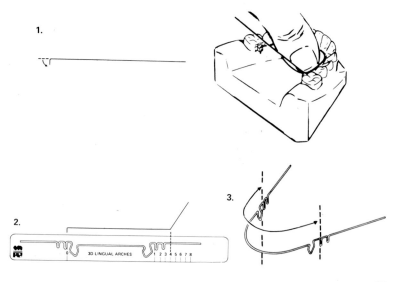

(F)

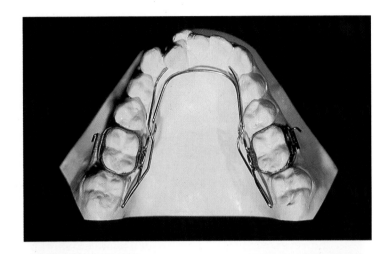

Figure 5-50A

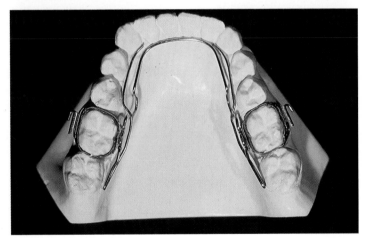

(B)

"If time aids thee to victory,
he will aid thy foe anon
to take full revenge."

al-Ma'arri AD *973–1057*
Arabian Poet, Teacher, Ascetic
Meditations, *VII*

RETENTION

Retention plays a more important role in lateral development of the arches than in any other aspect of FJO technique, with possibly the exception of anterior development of the premaxilla in Class II, Division 2 cases. Retention of cases of lateral development is important due to the amount of tissue and other structures moved during active therapy. The farther the teeth must be moved *laterally* and the more rapidly they are moved, the longer should be the period of retention. If a case is widened a short distance over a clinically long period of time with slow expansion, the chance of major relapse is minimal. If such occurs, it is usually related to recurrence of the improper muscle function, which caused the problem in the first place. If, however, a case is widened over a relatively short period of time with more clinically rapid technique, the chances of relapse after withdrawal of the appliance are increased. Slight overexpansion is then generally advisable also.

The amount of retention needed for a given case is dependent on many factors. In estimating the length of time needed for active retention, it is better to overestimate and be sure than underestimate and suffer possible relapse due to the withdrawal of the appliance too soon. As a general rule most cases should remain in active retention at least 6 months with the following withdrawal sequence.

First, with a small brass separating-wire or wire ligature, tie the central cylinders of the expansion screws to prevent them from back-turning on themselves and contacting the appliance during the long period of wear during the retentive phase. This method of tying the screws is better than sealing them up with quick-cure acrylic because if they are ever needed again for active use, they are immediately accessible.

After the 6-month active phase (constant wear) of retention is complete, begin phasing the patient out of retention. Instruct the patient to wear the appliance for most of the day and all night for about 2 months. This means the patient may leave it out during classes at school but should wear it after school and after dinner and all night during sleep. Then for the second 2-month period, have the patient wear it at night during sleep only. Then for the third 2-month period, the patient should wear it every other night or every third night for the remainder of time, keeping to that schedule until seen for the 6-month checkup. If at any time during this period the patient feels the appliance starting to get "tight," he should regress to more lengthy daily periods of active wear. Some clinicians feel that retention for this long of time is unnecessary and shorten the schedule by about 25% or so depending on the case.

Another factor to consider is the transition of one appliance to another. If a Schwarz plate is followed by a Sagittal, the latter will act as its own retainer during its phase of active treatment. If an arch-widening appliance is followed by a Bionator, however, the original active plate must be kept available to be worn as its own retainer whenever the Bionator is *not* being worn. Some patients will be in a treatment program, whereby they will wear the Sagittal, Schwarz, or Transverse plates at school or to work during the day and wear their Bionator or Orthopedic Corrector at night. In these cases the Bionator worn at night will retain the development gained by the active plates, but something more is needed during the day when the Bionator is out. This double appliance combination type of treatment is also another reason why the screws of the active plate are better off being secured with wires rather than being filled in with acrylic. Tying the expansion screws allows a certain amount of flexion to take place over the length and width of the expanded active plate. This is useful in that when the Bionator is being worn, certain changes in the shape of the maxillary arch may take place that require a certain amount of "give" in the active plate, especially Sagittals. This is possible if the screws are secured with only wire; whereas if they are "sealed shut with acrylic," the acrylic imparts a rigidity to the plate that may not be desired.

Also, if the premaxilla is being rotated down and in slightly with the Bionator, the acrylic of the active plate used to prepare the arches, and now acting as part-time retainer, must be adjusted so that the acrylic just lingual to the maxillary anterior teeth is reduced to prevent interference with the movement of these teeth in a lingual direction.

If the next appliance called for in the treatment of a case, after use of an arch-widening appliance, is a Straight Wire–type fixed bonded bracket system, a simple Hawley-type retainer may be used free of any labial bow and retained with simple ball clasps. This would expedite the transition of the case from removable to fixed appliances and would reduce the length of time needed for the wearing of the old active plate before going to the Straight Wire appliance. A thin and inoffensive palatal "turtle" may be used to prevent collapse of the upper arch during the initial phase of Straight Wire therapy provided it does not interfere with the movement of the teeth affected by the fixed appliance. Once it is obvious that the case has stabilized orthopedically, the palatal acrylic retainer may be withdrawn and the Straight Wire therapy continued without the benefit of the acrylic palatal retainer.

Regardless of which technique is used for Transverse expansion or the type or length of retention used, one must ultimately confront the fact that a certain amount of relapse is inevitable. This point was brought out by a study conducted by C. W. Schwarze[88] (not to be confused with A. M. Schwarz of active plate fame) while at the University of Cologne, West Germany. In a study of almost 500 patients who had varying degrees of active Transverse development of the arches, measurement of casts of these patients was made to decipher the amount of relapse occurring. The cases ranged from 3 to 20 years past treatment. When the average active Transverse expansion between the molars was approximately 3.65 mm, the average amount of relapse was 2 mm. In the canine region when the average inter-canine width was expanded 1.77 mm, the average relapse was 0.75 mm. Also there was no correlation shown between the length of retention and the amount of relapse! This problem is also compounded by the observation that over a 10-year period the first molars drifted mesially on the average 4.4 mm! This is partly responsible for some of the observed relapse, of course, since as the molars drift mesially, they move to a narrower part of the arch.

As you might imagine, here is where the importance of the extraction of the second molars comes into play as a key factor in Transverse appliance technique. We know that the powerful mesial thrust of the second molars lends to the crowding of teeth in the bicuspid, and even anterior regions.

As formerly discussed, with the elimination of this forward thrust by means of second molar extraction (where indicated), stability is gained in an anteroposterior direction. Now, from the previously mentioned study by C. W. Schwarze, it can be seen that a certain amount of stability may be gained for Transverse expansion also by means of second molar extraction. Without the forward thrust of the second molars present to push the first molars forward into a narrower position on the more anterior part of the arches, a certain amount of stability of a lateral nature is gained. This leaves only the purely Transverse component of relapse left to affect the case. But two other factors come into play here to help in this battle.

The first is the age of the patient. The younger they are, the greater the chances of stability in lateral development. As the appliance is opened, it will separate the palate gradually at the midpalatal suture. This allows for regeneration of the bone to close the suture incrementally with resultant stability. In older patients the problem becomes a little more difficult. Yet some expert clinicians report that as late as age 25, there is a 50% chance of still being able to open the midpalatal suture. After that the teeth may be subject to a little labial tipping.

The second concept to keep in mind is that of lateral "development" and not "expansion." By this is meant that the teeth are merely being brought out to their full genetic potential, not past the point where the limit of the basal bone has been genetically programmed. Altoona et al at the Univer-

---

Figure 5-51   The Cologne study, conducted by Dr C.W. Schwarze. **(A)** Diagrams showing that, according to Cologne study, when second molars are left intact in maxillary arch after transverse expansion, relapse is mesiolingual. Similar results are found in mandibular arch also. **(B)** When second molars are removed in maxillary arch, after transverse expansion relapse is distolingual. Same is true for mandibular arch. With second molars out after transverse expansion, relapse is distolingual.

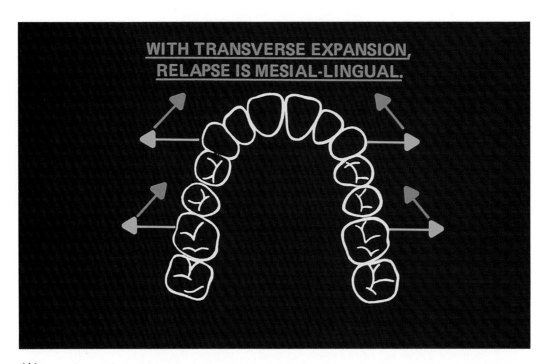

(A)

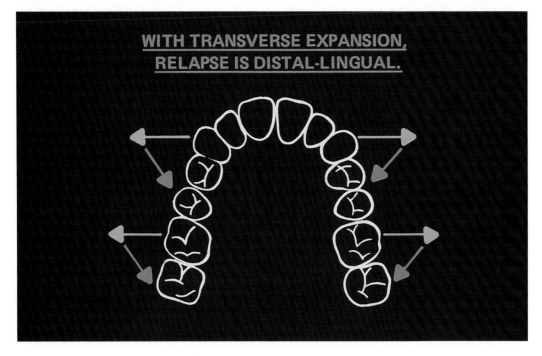

(B)

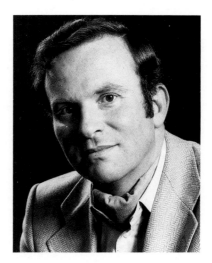

Figure 5-52   C.W. Schwarze

sity of Toronto have stated that though the *shape* of a bone may be affected by function, the *volume* is genetically predetermined. Expansion, in the truest sense of the word, of the teeth beyond the genetic limits of the basal bone is a perpetually unstable situation. That is why we refer to arch widening as "development," that is, taking the arch to its genetic ideal, and not "expansion," which would imply moving the teeth out past the basal supporting bone's genetic limit. Using the guidelines of the various facially corrected model analysis systems should prevent the clinician from "overexpanding" arches and stripping the teeth out beyond the arch limit. This helps in the battle for stability.

A third factor to be considered is the direction of the relapse of the first molars once the second molars have been extracted. After lateral development in conjunction with second molar extraction, the slight relapse that does occur is not in a mesiolingual but rather a distolingual direction. This in turn moves the teeth slightly posteriorly back on the wider part of the arch, thus helping offset the effect of the transverse relapse of the alveolar ridges themselves.

Thus we see that the best chance for lateral widening arch stability is to treat as young as possible, and where possible seriously consider extraction of the second molars!

Uphold us, cherish, and have power
to make
Our noisy years seem moments in the being
Of the eternal silence; truths that wake,
To perish never;

William Wordsworth 1770–1850
Ode "Intimations of Immortality From
Recollections of Early Childhood"

SUMMARY

What we have seen in this brief sojourn through the neighborhood of lateral expansion appliances are a few of the most commonly used methods and materials called upon by clinicians to effect the widening of dental arches. It is not intended, nor does it profess to be a complete survey of all possible techniques as that would take an entire separate volume. However, the "starting line-up" of the lateral expansion team has been adequately covered as well as some of the more important diagnostic aids used to assist in proper appliance selection.

But, more importantly, what has been shown here is a profound principle of orthodontics and orthopedics (or "orthopedia" if you will, a term signifying the combination of both principles), and that is the *importance of the integrity of the arch form!*[9,89-91] All of the appliances and techniques mentioned on the previous pages are devoted to the singular concept of producing an acceptable arch out of a group of teeth that may be anything less. Arches, nonextracted in the bicuspid area, correctly balanced, nonforeshortened, correctly positioned relative to their structural bases, correctly shaped relative to geometric considerations, correctly spaced and correctly aligned — arches are everything! Well, almost. But in all fairness to this extremely far-reaching concept, the development of dental arches with their full complement of bicuspids present is the talisman of the new direction modern orthodontics will take. Now admittedly, ideal arch production has always been a chief concern of traditional orthodontics, but up until now it has been viewed in a much different light.

Prior to the use of functional appliances in specific and the gross consideration of dental orthopedics in general, the treating clinician was faced with the problem of being forced to not only prepare, but also match up opposing arches *simultaneously,* with the mere use of fixed appliances. Often this represented an enormous challenge that required heroic efforts on the part of the operator and patient alike to correct. The chief and most fundamental underlying problem of the treatment regimens for Class II situations was that old onus of having to bring both arches into alignment, with proper overjet and overbite, at once!

Using only purely orthodontic techniques, this meant that to effect such simultaneous orthodontic interarch alignments often the risk would be great that orthopedics would suffer.[92-93] It did. Moving teeth alone orthodontically through bone to bring them into a compromised arch form from a Class II relationship while disregarding, by necessity, the orthopedics that may coincide with the malocclusion or even be the chief etiological factor, is merely the forcing of one technique to try to accomplish effects that are of essence out of its realm of authority. Fixed appliance therapy is the undisputed method of choice for purely orthodontic tooth movement of any considerable degree. Functional appliance therapy, supplemented by the much-appreciated helping hand of active plate mechanics, is very often the best way to solve purely orthopedic changes. Separating the malocclusion into these two components relieves the enormous burden from the shoulders of the fixed appliance of having to try to accomplish successful treatment of both problems at once. It frees the hands of the operator to use his skills to the fullest and in an uncompromised fashion to prepare the patient's arches singly, one at a time, totally independent of each other. He may prepare an orthopedically proper, orthodontically correct, beautiful upper arch without the disclaimers of bicuspid extractions. He may do the same in the lower arch with all but complete disregard for the occlusion and alignment arch to arch. The reason this is now possible, of course, is what is the key to the whole FJO philosophy—the Bionator. Once proper arch form is obtained for the Class II patient in each of the arches individually, without the restraints of matching the two arches to each other simultaneously, the Bionator may be inserted to bring the case out of Class II from its retruded deep overbite position into the full Class I relationship molar to molar, cuspid to cuspid, with all the benefits of a full beautiful broad smile line, pleasing facial contour, proper lower face height, and healthy unstrained temporomandibular joints. Assuredly, not all malocclusions are the Class II deep overbite, large overjet type. But many are. And for those that are, the treatment plans devised for them can now be changed from a theater of one of the more difficult to the realm of one of the easiest. No matter how perfectly shaped a pair of arches are, the key to their successful function is their proper arch-to-arch alignment. And arch-to-arch alignment in all three anatomical planes of reference is the main forte of the Bionator. But, as now may plainly be seen, the entire process of Bionator treatment is predicated on having proper arches to align. That means proper arch preparation, which in turn implies, sooner or later, the eventual use of active plates of one sort or another.

Active plates can be used to develop arches either sagittally or laterally. The type selected is a function of the *needs* of the case indicated by the respective model analysis aids. Sometimes both sagittal and lateral development are needed. But, as can be surmised from the information in this chapter, the proclivity of appliances for the lateral development component alone indicates several things. First, the need for widening narrow arches has long been recognized as an important component of correct orthodontic treatment. The attention paid to this problem, evidenced by both the history and number of appliances created to handle it, indicate that in the realm of the dental malocclusion, narrowness of the arches is quite ubiquitous throughout the population of patients. The variety of appliance designs also indicates that lateral development of the arches is a relatively easy task to accomplish. Though widely differing in designs from one end of the spectrum to the other, all members of the "Transverse family" have certain elements in common. They all have a means of internal force, either a spring, wire, or screw, etc, and a means of administering that force to the teeth and alveolus (and sometimes the midpalatal suture).

However, this does not mean the Transverse family of appliances may be leaned upon as a panacea for all arch-crowding problems. Lateral development is easy to obtain in the mixed dentition provided it is fortified with adequate periods of retention. But as the patient goes through puberty and starts proceeding farther down the road to adulthood, lateral development is subsequently more liable to the risks of instability. These factors must be considered in treatment planning to ensure a successful outcome. But with the incidence of arch narrowness being what it is (one almost never sees one too wide to begin with), and with the importance of proper arch form for the sake of properly finishing the cases now obvious, the clinician cannot avoid mastering the use of transverse-type appliances. Fortunately, due to the variety of appliances available for this purpose and their ease of manipulation, this is not difficult. Once the arches have been brought to their full genetic potential and have received the benefit of proper structural anatomy by means of the active plates, or "arch preparers," the operator may get on with the business of treating the orthopedics with the proper "arch aligners," the functional appliances. His cases will be slowly homing in on the goal of stability rather than drifting away from it because the excessive tooth movement required to close bicuspid extraction sites will not have been initiated in the first place. Also absent, in most cases, will be the gigantic forward thrust of the second molar and its arch-collapsing efforts at making room for the doddering third. His cases will also be moving toward the ideal of full and pleasing facial profiles and smile lines because all the teeth are present that are concerned with this notion, and the jaws with their teeth in the correct anatomical relationships are being matched to the face, not vice versa, ie, the shoehorn fitting of teeth into underdeveloped bone. This would be conversely forcing the face to match the teeth. And finally, the temporomandibular joints of the patient thus treated are given their best chance of a normal balanced existence and carefree life. But all this is totally dependent upon the acceptability of the arches for what the functional appliance is capable of giving. Hence the undisputed need for the use of active plates as both an orthodontic and orthopedic adjunct to the use of functional appliances in the long and arduous search for the best possible treatment that may be given the patient. And yet for all their strength, versatility, and importance, there are some aspects of arch preparation that require the finesse and refinement that the removable active plate repertoire finds difficult to effect. Hence, they alone cannot be totally relied upon to meet all the demands that might be made on a treatment plan to bring the case to its highest level of both orthodontic as well as orthopedic development. Some of the subtleties of purely orthodontic-type tooth movement require force delivery systems of the most exacting and exquisite variety. Fortunately for us, as if by some miracle of our modern technological age, just such a system stands ready and waiting in the wings!

REFERENCES

1. Harvold EP: The role of function in the etiology of malocclusion. *Am J Orthod* 1968;54:883–897.
2. Broekman RW: The influence of the tongue on the shape and development of the jaws and tooth position. *Ned Tijdschr Tandheelk* 1965;72:355–367.
3. Peat JH: A cephalometric study of tongue position. *Am J Orthod* 1968;54:339–351.
4. Brodie AG: Anatomy and physiology of head and neck musculature. *Am J Orthod* 1950;36:331–334.
5. Biourge A: The tongue and orthodontics. *Actual Odontostomatol* 1967;79:295–334.
6. Hansen ML, Logan WB, Case JL: Tongue-thrust in pre-school children. *Am J Orthod* 1970;57:15–22.
7. Thoma KH: Principle factors controlling the development of the mandible and maxilla. *Am J Orthod Oral Surg* 1938;24:171–179.
8. Cohen JT: Growth and development of the dental arches in children. *J Am Dent Assoc* 1940;27:1250–1260.
9. Hawley CA: Determination of the normal arch and its application to orthodontia. *Dent Cosmos* 1905;47:541–552.
10. Stanton FL: Arch predetermination and a method of relating the predetermined arch to the malocclusion to show the minimum tooth movement. *Int J Orthod* 1922;8:757–778.
11. Goldstein MS, Stanton FL: Changes in dimensions and form of the dental arches with age. *Int J Orthod* 1935;21:357–380.
12. Chapman H: The normal dental arch and its changes from birth to adult. *Br Dent J* 1935;58:203–229.
13. Brader AC: Dental arch form related with intraoral forces: PR=C. *Am J Orthod* 1972;61:541–561.
14. White LW: Individual ideal arches. *J Clin Orthod* 1978;12:779–787.
15. Ricketts RM, Roth RH, Chaconas SJ, et al: *Orthodontic Diagnosis and Planning.* Rocky Mountain/Orthodontics, 1982, vol 1, p 231.
16. MacConaill MA, Scher EA: The ideal form of the human dental arcade, with some prosthetic application. *Dent Rec* 1949;69:285–302.
17. Scott JH: The shape of dental arches. *J Dent Res* 1957;36:996–1003.
18. Lu KH: Analysis of dental arch symmetry, abstract. *J Dent Res* 1964;43:780.
19. Currier JH: A computerized geometric analysis of human dental arch form. *Am J Orthod* 1969;56:164–179.
20. Garn DH: Human dental arch form determination from cranial anatomy through ionic section geometry, thesis, Temple University, Philadelphia, 1968.
21. Schwarz AM, Gratzinger M: Removable Orthodontic Appliances. Philadelphia, WB Saunders Co, 1966.
22. Ricketts RM, Roth RH, Chaconas SJ, et al: *Orthodontic Diagnosis and Planning.* Rocky Mountain/Orthodontics, 1982, vol 1, pp 24–143.

23. Tweed CH: Indications for extraction of teeth in orthodontic procedure. *Am Assoc Orthod Trans* 1944,22–45.

24. Williams R, Hosila FJ: The effects of different extraction sites upon incisor retraction. *Am J Orthod* 1976;69:388–410.

25. Posen AL: The application of quantitative perioral assessment to orthodontic case analysis and treatment planning. *Angle Orthod* 1976;46:118–143.

26. Riedel RA: A review of the retention problem. *Angle Orthod* 1960;30:179–194.

27. Steadman SR: Changes of intermolar and intercuspid distances following orthodontic treatment. *Angle Orthod* 1960;31:207–215.

28. Walter DC: Changes in the form and dimension of dental arches resulting from orthodontic treatment. *Angle Orthod* 1953;23:1–18.

29. Nord CFL: Loose appliances in orthodontia. *Trans Eur Orthod Soc* 1929.

30. Skieller V: Expansion of the midpalatal suture by removable plates, analysed by the implant method. *Trans Eur Orthod Soc* 1964;143–157.

31. Lebret LML: Changes in the palatal vault resulting from expansion. *Angle Orthod* 1965;35:97–105.

32. Jackson VH: Some methods of regulating. *Dent Cosmos* 1887;29:373–387.

33. Hockel JL: *Orthopedic Gnathology.* Chicago, Quintessence Publishing Co, 1983, p 47.

34. Crozat GB: Possibilities and use of removable labio-lingual spring appliances. *Int J Orthod Oral Surg* 1920;6:1–7.

35. Gore SD: Treatment of Class II malocclusion in the mixed dentition with the use of removable appliances. *Am J Orthod* 1954;40:359–363.

36. Lamons FF: The Crozat removable appliance. *Am J Orthod* 1964;50:265–292.

37. Dewey M: Application of spring force from gold and platinum appliances. *Int J Orthod* 1923;9:512.

38. Wiebrecht A: *Crozat Appliance in Maxillo-facial Orthopedics.* Menomonie, Wis, E.F. Schmidt Co.

39. Wiebrecht A: The application of the Crozat removable appliance for the development of the arches in orthodontia. *Fort Rev Chicago Dent Soc* July 1961, p 13.

40. Sheppe JH: The construction and use of a Crozat appliance. *Int J Orthod* 1971;9:192–201.

41. Angell EH: Treatment of irregularities of the permanent or adult teeth. *Dent Cosmos* 1960;1:540–544, 599–600.

42. McQuillen JH: Treatment of irregularities of the permanent or adult teeth, review. *Dent Cosmos* 1960;1:540–544, 599–600.

43. Farrar JN: *Irregularities of the Teeth and Their Correction.* New York, International News Co, 1888, vol 1, pp 182–185.

44. Cryer MH: The influences exerted by the dental arches in regard to respiration and general health. *Dent Items Interest* 1913;35:16–46, discussion 94–115.

45. Federspiel NM: Development of the maxillae with reference to opening the median suture. *Items Interest* 1913;35: discussion 271–282.

46. Kemple F: The pathologic and therapeutic possibilities of upper maxillary contraction and expansion. *Dent Cosmos* 1914;56:215–222.

47. Angle EH: Bone growing. *Dent Cosmos* 1910;52:216–267.

48. Case CS: Expansion of the dental arch. *Dent Rev* 1893;7:207–217.

49. Dewey M: Development of the maxillae with reference to opening the median suture. *Items Interest* 1913;35:189–208, discussion 271–282.

50. Ketcham AH: Treatment by the orthodontist supplementing that by rhinologist. *Dent Cosmos* 1921;54:1312–1321.

51. Korkhaus G: Present orthodontic thought in Germany. *Am J Orthod* 1960;46: 187–206.

52. Haas AJ: Rapid expansion of the maxillary dental arch and nasal cavity by opening the midpalatal suture. *Angle Orthod* 1961;31:73–90.

53. Haas AJ: The treatment of maxillary deficiency by opening the midpalatal suture. *Angle Orthod* 1965;35:200–217.

54. Haas AJ: Palatal expansion: just the beginning of dentofacial orthopedics. *Am J Orthod* 1970;57:219–255.

55. Isaacson RJ, Murphy TD: Some effects of rapid maxillary expansion in cleft lip and palate patients. *Angle Orthod* 1964;34:143–154.

56. Isaacson RJ, Wood JL, Ingram AH: Forces produced by rapid maxillary expansion. *Angle Orthod* 1964;34:256–270.

57. Thorne NAH: Expansion of maxilla; spreading the midpalate suture; measuring the widening of the apical base and nasal cavity on serial roentgenograms, abstract. *Am J Orthod* 1960;46:626.

58. Finring JF, Isaacson RJ: Forces produced by rapid maxillary expansion. *Angle Orthod* 1965;35:178–186.

59. Wertz RA: Skeletal and dental changes accompanying rapid midpalatal suture opening. *Am J Orthod* 1970;58:41–66.

60. Wertz RA: Changes in nasal air flow incident to rapid maxillary expansion. *Angle Orthod* 1968;39:1–11.

61. Wertz R: Midpalatal suture openings: a normative study. *Am J Orthod* 1977; 71:367–381.

62. Krebs A: Expansion of the mid-palatal suture studied by means of metalic implants. *Eur Orthodont Soc Rep* 1958;34:163–171.

63. Starnbach HK, Cleall JF: Effects of splitting the midpalatal suture on the surrounding structures. *Am J Orthod* 1964;50:923–924.

64. Hershey HG, Stewart BL, Warren DW: Changes in nasal airway resistance associated with rapid maxillary expansion. *Am J Orthod* 1976;69:274–284.

65. Stockfish H: Rapid expansion of the maxilla—success and relapse. *Trans Eur Orthod Soc* 1969;469–481.

66. Timms DJ: Long-term follow-up of cases treated by rapid maxillary expansion. *Trans Eur Orthod Soc* 1976;211–215.

67. Linder-Aronson S: The skeletal and dental effects of rapid maxillary expansion. *Br J Orthod* 1979;6:25–29.

68. Brown GVI: The application of orthodontic principles to the prevention of nasal disease. *Dent Cosmos* 1903;45:765–775.

69. Black NM: The relation between deviation of the nasal septum and irregularities of the teeth and jaw. *JAMA* 1909;52:943–945.

70. Dean LW: The influence on the nose of widening the palatal arch. *JAMA* 1909; 52:941–943.

71. Willis FM: Rapid separation of the superior maxillary bones to relieve deflected nasal septum and contracted nares. *Dent Cosmos* 1911;53:784–786.

72. Wright GH: I. A group of deformities of the nasal respiratory tract, coincident with dental irregularities, II. A new instrument for comparative studies. *Dent Cosmos* 1912;54:261–269.

73. Biederman W: Rapid correction of Class III malocclusion by midpalatal expansion. *Am J Orthod* 1973;63:47–54.

74. Hilger DC: A synopsis of seven current concepts and procedures of maxillary palatal expansion and posterior-anterior cephalogram standardization and utiliza-

tion. Read before the Annual Meeting of the American Association of Orthodontists, Miami, April 1969.

75. Epker BN, Wolford LM: *Dentofacial Deformities: Surgical Orthodontic Correction,* St Louis, CV Mosby Co, 1980, pp 320–331.

76. Witt E, Gehrke M: Leitfaden der Kieferorthopädischen Technik. Berlin, Quintessence, 1981, pp 95–99.

77. Pollock HC: An orthodontic appliance, being a combination of principles involved in the lingual appliance, ribbon arch, and expansion arch. *Int J Orthod* 1920;6:573–578.

78. Pollock HC: Personal communication, July 1976.

79. Pollock HC: Elementary orthodontic technic. *Int J Orthod* 1923;9:120–121, 207–210, 282–287, 364–369, 453–459, 527–531, 770–772, 840–846, 929–936; 1924;10:38–41, 166–171, 364–369.

80. Pollock HC: Modification of the fixed removable type of orthodontic appliance. *Int J Orthod* 1930;16:737–743.

81. Pollock HC: History repeats itself – Part I and Part II. *Am J Orthod* 1968;54:536–539, 561–565.

82. Dukes HH: The Pollock appliance. *Am J Orthod* 1969;55:734–738.

83. Ricketts RM: *Development of the Quad Helix Appliance. Features of the Bioprogressive Therapy.* Rocky Mountain/Orthodontics, 1973, No. 14, pt 8, pp 33–36.

84. Wilson WL, Wilson RC: *Modular Orthodontics.* Rocky Mountain/Orthodontics, 1982.

85. Mershon JV: The removable lingual arch as an appliance for the treatment of malocclusion of the teeth. *Int J Orthod* 1918;4:578–587.

86. Mershon JV: The removable lingual arch appliance. *Int J Orthod* 1926;12:1002–1026.

87. Mershon JV: A practical talk on why the lingual arch is applicable to the orthodontic problem. *Dent Rec* 1926;46:297–301.

88. Schwarze CW: Expansion and relapse in long follow-up studies. *Trans Eur Orthod Soc* 1972;263–274.

89. Stanton FL: A consideration of normal and abnormal dentures as a problem of three dimensional space, etc. *Int J Orthod* 1922;8:185–204.

90. Baume LJ: Physiological tooth migration and its significance for the development of the occlusion. III. The biogenesis of the successful dentition. *J Dent Res* 1950;29:338–348.

91. Sillman JH: Dimensional changes of the dental arches: Longitudinal study from birth to 25 years. *Am J Orthod* 1964;50:824–842.

92. Moore AW: Orthodontic treatment factors in Class II malocclusion. *Am J Orthod* 1959;45:323–351.

93. Meach CL: A cephalometric comparison of bony profile changes in Class II, division 1 patients treated with extra oral force and functional jaw orthopedics. *Am J Orthod* 1966;52:353–369.

CHAPTER 6
The Bionator II, III

The Bionator II is an anterior premaxillary arch-*leveling* appliance. Often referred to as a "Bionator to close an open bite," a cumbersome name at best, the Bionator II is mainly used to close down the open bite created in the anterior region due to a protruding premaxilla with labially flared maxillary central and lateral incisors. Although used primarily for this purpose, it may also be used to increase the vertical eruption of the lower incisor arch in an effort to help close the anterior open bite. Another simple modification allows this appliance to advance the mandible when needed. But by virtue of the acrylic bite blocks of the appliance that fill in the interocclusal space between the upper and lower posterior teeth, this appliance is totally neutral with respect to changes in vertical dimension. The vertical dimension of occlusion is totally unaffected by this device. Thus in some ways the Bionator II is similar to the more conventional standard Bionator in design and effect, and yet in other ways it is radically different.

Its similarities in appearance to the standard Bionator are in its two vertical acrylic plates or "wings" that fit snugly against the lingual surfaces of the upper and lower posterior segments. These wings are held together posteriorly by means of the standard Coffin spring. Anteriorly, the two halves of the appliance are connected by an acrylic lingual bar, usually bear-

419

ing an expansion-type jackscrew at the midline, a lingual wire, and the conventional labial bow.

But where the appliance differs is in the acrylic bite blocks or "pads" that fill in the interocclusal spaces posteriorly. The pads have the indentations of the occlusal surfaces of the upper and lower posterior teeth reproduced on their respective upper and lower surfaces. These pads are approximately 2 mm thick and the upper and lower posterior teeth interdigitate with them while the appliance is being worn in the mouth. There may or may not be an incisal acrylic cap processed onto the appliance depending on whether or not incisal eruption is desired in the mandible. This same principle is why the appliance remains neutral relative to the vertical. The acrylic pads on the posterior teeth prevent eruption in this area as increasing the vertical in anterior open bite cases is contraindicated.

Like the conventional Bionator, the Bionator II has a nearly identical sister appliance, the Orthopedic Corrector II. Its actions and design are similar to the Bionator II except that it has expansion screws mounted in the sides of the appliance which, when opened, advance the lower anterior cap and thus advance the mandible in cases where the anterior open bite is complicated by a severely retruded Class II-type mandible. Adjustments of this modified appliance, when activating the side screws, are similar to those used when treating with the standard Orthopedic Corrector I.

When properly used for the types of cases for which they were originally designed, these appliances quickly and easily bring a protruded premaxilla with its flared or infraerupted maxillary lateral and central incisors back down and into their correct positions on the level occlusal plane. They are also helpful in correcting the tongue thrust or thumb-sucking habits

---

Figure 6-1 Basic Bionator II appliance, often referred to as a "Bionator to close an open bite." It's primary function is to close down an anterior open bite, rotate premaxilla down and in, and intercept both tongue thrust and thumb- or finger-sucking habits that are most likely etiological agents of such a condition. The action of this appliance in the late mixed and early adult dentition is greatly enhanced by extraction of second molars. (*Courtesy of Ohlendorf Co, St Louis, MO.*)

Figure 6-2 **(A)** Lateral view and **(B)** frontal view of fit of Bionator II in typical anterior open bite case. Note high course of labial bow as it traverses anterior maxillary area. In Bionator II technique, it is always kept in contact with labial surfaces of maxillary anteriors. **(C)** Viewed from inferior aspect, midline expansion screw is clearly visible as are **(D)** the interocclusal acrylic pads. (Note: these particular appliances do not possess either lingual wire or lingual "tongue retraining" loops that are common additions to this type of appliance.) (*Courtesy of Ohlendorf Co, St Louis, MO.*)

Figure 6-3 **(A)** Basic Orthopedic Corrector II appliance. **(B)** Note location of expansion side screws that advance lower cap, and as a result entire mandible, similar to Orthopedic Corrector I technique.

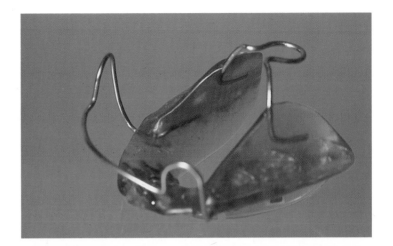

Figure 6-1A

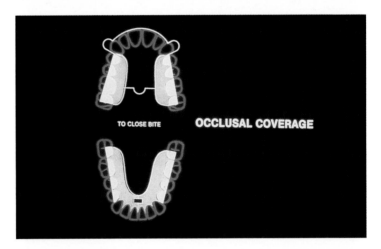

TO CLOSE BITE   OCCLUSAL COVERAGE

(B)

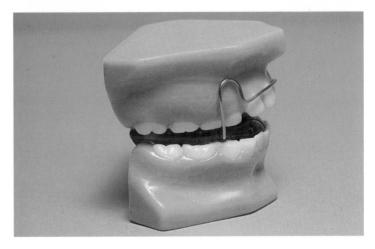

Figure 6-2A

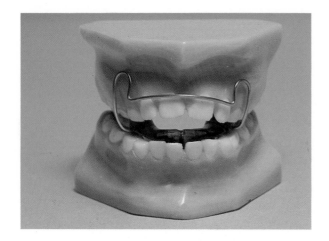

(B)

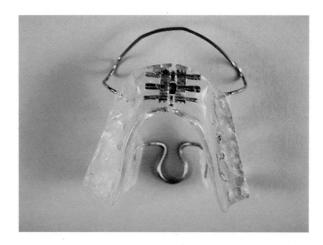

(C)

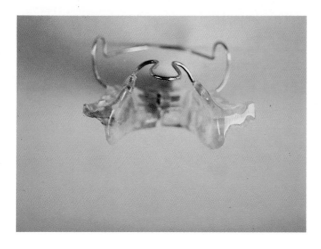

(D)

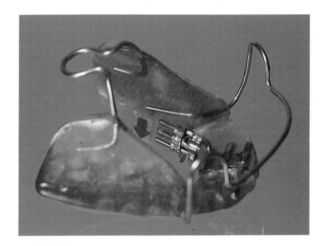

Figure 6-2E

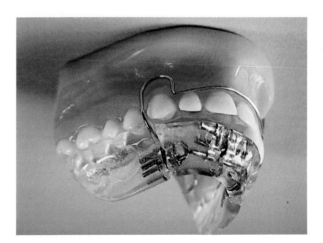

Figure 6-3A

(B)

ORTHOPEDIC CORRECTOR II
Patent Pending

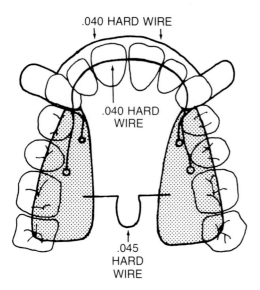

.040 HARD WIRE

.040 HARD
WIRE

.045
HARD
WIRE

INDICATIONS:
1) Class II to Class I without vertical growth
2) Decrease vertical in mixed dentition
3) Correct open bites in mixed dentition from thumb sucking, tongue habits, etc.
4) To achieve forward growth of the mandible in open-bite tendency cases (clock-wise growers).
5) In the mixed dentition:
   a) Enlarges the dental arches, without tipping of teeth, in case of arch length deficiency (crowding).
6) TMJ PAIN PATIENTS: For repositioning of the mandible without increasing the vertical, the Orthopedic Corrector II is unexcelled.

Note 1:
   To this appliance can be added several modifications for specific tooth movement, rotations, tongue training, space closure, etc., depending on the case. These are taught in the advanced technique seminars.

Note 2:
   This appliance will treat the above indications to the finest, most stable results, in the shortest period of time, of all orthopedic or functional appliances in use today.

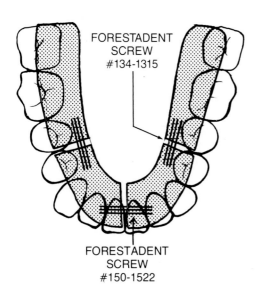

FORESTADENT
SCREW
#134-1315

FORESTADENT
SCREW
#150-1522

Figure 6-3C

which are usually the etiologic agent responsible for many anterior open bite cases.[1-4] By virtue of their relatively short treatment time and the visually dramatic results achieved, they are very popular appliances for both patient and doctor. Parents are very happy to see the improved appearances of their child during the course of treatment as the unesthetic anterior open bite closes down nicely. The patients are very happy when they realize they do not have to wear external headgear or be in fixed appliances for years to obtain the desired results. They are also happy that the appliance helps those who deal with prolonged thumb-sucking problems to break the habit. Having the appliance in their mouths satisfies much of the sucking urge for many children, especially during sleep. The patients are also happy that the very pleasing results come quickly and with little or no pain or discomfort. The doctor is also happy to see such excellent progress come so easily and with such pleasant effects. He is also pleased with the practice-building ramifications of treating these types of cases. These appliances inspire gratitude, confidence, and satisfaction for parent, patient, and doctor alike.

CONSTRUCTION BITE

The construction bite may be taken in one of several ways depending on the type of case being treated. There are two basic categories: anterior open bite cases where the molars and cuspids are already in a satisfactory Class I position, and open bite cases with concomitant moderate or severe Class II jaw relationships.

For the Class I cases, the bite is usually taken in a normal centric relationship with possibly some slight advancement of the mandible into a super-Class I position. The wax sheets, or preformed bite blocks, must be heated thoroughly in 140°F water until soft. The wax is placed on the lower posterior teeth far enough away from the anteriors to allow good visibility of the front teeth to permit judgment of the thickness of the bite. The patient is asked to close his teeth in either their normal or *slightly* protruded position until the posterior teeth are biting into the wax with an interocclusal separation of about 2 mm. Two aspects of this procedure are critical to the successful and correct construction of the appliance. First, the wax must be thoroughly heated so as to be soft enough to allow the patient to bite into it with little effort. If the wax is too firm, the pressure required to bite into it combined with the resistance of the wax against the teeth and gum tissue as these push through the wax causes a slight dislocation of the condyle in the glenoid fossa in an inferior direction. If such a bite is used to relate two models to one another in the laboratory during construction, the resultant appliance will come back with acrylic that is too thick posteriorly and when the appliance is inserted into the mouth, and the patient told to bite on it, the extra thickness over the posteriors will cause the bicuspids farther forward in the arch to appear to be open, out of occlusion with the acrylic. This necessitates bothersome reduction of the extra acrylic posteriorly with acrylic burs, etc, until the occlusion is even throughout the appliance front to back.

This is true for *any* appliance that has acrylic between the occlusal surfaces of the posterior teeth. To prevent uneven anterior open occlusion on appliances with interocclusal acrylic, keep the wax *soft*.

The second critical factor to keep in mind concerning the construction bite for this appliance is its thickness. Two millimeters interocclusal distance is ideal. Four millimeters is the outermost limit tolerable for appliances of this sort. If a bite is registered greater than 4 mm in thickness, it causes the bite blocks of the finished appliance to be so thick that they produce an "unloading" effect on the condyle similar to the action of a conventional Bionator and thereby stimulate condylar growth, an undesirable effect for Class I anterior open bite cases. This is especially true in patients who exhibit "counterclockwise" or predominantly horizontal growth tendencies, flat occlusal planes, and low facial axis angles. The unwanted condylar growth stimulated by too thick a construction bite would tend to increase the Class III tendencies, already a problem in "counterclockwise" horizontal growers in Class I relationships. For the patient with anterior open bites and Class I molars, remember: Keep the construction bite *soft* and *thin*.

For the Class II anterior open bite case, a slightly different construction bite is taken. Here mandibular advancement *is* desirable. The acrylic bite plates or pads will prevent an increase in vertical, but this is usually not a problem to begin with in open bite cases. Yet the mandible still may be advanced as a whole, keeping its vertical constant by means of taking the construction bite with the lower jaw in a protruded position similar to that of a conventional Bionator construction bite. In the younger patient of either the mixed or early adult dentition stage, the bite may be taken with the mandible protruded enough to cause a super-Class I or even slight Class III relationship to the molars. This is not as easy as it sounds. Ideally, it would be such that if the upper anteriors were down in their normal posi-

---

Figure 6-4 Case study: Classic Bionator II case early mixed dentition. This patient presented at age 8 years, 10 months with skeletal Class II, Division 1 anterior open bite. She was 6.5 mm short of arch width according to Schwarz index and suffered from 7 mm open bite and 6.75 mm overjet in anterior region. Her anterior open bite and skeletal Class II narrow arch condition was concomitant with retained thumb-sucking habit and adaptive tongue thrust during swallowing. Entire case was treated with Bionator II appliance. Not only did it close down anterior open bite and retrain adaptive tongue thrust to more proper swallowing pattern, but midline screw and Coffin spring were utilized to regain deficient arch width. Treatment time was 18 months. **(A)** Pretreatment frontal facial views. **(B) (C)** Pretreatment study models exhibiting severity of anterior open bite. **(D)** Posttreatment facial view. **(E)** One year after withdrawal of appliance, no retention. Note how cuspids have fully erupted, arch form remains stable, and overbite is increased to 2.5 mm as bite settles in. **(F)** Overlaying cephalometric tracings divulge true anatomical nature of total correction of case.

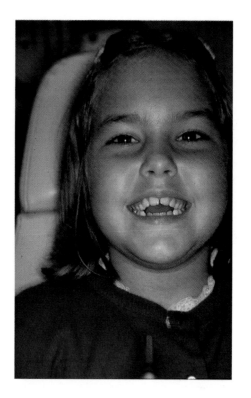

(A)

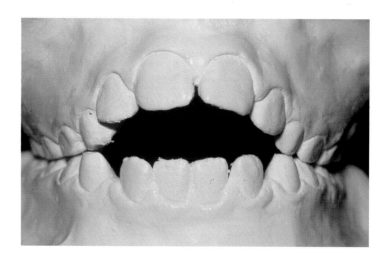

(B)

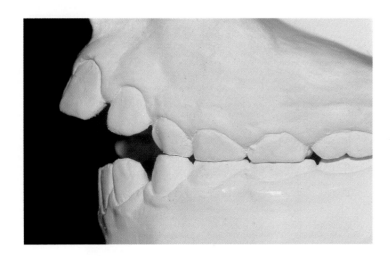

(C)

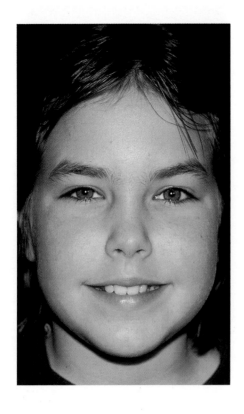

(D)

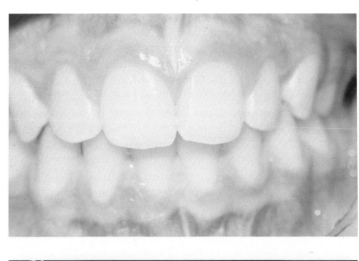

(E)

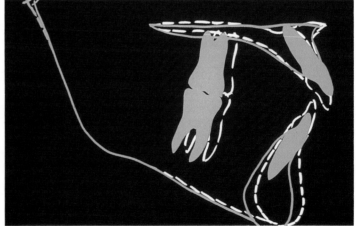

(F)

tion level with the occlusal plane, the lower incisors would be about 2 mm past the uppers anteriorly. But the upper anteriors are nowhere near the occlusal plane due to the open bite situation. They may be high up in a protruded premaxilla or flared forward anteriorly or in a state of semicomplete eruption. This makes judging their imaginary correct position when finished difficult at times. Not only is the amount of mandibular advancement important, but one must also take the bite with a degree of thickness that would correspond to an interincisal distance of, again, about 2 mm, *if* the anteriors were in their final correct position. Since 1 to 2 mm overbite anteriorly is desirable and the minimum thickness for acrylic pad strength and proper interdigitation with teeth is 2 mm, the standard 2-mm thickness interocclusally will do. But even with the upper anteriors up and out of the plane of occlusion, the simple observation of where the lower cuspid is relative to the upper cuspid when the bite is taken will offer adequate evidence of sufficient advancement and thickness to bring about proper condylar growth and mandibular advancement from Class II to Class I. If after the bite closes down anteriorly, the mandible is insufficiently advanced from Class II to Class I, a new more accurate construction bite may be taken, now that the incisors are in their correct position to be used as a guide in the conventional manner. Then either the appliance may be relined on the lower inner surface to keep the mandible in a newer more protruded position, or an entire new appliance may be constructed. If the operator anticipates difficulty in judging the sufficiency of advancement of the mandible in a construction bite for a case with a severe Class II retruded mandible, he can avoid the chances of needing two appliances by merely having an Orthopedic Corrector II constructed instead. Then, should mandibular insufficiency still be evident after the bite closes down anteriorly, the side screws may be activated and the lower occlusal and interdental acrylic reduced in the conventional manner. The mandible then may be advanced steadily until it achieves the correct Class I position.

For the late teen and early adult patient a greater thickness interocclusally and slightly more protrusion of the mandible for the construction bite is indicated. The older the bone, the more intense the stimulation must be to cause change. For these cases in Class I, 3 mm thickness interocclusally will do. If mandibular advancement is also needed, alignment of the cuspids in Class I or just past, to the position of super-Class I, can act as a guide. Or again, the clinician may merely take the bite in some degree of protrusion and if need be allow the expansion screws of the Orthopedic Corrector II to pick up the difference. In all cases concerning the anterior open bite, it must be remembered that the problem facing the clinician is where to put the mandible when taking the construction bite. It must be kept in mind that the upper anteriors are not the guide; they can be anywhere, and they usually are.

After obtaining an accurate set of plaster casts and the correct construction bite, the models and bite are sent to the laboratory for appliance fabrication.

ADJUSTMENTS

The first thing the clinician will notice upon receiving a Bionator II back from the laboratory is that, upon initial inspection, the labial bow appears to have been distorted somehow during transit as it is bent far superiorly up and away from the normal plane of occlusion. But this is its correct position. The worse the case is, the higher the bow will be. It is designed to contact the labial surfaces of the maxillary anterior central and lateral incisors at about the gingival third of their crowns. Once inserted in the mouth, it will be observed that the bow almost always traverses across the maxillary anterior arch in this exact position.

The usual procedures are followed upon insertion of the appliance in the mouth. First, it is checked for acrylic bubbles or rough spots. Then after insertion, the patient is informed of the normal effects to be expected upon trying to accommodate to the new appliance such as mouth watering, difficulty in speech, and the awkward feeling of "having a mouthful."

The labial bow must be carefully examined to make sure it is contacting the teeth properly. Unlike the more standard Bionator I and Orthopedic Corrector I, the labial bow of the Bionator II is designed to contact the labial surfaces of the maxillary anteriors immediately upon insertion. It should not impinge on the gingival tissues anywhere as this would produce ulceration, but it should fit snugly against the enamel surfaces of these upper front teeth. If it fails to do so upon insertion, adjust the bow in the conventional manner until it does so. It should not be free and away from these teeth as is the case with the standard Bionator. This allows the full pressures of the weight of the upper lip and the stretched muscles to be brought to bear against the protruded premaxilla.[5-6] This along with other factors, discussed later, are the prime factors that bring about the reduction of the open bite. The labial bow is to be kept in this position continually during treatment. This requires that it be readjusted at the periodic checking appointments, about every 3 to 5 weeks, to maintain contact. As the premaxilla rotates down and away from the bow, a small space starts opening between the bow and the labial surfaces of the teeth. This space is closed by tightening the bow at the routine appointments.

The other important adjustment to be performed is the cutting of the lingual retention wire. This wire acts to prevent lingual movement past a certain point in the standard Bionator and Orthopedic Corrector I. But it serves an entirely different function in the Bionator II. Here it acts as a tongue trainer. Two of the major causes of anterior open bite are the tongue and the thumb.[7,8] When either one occupies a place in the premaxillary region for more than a minimal amount of time, the age-old battle between bone and muscle ensues and, as usual, bone loses.

If the tongue is the chief offender, it is so by means of a deviant swallowing pattern involving an anterior tongue thrust. The true tongue thrust of an endogenous neuromuscular origin is somewhat rare. Most are of the simpler adaptive type.[9-11] The endogenous or neuromuscular tongue thrust is a little more difficult to deal with. During the abnormal tongue-thrust swallowing pattern, the tip of the tongue is thrust forward and slams against the anterior palatal area and lingual surfaces of the upper, and sometimes even lower, anterior incisors.[12] At 1500 to 2000 incidents per day,[13] the average number of swallows in a 24-hour period, it doesn't take long before the pliable growing cancellous bone of the premaxilla gives way to the unrelenting albeit intermittent muscular pressures. Improper function soon results in improper form.

To help counteract this action and assist in retaining the tongue, the lingual retention wire that arcs across the anterior section of the appliance may be cut at the midline and each free end bent back distally. Some clinicians substitute actual "tongue-training" wire loops for the cut lingual wire. Either produces a tactile sensation to the tongue that is just unpleasant enough to cause it to seek out a more comfortable portion on the vault of the palate while forming a seal during swallowing. It also acts as a physical reminder for the patient to remember to concentrate on proper tongue positioning and make a conscious effort to swallow correctly. It is a more efficient and humane replacement for tongue-training devices of former times that ranged all the way from simple soldered wire band loops to sharpened "hay rakes" that could have been designed by the Marquis de Sade! The younger the patient, the more prone to success this process is. In the teen or early adult patient, tongue habits are more difficult to correct and the clinician may want to refer the patient for myofunctional therapy. Left un-

---

Figure 6-5 **(A)** Infants are normally born skeletal Class II, closed bite (a bit of a misnomer, since they usually have no teeth), with relatively flat palatal vaults. This necessitates that they have slight forward component of thrusting with tongue as they swallow, ie, the infantile swallowing pattern. Even though teeth may not be present at birth, within 6 months they begin to appear. **(B)** It has long been known that when teeth are erupting they are most sensitive to directional pressures that affect their path of eruption. **(C)** Likewise, the young growing alveolar process through which these teeth erupt is also highly sensitive to pressures and shaping forces of the muscular environment. The teeth and alveolar process in which they reside usually occupy the neutral zone between forces pushing out (tongue) and forces pushing in (perioral musculature).

Figure 6-6 **(A) (B)** Thumb- and finger-sucking habits, if constant enough, may easily tip balance of forces in favor of those pushing out, especially in highly bioplastic anterior alveolar area. **(C)** Classic anterior skeletal and dental open bites are all but pathognomonic for this circumstance. **(D)** Adaptive tongue thrusts or retained infantile swallowing patterns reinforce this condition. Notice how the tongue (always hungry for space) thrusts forward to seal during swallowing. (*Courtesy of Dr Waldemar Brehm.*)

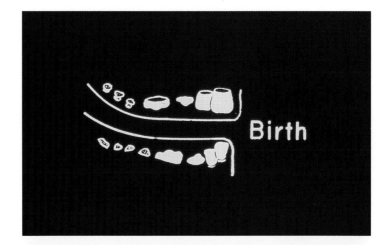

(A)

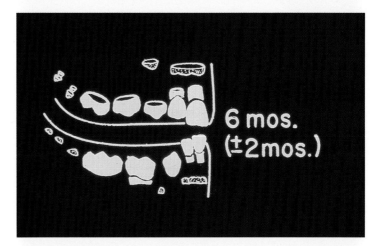

(B)

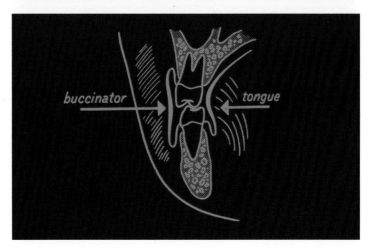

(C)

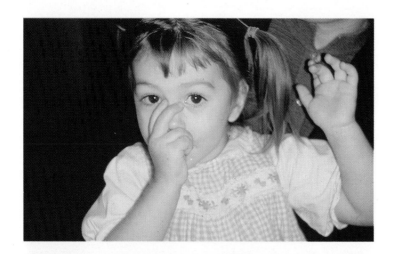

Figure 6-6A

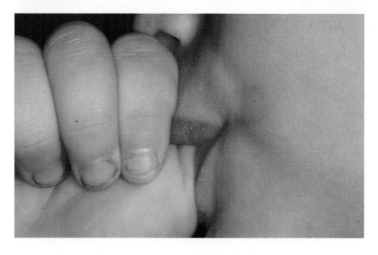

(B)

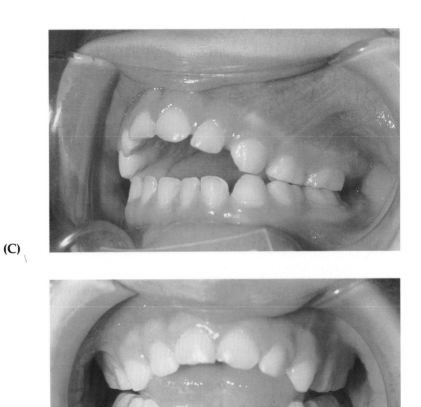

(C)

(D)

treated, the tongue thrust in the older teen or young adult patient may remain to undo the work of the orthopedic appliance.

Less severe forms of forward positioning of the tongue during swallowing are referred to as "adaptive swallowing." A variation of the adaptive tongue thrust is known as the retained infantile swallowing pattern. All infants are born skeletal Class II deep bite and swallow with a forward tongue thrust to obtain proper seal due to the lack of vault to the infantile palate. They convert to the adult swallowing pattern at age 4 to 5 years but may convert as late as age 8. Beyond this, the retained infantile swallowing reflex is considered a major etiological agent in the development of pointed gothic maxillary arches and/or anterior open bite. However, the difference between the adaptive tongue thrust and a retained or lingering infantile swallowing pattern is mostly one of semantics. These cases[14] respond very well to Bionator II therapy and little effort is required to retrain the tongue. Once the teeth have been repositioned, the mild anterior thrusting, adaptive swallowing pattern ceases. The tongue may also bring about an open bite by means of habitually resting in the anterior area. This is referred to as adaptive postural positioning of the tongue. This is also a relatively innocuous condition and responds well to treatment.

Figure 6-7 **(A)** Normal interincisal angulations, overbite and overjet relations in adult and primary anterior teeth. **(B)** Teeth occupy neutral zone between forces pushing out and forces pushing in. In anterior incisor area, these forces are represented by (1) the tip of the tongue and its posture during rest; its main seal point during swallowing (the recipient of its thrusting forces), and (2) the perioral labial musculature, its consistency and tonicity. **(C)** Chronic thumb- or finger-sucking habits quickly throw equilibrium of these forces of muscular balance in favor of tongue's anterior component. With resultant deformation and propensity for forward posturing and thrusting of tongue, lateral forces of external musculature and buccal tissues often bring about shift in equilibrium in posterior areas, and narrow arch forms will often result. **(D)** In sucking action, forces against lower arch, especially lower anterior teeth, are greatly enhanced.

Figure 6-8 Muscle tonicity, balance, and lip seal. **(A)** Schematic representation of muscle fiber direction and balance required for normal lip seal in orbicularis oris group, the superior and inferior incisive, the levator anguli oris, depressor anguli oris, and anterior most fibers of the buccinator. **(B)** Normal perioral muscular balance, tonicity, and unstrained lip seal. **(C)** Imbalanced hypotonic perioral musculature with concomitant insufficient lip seal. Such conditions often occur in skeletal Class II deep bite cases and are also often accompanied by hyperactive or hypertonic mentalis, especially during swallowing. This may often be observed in patient exhibiting "peach-stone chin" during swallowing or strained lip seal.

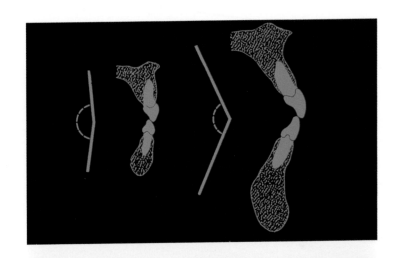

(A)

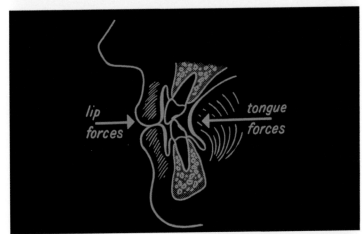

(B)

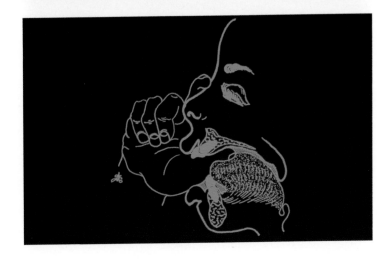

(C)

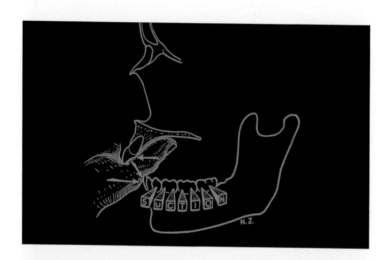

(D)

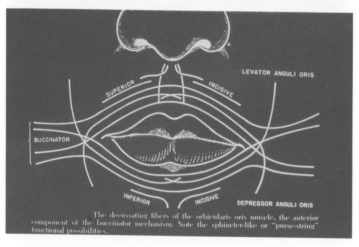

The decussating fibers of the orbicularis oris muscle, the anterior component of the buccinator mechanism. Note the sphincter-like or "purse-string" functional possibilities.

Figure 6-8A

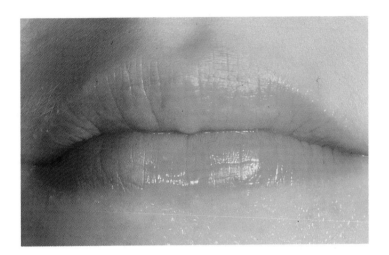

(B)

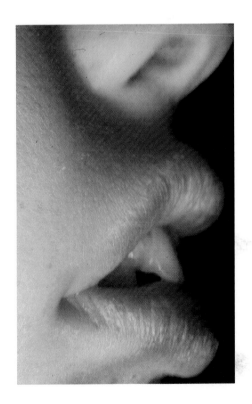

(C)

Since both adaptive swallowing and true endogenous neuromuscular tongue-thrusting are capable of producing the same effect of anterior open bite, it would greatly assist the clinician to be able to determine which is prevalent in a given case. This may be difficult at best. However, certain clinical signs may be noted that would act as clues as to which type of problem is present. First, observe whether or not there is a distinct lisp associated with the patient's speech or in the speech patterns of either of the child's parents. If so, this is an indication that the patient might be suffering from true neuromuscular tongue-thrusting as the lisp is often associated with this type of thrust. Also, the extent of the open bite tends to be of a wider nature across a greater extent of the anterior arch in neuromuscular type thrusting. But these signs are not by any means pathognomonic for this condition. Experience and judgment must also be called upon in evaluating which condition exists with a realization that some cases might tend to fail in spite of both orthodontic and myofunctional efforts, especially in the older patient. Fortunately, these types of circumstances are relatively rare.

If instead the thumb is the original offending agent, the lingual wire of the appliance may still be cut and bent back in a similar manner or lingual "training loops" may still be employed. If excess volume exists in the premaxillary area, the tongue may have a tendency to slip farther forward as a consequence, thus reinforcing the damage caused by finger- or thumb-sucking. Think of the tongue as always being "space-hungry." The action of the cut and recurved lingual wire helps prevent the tongue from developing a secondary, or pseudothrust (adaptive), as a result of the acquired habit of moving forward and sealing itself in the open space anteriorly.

The appliance is worn at all times except when eating and during active sports. As the case approaches completion, after 9 to 12 months or so, as with all forms of orthodontic and orthopedic movement of this type, overcorrect slightly. This means the appliance should be worn until the bite is closed down to a 1- to 3-mm overbite.

During therapy, the midline expansion screw may be utilized, if need be, to help relieve any lower anterior crowding that may be present in the case. One quarter turn of the central cylinder of the expansion screw every week is the usual frequency. This widens the two halves of the appliance by the standard 0.25 mm. Of course, as the appliance expands laterally in

Figure 6-9 Tongue thrust and deep bite. **(A)** In addition to anterior open bites, tongue thrusts may contribute to deep bite problems also. Since tongue thrusts forward improperly in many Division 1-type cases because of convenience of having extra space anteriorly, being of limited volume it exerts less lateral arch developing forces also. It will also frequently have tendency to flatten out slightly over top of lower posterior segments (possibly as reaction to narrower arch form—a "vicious cycle"). **(B)** This retards alveolar eruption and inhibits normal development of vertical.

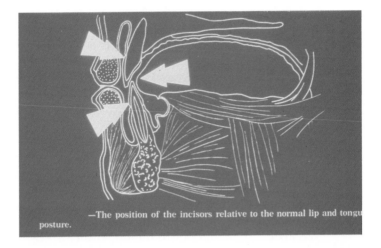

(A)

—The position of the incisors relative to the normal lip and tongue posture.

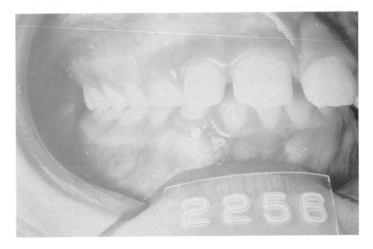

(B)

the anterior region, the Coffin spring must be adjusted periodically to relieve tension in this area. This may cause slight widening in the posterior segments, but this is usually very easily tolerated.

If the lower anteriors are below the plane of occlusion and are in need of vertical eruption to complete the closing of the bite, the appliance is processed without the conventional acrylic incisal cap. If the lower incisors are already at an adequate vertical, the cap is left on as the lip that rides over the incisal edges will hold these teeth in their present position and prevent unwanted further eruption.

If an Orthopedic Corrector II is being used, the side screws may be activated after about 3 months of wear. At this time the mandible has advanced about as far forward as is possible with the appliance constructed in the unexpanded position. If more advancement is needed to bring the case from Class II to Class I, the expansion screws may now be opened to produce the necessary additional forward repositioning of the mandible. As with the conventional Orthopedic Corrector I, the acrylic projections must be removed from the lingual acrylic adjacent to the lower posterior teeth. In the case of the Orthopedic Corrector II, the acrylic on the inferior surface of the bite blocks is to be flattened also to permit smooth advancement of the mandibular teeth along the lower sides of the appliance. Three-quarter turns of the screws on each side every week is usual until the lower incisors are about 2 mm anterior to the upper incisal edges. These upper incisors are usually starting to come near their final correct position by this phase of the treatment time line. (Note: In the early full adult dentition, the clos-

Figure 6-10 **(A)** Tongue retraining devices of former times ranged from soldered wirefence-type affair to such things as **(B)** the hayrake, with its auxilliary spurs.

Figure 6-11 Case study: Class I, anterior open bite, late mixed dentition stage. In this late mixed dentition case, malocclusion originated from prolonged thumb habit supported by adaptive anterior tongue thrust. Treatment required only closing down of anterior open bite because case was already Class I with good arch form. Treatment was initiated at 10 years, 6 months of age and lasted 1 year with a 2-month break two thirds of way through year, when patient lost appliance while on a 3-month summer visit. At completion of treatment, appliance was withdrawn gradually with patient wearing it only at night for 6 months. **(A)** Intraoral view of malocclusion. Note good arch form and adequate arch width of upper and lower arches. Also note eagerness of tongue (always hungry for space) to fill extra space in anterior portion of arch, represented by open bite, during swallowing. **(B)** First Bionator II appliance inserted—worn for only 9 months before being lost. After 2 months of not wearing appliance, 9 months into treatment a second appliance was made **(C)** and inserted for remainder of treatment until bite closed rest of way down. **(D)** Final closure.

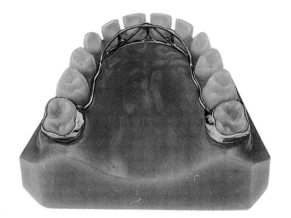

(A)

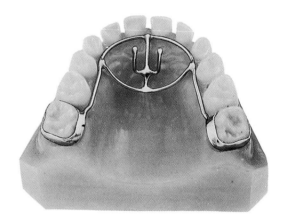

(B)

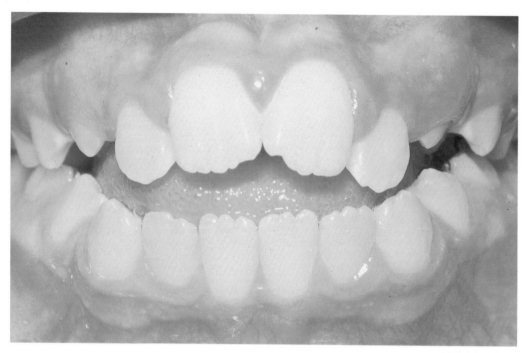

Figure 6-11A

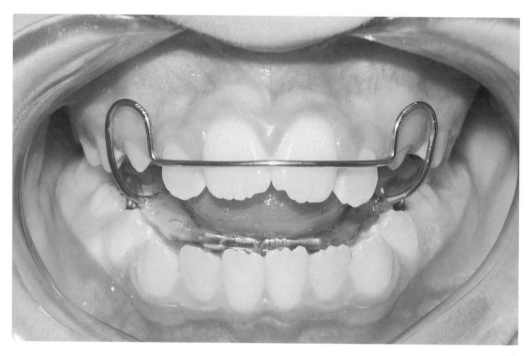

(B)

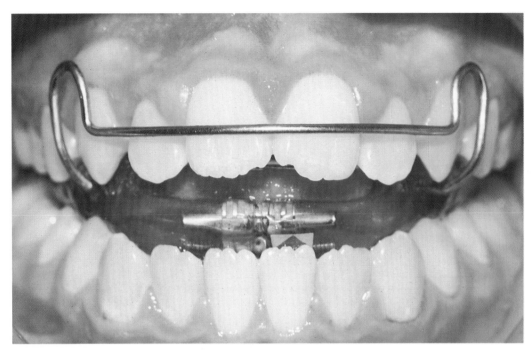

(C)

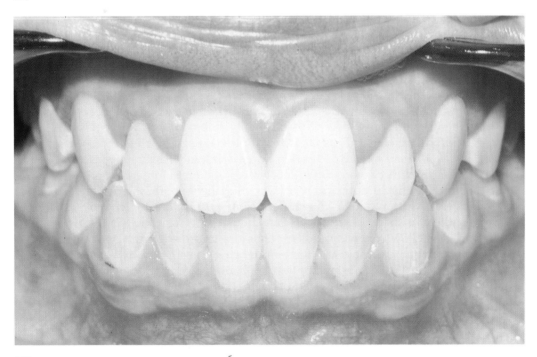

(D)

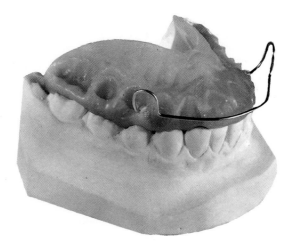

Figure 6-12   Original design of prototype Bionator III.

Figure 6-13   Case study: Bionator III, mandibular advancement only. Retraining Class II neuromuscular sling. **(A) (B)** This adult dentition presents one of the more uncommon examples of a case requiring Bionator III treatment. Displacement of mandibular condyles in superior posterior direction within TMJs bilaterally accompanied malocclusion. Reciprocal clicking and usual TMJ symptomatology also were present. However, there already exists ideal arch form and adequate vertical dimension of occlusion. Only deficient component is interarch alignment. Bionator III appliance **(C) (D)**, which holds both anterior and posterior vertical dimensions of occlusion constant but merely advances mandible, is inserted and holds mandibular arch forward. **(E) (F)** Note that labial bow contacts maxillary anteriors to provide extra anchorage to prevent any "headgear effect" from being transmitted to maxillary arch by tension of musculature on appliance. After period of months (varying with age, severity, and compliance of patient), neuromuscular sling that cradles and suspends mandible has been retrained and patient habitually both carries and occludes with mandible in advanced, corrected position. **(G) (H)** This eliminates TMJ symptoms. Bicuspids and molars must merely "settle in" a millimeter or so to lock in to new position.

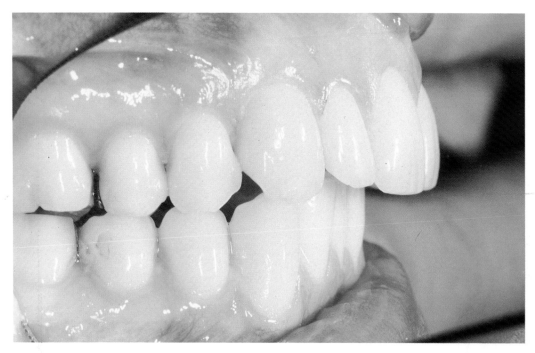

(A)

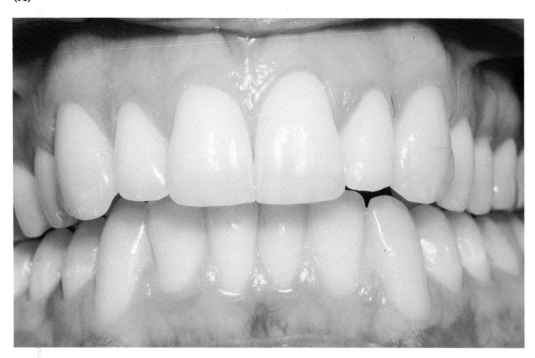

(B)

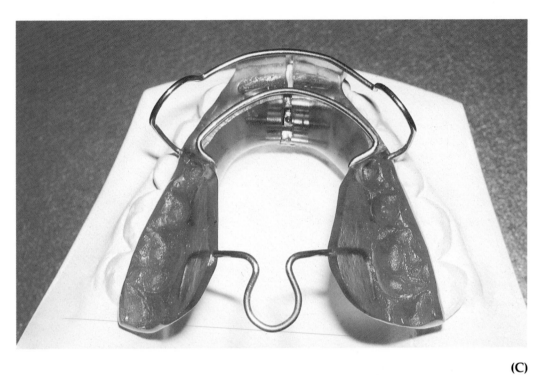

(C)

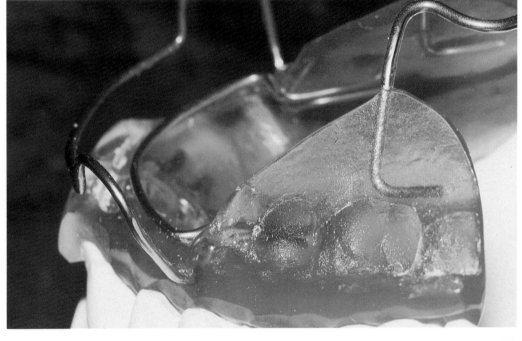

(D)

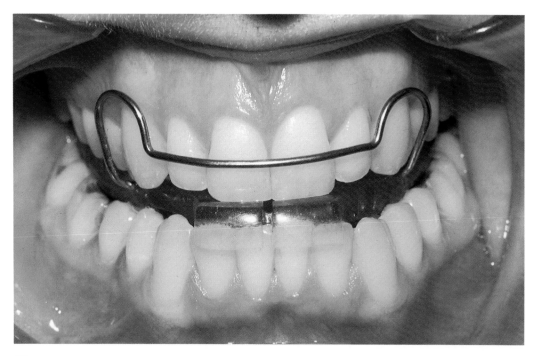

(E)

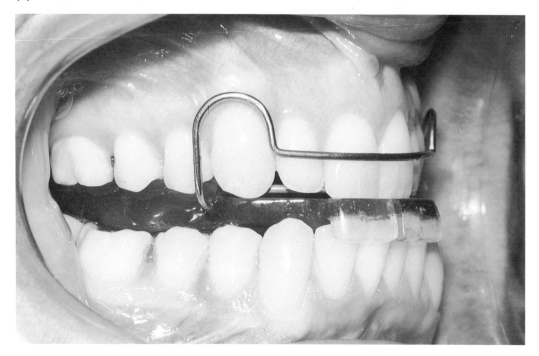

(F)

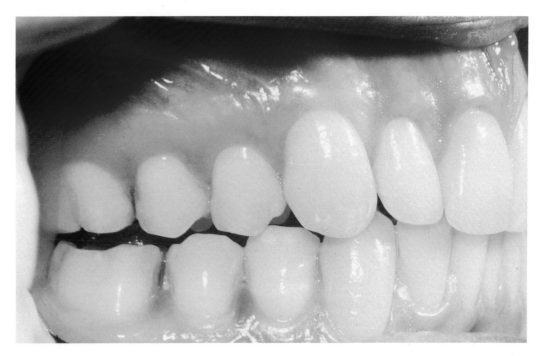

(G)

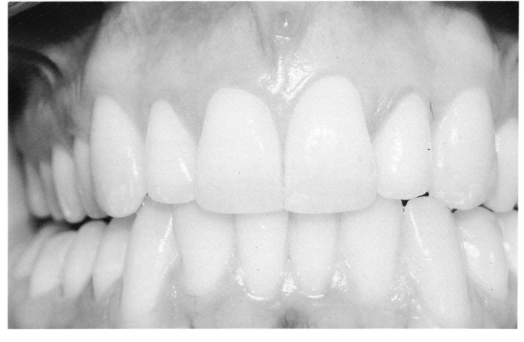

(H)

ing down of the anterior open bite with Bionator II- or Orthopedic Corrector II-type treatment is *enormously* facilitated by second molar removal.)

Retention is unnecessary for most cases once the bite is adequately closed. For the rare cases of neuromuscular or endogenous tongue-thrusting, care must be used in withdrawing the appliance abruptly before it is certain whether or not the tongue has been fully restrained. Phasing the appliance out gradually by means of nighttime wearing only may be indicated in these cases.

THE BIONATOR III

The Bionator III is a lower arch-advancing appliance. It is totally neutral with respect to the vertical and leaves that dimension completely unaffected. Its sole purpose is to advance a mandible from a Class II to a Class I relationship and retrain the Class II neuromuscular sling! It is not intended to change anything else.

Occasionally, certain patients will present with a Class II malocclusion and retruded mandible whose arches are of proper form and shape and whose vertical dimension of occlusion is also quite satisfactory, but who still suffer from the Class II condition with its concomitant mandibular retrusion. All that is needed is a simple advancement of the mandible from Class II to Class I without any increasing of the vertical. The appliance used for this, the Bionator III, looks like a cross between the Bionators I and II. It has the complete trappings of the Bionator I, labial bow, Coffin spring, acrylic cap, vertical wings, etc, but it also has the acrylic pads of the Bionator II. These pads keep the vertical in the posterior area constant; and the full acrylic cap in the anterior region, upon which both the upper and lower incisors articulate, keeps the overbite in that area constant. The only thing changed by this appliance is the position of the mandible.

The construction bite is even the same as the standard Bionator I. Have the patient bite into the softened wax such that the lower incisors are 2 to 3 mm past the upper incisors with an interincisal distance of about 2 to 3 mm. There are no adjustments to this appliance other than those to insure correct and comfortable fit.

REFERENCES

1. Straub WJ: Malfunction of the tongue, Part I. The abnormal swallowing habit: its cause, effects and results in relation to orthodontic treatment and speech therapy, *Angle Orthod* 1960;46:404–424.
2. Graber TM: The "three M's": Muscle, malformation and malocclusion, *Am J Orthod* 1963;49:418–450.
3. Kydd WL, Adamine JS, Mendel RA, et al: Tongue and lip forces exerted during deglutition in subjects with and without an anterior open bite. *J Dent Res* 1963; 42:858–866.

 4. Wildman AJ: Analysis of tongue, soft palate, and pharyngeal wall movement. *Am J Orthod* 1961;47:439–461.
 5. Kydd WL: Maximum forces exerted on the dentition by the perioral and lingual musculature. *J Am Dent Assoc* 1957;55:646–651.
 6. Weinstein S, Haack DC, Morris LY, et al: An equilibrium theory of tooth position. *Angle Orthod* 1963;33:1–26.
 7. Swindler DR, Sassouni V: Open bite and thumbsucking in Rhesus monkeys. *Angle Orthod* 1962;32:27–37.
 8. Graber TM: *Orthodontics: Principles and Practice.* Philadelphia, WB Saunders Co, 1961, pp 235–257.
 9. Barrett RH: One approach to deviate swallowing. *Am J Orthod* 1961;47:726–736.
10. Brauer JS, Holt TV: Tongue thrust classification. *Angle Orthod* 1965;51:106–112.
11. Heath JR: Some dental deformities caused by abnormal muscular behavior patterns. *Oral Top* 1956;73:172–173.
12. Hanson ML, Logan WB, Case JL: Tongue thrust in preschool children. *Am J Orthod* 1969;56:60–69.
13. Lear CSC, Flanagan JB, Moorrees CFA: The frequency of deglutition in man. *Arch Oral Biol* 1965;10:83–99.
14. Richardson A: Facial growth and the prognosis for anterior open bite. *Trans Eur Orthod Soc* 1971;149–157.

CHAPTER 7

The Straight Wire Appliance

The Straight Wire* custom preangulated bonded bracket system is an arch- *perfecting* appliance. At least that is the level at which it will be discussed here. But actually, it represents much more than that. It has the capability of being extended to the point where it is capable of performing all the necessary tooth movements required of a fixed orthodontic system and comprises state-of-the-art mechanics in modern-day orthodontic therapy. Straight Wire fixed appliance therapy allows the clinician to quickly and eas-

---

*The term "Straight-Wire® Appliance" is a registered trademark of "A"-Company of San Diego, Calif. "A"-Company was the first corporation to commercially develop the appliance according to the theories and specifications of its originator, Dr Larry Andrews.

ily bring about the final perfection of his cases by virtue of its ability to *level*, *align*, and *rotate* individual teeth in the dental arch. Once the orthopedics has been completed by means of active plates and/or functional appliances, the Straight Wire system gives the quickest form of orthodontic "touch-up" that is required to bring the case to completion.

Functional appliances and active plates can be used for individual tooth movements, but these consist mostly of the tipping of teeth. Rotations, root torque, extrusion, intrusion, and various other types of individual, purely orthodontic movements of teeth are not exactly their main forte. But that is where the Straight Wire Appliance (SWA) is right at home.

Consummate skill has always been required to manipulate conventional fixed band orthodontic appliances.[1-7] That is because the principle upon which they operate is somewhat complicated. The idea was that if one were to band a particular tooth with a metal band that had a bracket soldered to the band to which an arch wire could be attached, by simply bending the wire before attaching it to the bracket, the tooth could be moved in the direction dictated by the bend in the wire. A sound principle, but far from simple. Consider the case where only one tooth is to be moved. First, it must be isolated so the force system might be delivered to it in some way.[8-19] This means placing a band on the tooth with a bracket attached. The force system will be a resilient wire in this instance. It is bent in such a way as to cause tension in the wire when it is ligated to the bracket. This tension is the source of energy that accomplishes the desired orthodontic movement of the tooth in the direction programmed into the wire by the nature of its bend. But now the wire itself must be anchored to the two teeth on either side of our sample tooth to be moved. This also requires a banding and wire attachment process. But when the wire, with its tension-producing bend in it, is attached to all three teeth, namely the tooth to be moved and the two anchor teeth on either side of it, not only is the tension of the wire delivered to the middle tooth, but also a reciprocal force is generated which must be absorbed by the anchor teeth. Now these anchor teeth are unconcerned with the fact that they are supposed to be rigid anchors and are supposed to remain unmovable, so they also start to drift slightly in response to the forces they in turn feel from the wire. Thus what you now have in our hypothetical example is three teeth moving all at once instead of one.

Figure 7-1 The Straight Wire appliance. **(A)** Once final rectangular wire used in course of treatment has its way, because of its precision fit in corresponding rectangular bracket slots of each custom preangulated bracket, all tip, torque, crown, and root angulations are produced according to predetermined standards programmed and engineered into bracket bases. **(B)** At conclusion of treatment, final wire will be perfectly horizontally level or "straight," hence the name. Tooth crown and root positions are determined by bracket base and slot angulations, not by bends in wire. (*Courtesy of "A"-Company, Inc., San Diego, CA.*)

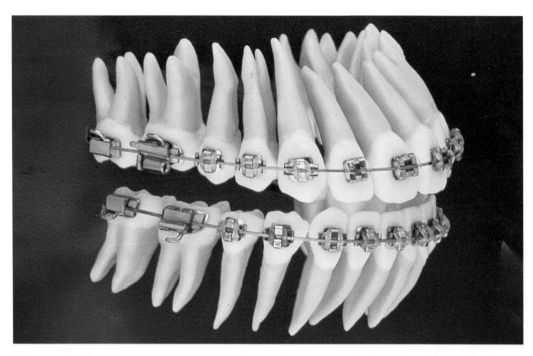

(A)

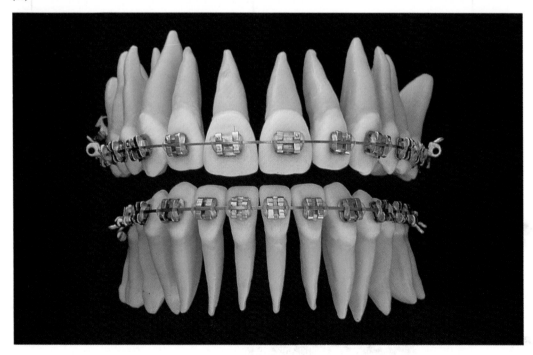

(B)

Now, let us look at the problem from a different viewpoint. Let us take a perfectly formed arch of 14 ideal teeth, each with a band and soldered edgewise bracket flush on it with the central horizontal slot perfectly parallel to the widest mesiodistal axis of each tooth through the contact points. Thus the bracket slots on these hypothetically perfect teeth would be perpendicular to the long axes of each of the teeth. Now, if we were to place a perfectly shaped, but unbent rectangular arch wire next to this setup, the general form of the dental arch and the arch wire would be the same. But the facial surface enamel of each tooth and therefore the band and parallel bracket over it would be slightly askew relative to the perfectly shaped arch wire. At each site of alignment of tooth-band-bracket, there would be an individualized, irregular space in a three-dimensional plane between the arch wire and the bracket slot. Now, let's say we wanted to attach the arch wire to each and every tooth in our perfectly shaped dental arch by fitting the unbent wire into the bracket slot on each band. Since the varied anatomical facial surfaces of each individual tooth would go in and out when viewed from the occlusal as we travel around the arch due to the individual anatomy of each tooth, their corresponding brackets with their wire slots would conform to the same in and out pattern of variations. Thus if we wish to attach the arch wire to each of these bracket slots, the arch wire must be bent so as to lie passively in each slot. This would necessitate reproducing these in-and-out bends at each tooth position in the arch wire so the wire could be put into the slot passively without exerting any tension whatsoever to the bracket, which would move our teeth out of their perfect arch shape. These ad-

---

Figure 7-2   (A) In-and-out compensation. It would be necessary to place in-and-out bends in arch wire to bring wire flush with facial surface of each tooth in dental arch because these facial surfaces each have their own degree of variance when viewed from occlusal or incisal aspect. **(B)** First-order bends, or in-and-out bends, must be placed in arch wire at each wire–bracket–tooth surface interface when using conventional noncompensating brackets. This may be seen on left, whereas this is not necessary when brackets are preangulated as in Straight Wire-type appliance (right). **(C)** Second-order bends or root tip must also be bent into arch wire at each tooth–bracket–wire juncture also when using noncompensating brackets to compensate for individual tooth long axis angulation. This also is eliminated in Straight Wire-type appliance brackets as slot tip is programmed into bracket by virtue of angulation of slot. **(D)** Third-order bends or root torque (crown torque) must also be placed in rectangular arch wire by means of torquing it about its own long axis when using noncompensating conventional brackets—even this third dimension is taken care of by slot torque built into bracket in Straight Wire-type bracket. First-, second-, and third-order bends are custom preangulated and individualized into each respective Straight Wire-type bracket base and slot. (*Courtesy of "A"-Company, Inc., San Diego, CA.*)

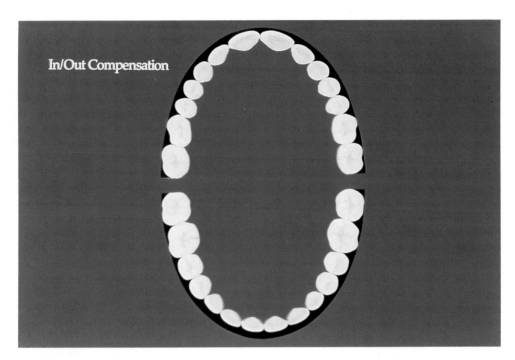

(A)

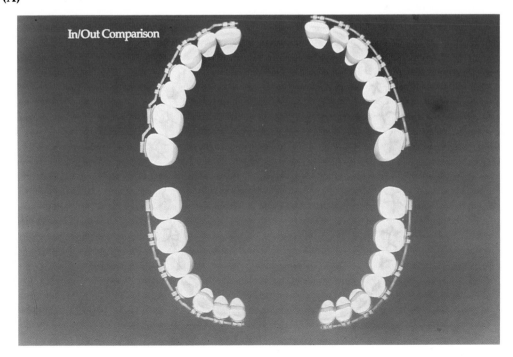

(B)

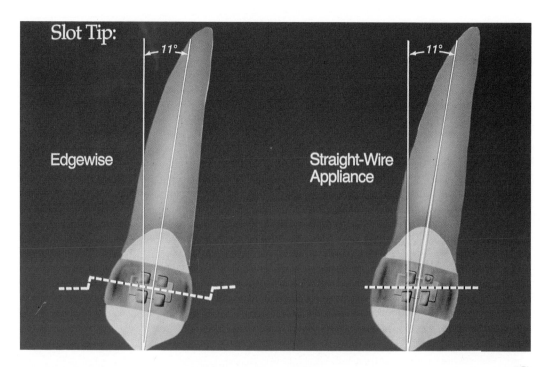

(C)

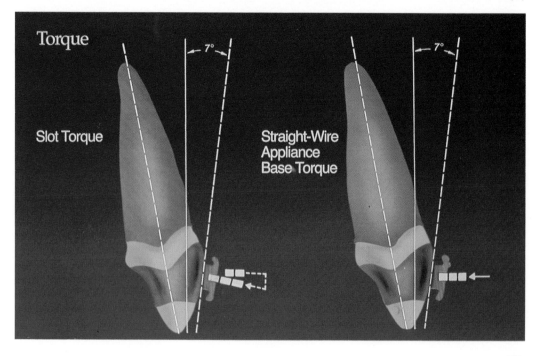

(D)

justments of the wire to compensate for the in-and-out positioning of each tooth's facial surface-band-bracket combination are referred to as first order bends. There are 14 per arch!

But the wire so adjusted with its 14 first order bends will not yet rest passively in the slot of the bracket of each banded tooth, even with each of the 14 bends perfectly executed. Our arch wire is still flat (theoretically) with respect to the horizontal plane. But, alas, our teeth with their in-and-out bracket slots are not. Each bracket slot via its soldered position on the band is positioned on the tooth perpendicular to the long axis of its root and crown. Each tooth has a different naturally occurring angulation of its long axis relative to the horizontal. This means each facial surface-band-bracket slot combination is angled differently relative to the horizontal. Our original arch wire, now proudly sporting its 14 in-and-out bends, is still perfectly flat relative to the horizontal plane, unlike all the slots we are trying to fit it into. We want the wire totally passive in each slot. Therefore, it at once becomes obvious that we must place 14 more bends in the wire at each tooth-bracket site to compensate for the deviation in angulation relative to the *vertical axis* of the long axis of each tooth and its corresponding bracket slot relative to the mesiodistal dimension: upper centrals, 5 degrees; lateral, 9 degrees; cuspids, 11 degrees; bicuspids, 2 degrees; molars, 5 degrees; and on the lower everything 2 degrees mesially except for the cuspid which is 5 degrees. Again, 14 more bends are added to compensate for long axis variation of each tooth. These are referred to as second order bends. Thus we have now put 28 separate bends in our original arch wire. But we are not yet ready for attachment to all the bracket slots. There is still one more dimension to contend with before our wire can lie passively in all 14 slots at once.

Each tooth also has a vertical torque angulation of its roots relative to the long axis of its crown-root length. This represents the rotation labiolingually of the tooth about a *horizontal axis* running mesiodistally. Now, if our bracket slots are square (which they actually are) and if our wire is square (which it sometimes is, especially at the end of treatment), this means the wire also has to be twisted, or torqued, about its own long axis at each tooth-bracket slot site to fit passively flush against the base of the square bracket slot. So our wire is again adjusted (twisted) for torque 14 times at each tooth-bracket slot site! These are referred to as third order bends (torque). Thus we have now bent or torqued our original arch wire 42 times! With the tip, torque, and angulation now expertly and precisely placed in the arch wire, it may be placed in the bracket slots of all 14 teeth of our perfect dental arch with complete undistorting passivity, resting there in full three-dimensional harmony of rectangular wire in rectangular bracket slot. Try it!

Two bends into an effort to accomplish this immediately reveals to the novice as to why men are called to such a specialty as orthodontics and why entire careers are devoted to the intricacies of manipulating arch wires in fixed edgewise mechanics. Such skilled individuals are masters in their field—eclectic, restrictive, celestial. A great deal of respect was the due to men who mastered this highly refined and cultivated discipline.

But times change and with the modernization of almost every aspect of technical subjects comes newer, more streamlined and efficient mechanisms. Orthodontics has not been spared this modernizing process. Much of the tedious work of arch wire bending has now been eliminated. The secret is in the "preangulation" of bracket bases!

A new idea to simplify orthodontic mechanics has been postulated. Let us again take our perfectly shaped dental arch of the hypothetical example. We will also take an unbent, untorqued rectangular arch wire that coincides in arch form exactly to this perfect arch of teeth. But this time we will do something quite different. Instead of placing the brackets on the teeth, we position all the brackets with their rectangular horizontal slots directly on the perfectly flat rectangular arch wire with each of the 14 brackets positioned such that its exact dead center of the bracket base corresponds with the exact dead center of the clinical crown of its respective tooth. With brackets only on the arch wire, bands are eliminated. But the brackets are not in full contact with the teeth yet; they are merely held very close to or in light contact with the teeth by their attachment to the arch wire. The arch wire is still unbent, untorqued, and passive. Teeth are still unmoved or unstressed. All of the brackets are securely and completely seated against the snugly fitting rectangular arch wire in close proximity to the teeth center on center. The brackets are flush on the wire, not the teeth. Now, what we have is a perfectly set and straight arch wire, perfectly aligned slotted brackets, whose slots are all in line along the arch wire that passes through each of them, and our aforementioned set of hypothetically perfect teeth in this arch are in close proximity to the backsides of the bases of these arch wire–held brackets center on center. Now, if we could imagine that all the little irregular three-dimensional spaces between the back sides of the brackets and the facial surfaces of the clinical crowns of their respective adjacent teeth were to fill up with bracket-base metal so the backside of each bracket base would become equally irregular and the mirror image of the adjacent respective facial surface of enamel, these brackets then would all be able to make full surface-to-surface contact between their bracket base backsides and their adjacent teeth. The arch wire is still perfectly straight, perfectly passive, and yet by means of our newly created individualized *custom base brackets*, it is in full contact with a perfectly shaped dental arch with all its teeth at their ideal tip, torque, and root and crown angulation. If we continue to imagine that we gently glue the brackets to the teeth center

---

Figure 7-3 **(A)** First-order (in-and-out) angulations may be individualized and idealized for facial surface of each tooth by custom preangulated Straight Wire-type bracket base. **(B) (C)** Same may also be done for angulation of each tooth (tip) by individualized slot tip calculated for each tooth bracket **(D)** as well as root and crown inclination (torque), which is compensated for by slot torque of each individualized tooth bracket. This allows for level slot alignment at completion of treatment. (*Courtesy of "A"-Company, Inc., San Diego, CA.*)

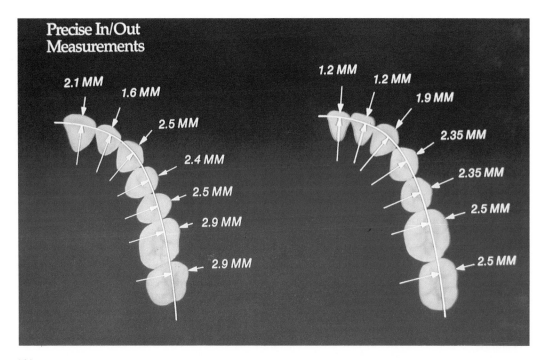

(A)

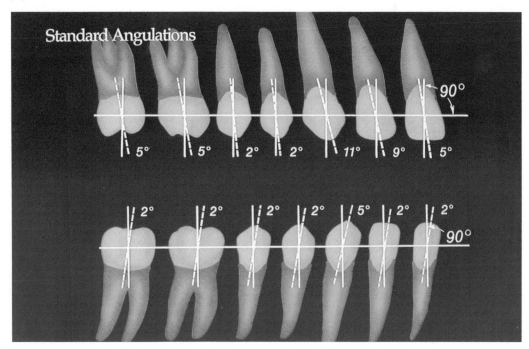

(B)

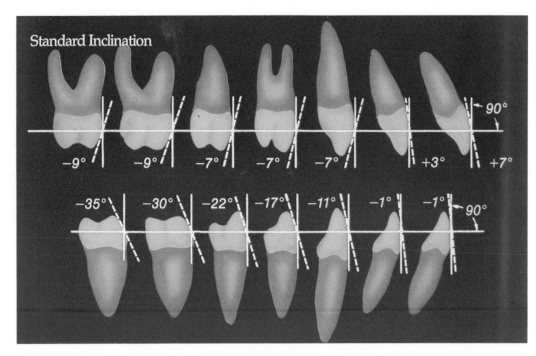

(C)

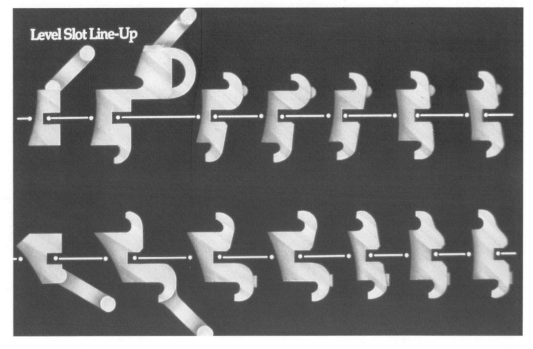

(D)

on center, the whole system is locked into perfect arch form. Now, leaving the brackets on the teeth but removing the rectangular arch wire will reveal the slots of each tooth bonded bracket line-up in a perfect line of sight down the buccal surfaces of the posterior quadrants from cuspid to second molar like a trough. With the tip, torque, and in-and-out all precalculated and anatomically built into the bracket bases, the bracket slots in turn may be seen to follow a straight unbroken line of sight around the arch, front to rear along a path perfectly horizontally straight. Now as a final step, imagine that the mesial and distal edges of the bracket bases are cut parallel to the long axis of the crowns. This is the principle upon which the first Straight Wire bracket base was conceived. All tip, torque, and in-and-out angulations are predesigned and engineered right into the bracket itself. In actual clinical situations, teeth are not perfectly positioned. So by merely bonding such a designed bracket to the tooth with modern composite acid etch bonding techniques (the backsides of the bracket bases are meshed to improve retention with bonding composites) so that the exact center of the bracket base aligns with the exact center of the clinical crown of the tooth so the square vertical edges of the bracket base are parallel to the long axis of the tooth, a resilient arch wire may be secured to the irregularly positioned teeth and their respective irregularly positioned slotted brackets such that as it seeks to regain its original straight shape, it continuously applies the appropriate forces until the teeth, bracket slots, and wire are all once again perfectly aligned and straight. Hence the name, principle, and genius of the Straight Wire appliance. Because of its ease of manipulation, high-quality results, consistency of performance, and unlimited capabilities, the Straight Wire appliance has revolutionized the traditional practice of fixed appliance orthodontic technique. The difficult days of the multiple bending, twisting, and shaping of arch wires by hand are over.

The essence of basic Straight Wire appliance therapy consists of bonding the brackets onto the teeth and sequentially attaching a consecutive series of progressively less resilient arch wires whereby the first ones used have the maximum flexibility. This is because the teeth are each individually misaligned in the arch at their maximum amount as treatment is initiated. Therefore, the first arch wire used must be flexible enough to traverse the highly irregular path through all the various bracket slots of the teeth and yet remain resilient enough to initiate orthodontic tooth movement. Then the wires are changed periodically to stiffer and progressively less flexible wires as the denture approaches more and more perfect arch form. The final wires are very stiff and tolerate little distortion, but by the time they are inserted, the teeth are nearly in perfect alignment. As might be surmised, the key to successful Straight Wire therapy is proper bracket placement on the tooth. When the wire has finally expressed itself, it will be straight, as will all the consecutive bracket slots attached to it. Though the brackets will then line up according to the dictates of the wire, if they are not placed dead center on the facial surface of each tooth, the teeth on which they are mispositioned will be malaligned by the corresponding amount. Bracket placement is critical. However, sometimes this may be used to an advantage. In the case where a tooth is so poorly positioned as to prevent proper bracketing, the bracket may be placed on as advantageous a spot as possible until the action of the arch wire pulls it part of the way into the correct position, thus exposing more of the facial surface of the tooth. At that time the individual bracket may be removed and reattached in the correct anatomical location. The arch wire may then be ligated again to the bracket to finish the desired movement.

HISTORY AND DEVELOPMENT

The eventual end results of the Straight Wire concept began with the search for an anatomical standard. For years the orthodontic community had used the guidelines of E. H. Angle as a reference point for orthodontic treatment.[20] His standards, laid down at the turn of the century, were held up as the goal for what constituted a proper occlusion. Angle's main criterion for acceptability was that the mesiobuccal cusp of the upper first permanent molar should occlude with the groove between the mesial and middle cusps of the lower first permanent molar. This standard acted as a guide for clinicians for over half of a century. But years of careful observation by keen eyes gradually revealed the fact that this criterion was insufficient to act as the true measure of correct and ideal occlusion. Too many cases that exhibited this trait, even after orthodontic treatment, were still inadequate as to what could be judged as satisfactory. What was wrong could be easily determined on an individual case-by-case basis. What was needed was a way of determining what was *right* on a general basis that could be applied to all cases and act as a positive, definitive measuring rod against which all future results could be judged. Thus a search for a new standard began.

The search was organized under the leadership of a true genius of the orthodontic world, Dr Lawrence F. Andrews of San Diego, and took approximately 4 years to conduct (1960–1964). The results of this survey were compiled and published in what has now become a classic and monumental paper, "The Six Keys to Normal Occlusion."[21] What Andrews did was to collect a series of records and models of 120 nonorthodontically treated cases that were as near perfect examples of "normal" occlusion as possible. These were all cases of full adult dentition that had not received orthodontic treatment of any kind and were judged to be of such a level of anatomical

---

Figure 7-4 **(A)** Flexible wires of braided or round variety may be inserted into properly positioned Straight Wire-type brackets, and as they exert their force in individual bracket slots they level, align, and rotate each tooth. **(B)** Final torquing of roots is accomplished by finishing rectangular wires, which produce individual torquing by virtue of action of rectangular wire held flush in its respective rectangular bracket slots.

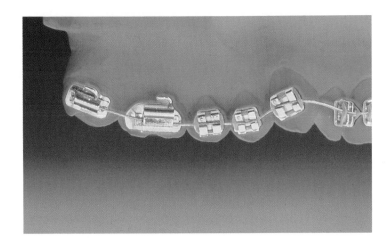

(A)

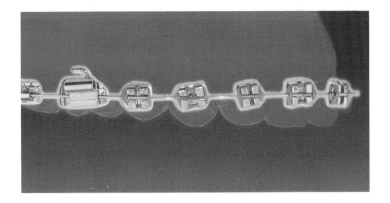

(B)

excellence that none would benefit in any way from any sort of orthodontic intervention or treatment.

Careful and detailed analysis of these nonorthodontic normals revealed that Angle's original cusp/groove relationship of the upper and lower first permanent molars and upper and lower cuspid relationships still held up, but another equally important anatomical relationship relative to the upper first molar and lower second molar emerged also, as well as important relationships of the other teeth. The six key factors he discovered on these cases are as follows:

1. *Molar relationship.* The mesiobuccal cusp of the upper first permanent molar occluded with the groove between the mesial and middle cusps of the lower first permanent molar, but also and with equal importance, the distobuccal cusp of the upper first permanent molar occluded with the mesial slope of the mesiobuccal cusp of the lower second permanent molar.

2. *Crown angulation (mesiodistal tip).* What is meant by "crown angulation" is the angulation of the long axis of the clinical crown of the tooth, *not* considering the root. The long axis of the crown is considered for anterior teeth and bicuspids to be the height of contour of the middevelopmental ridge running through the most prominent vertical portion of the facial surface of the crown. It was observed that for each tooth this long axis of the clinical crown was tipped so as the gingival portion was more distal than the incisal portion. All teeth of the 120 nonorthodontic normals had their crowns tipped distally at the gum line. The amount of distal tip of the gingival portion of the long axis of the clinical crowns are as follows:

	Upper	Lower
Centrals	5°	2°
Lateral	9°	2°
Cuspids	11°	5°
Bicuspids	2°	2°
First molar	5°	2°
Second Molar	5°	2°

3. *Crown inclination (torque).* Again, this refers to the inclination, or torque, in a labiolingual (buccolingual) direction of the clinical crown of each tooth, *not* the entire tooth. These inclinations of the 120 ideal nontreated cases fell into the following pattern:

a. Anterior teeth: Inclination was sufficient to prevent supraeruption and allow proper contact mesiodistally.

b. Inclination of all upper posterior teeth was lingual with the facial surfaces of the molars slightly more lingually inclined gingival to occlusal.

Figure 7-5 (A) Dr Lawrence F. Andrews, father of the Straight Wire-type appliances.

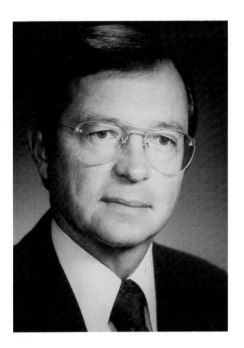

(A)

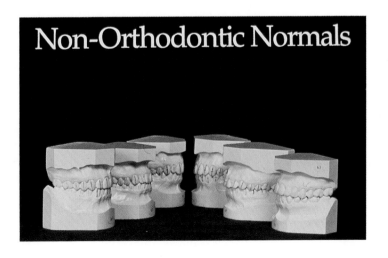

(B)

c. Inclination of all lower posterior facial surfaces followed the same pattern as the uppers, lingual crown inclination with molars slightly more pronounced.

4. Rotations. There were no improperly rotated teeth.
5. Spaces. There were no open contacts.
6. Occlusal plane. The occlusal plane showed some variation ranging from totally flat to a slight exhibition of a curve of Spee.

It is these criteria which Andrews deemed worthy of adoption as a new standard by which all orthodontically treated cases should be judged. But he was also willing to admit there would often have to be some compromises. But with these six keys acting as a goal, the clinician is given the very highest of standards to measure against, the very best Nature has to offer by Her own hand. It is these standards that serve as the model for which the Straight Wire system of brackets was designed to reproduce. It is this anatomical ideal that they are engineered to duplicate.

THE BRACKET

The essence of the Straight Wire system is the bracket. By virtue of the precalculated angulations of each respective bracket base and wire slot, the ultimate treatment goal may be consistently and accurately reproduced, case after case. The difficulties of manual wire bending have been all but totally eliminated, and when preceded by treatment with functional appliances and active plates, arch perfecting or "finishing" treatment usually consists of nothing more than gradually changing the arch wires from the more flexible round or braided ones used at the beginning to the more rigid rectangular ones used at the conclusion. As previously stated, an entire theater of more advanced treatment techniques is also possible. Since the wires used are free to exert their pressures in all three anatomical planes at once, slot alignment occurs simultaneously throughout the arch. This brings the designed buccolingual (in and out), crown angulation (tip), and crown inclination (torque) factors built into the bracket base to fruition as the case approaches conclusion. Thus the anatomical ideals of Andrews are realized.

Brackets, of course, are nothing new to the field of orthodontics as indicated by the plethora of various types that have become available over the years. There is the old standard family of edgewise brackets that go back to the days of E. H. Angle. This group is comprised of numerous offspring. Besides the standard edgewise brackets there are: the Broussard vertical slot edgewise bracket, the Steiner push-pull bracket, the Steiner bracket with rotation wings, the Lewis and Lang single wing brackets, the Ricketts bio-progressive bracket system, the combination Fogel-Magill edgewise bracket, not to mention entire other families of brackets such as the Begg, light-wire differential bracket of Jarabak, the Johnson twin-tie channel bracket, the Ford lock bracket, the Mexican Universal, the Mollin twin ties, and the Kessler! To compound this situation is the fact that various members of this roll call of hardware may be obtained in varying degrees of torque from 0 degrees on up! Straight Wire brackets are simple—and replace all of them. But even these highly advanced, sophisticated, and simplified Straight Wire bracket systems are not without some degree of their own variance, as we shall discuss later.

The Straight Wire brackets are of two basic production types, either cast, like an inlay, or milled. At present, two major companies produce these brackets, and both are of irreproachable quality. One has a mesh foil base while the other has a milled grid. Both interlock with the bonding composite equally well. Both companies also have individualized marking systems so that each bracket may be easily identified as for which tooth it has been designed, upper or lower, right or left.

The bracket slot angulation, or slot tip, is responsible for the angulation of the crown in the completed case. With the slot angled, instead of angling the entire bracket, much better tooth surface contact is maintained and band distortion with its resultant bracket rock is eliminated. The vertical long axis of the bracket, the tie wings, and the bracket base are made to coincide with the long axis of its respective clinical crown. Maintaining proper tip on each tooth insures correct contact point alignment.

Base torque is a product of the rotation of the slot about its horizontal axis. This brings about the correct crown torque once the final, or finishing rectangular wire is ligated into the rectangular slot of the bracket. *In brackets manufactured by "A"-Company* the center of the bracket slot is in the middle of the bracket base, which allows the uniform horizontal alignment of each and every bracket without varying the bracket height.

The variations in the thickness of the bracket base give the correct in-and-out relationships of all the facial surfaces of the teeth in the arch as viewed from the occlusal or incisal.

The twin tie wings are designed to allow both ease of ligation and freedom from occlusal interferences or tissue irritation. The tie wings are parallel to the long axis of the bracket base and therefore the long axis of the clinical crown. This acts as an aid in bracket placement.

Illustrations—Following Page

Figure 7-6 Identification systems. All preangulated direct-bond brackets would look alike if not for a means of identifying brackets one from another for sake of placing correct bracket on correct tooth. The identification system developed by "A"-Company for its brand of Straight Wire brackets is as follows: Dot placed on tie wing signifies bracket for upper tooth, whereas dash on tie wing signifies bracket for lower tooth. Dot or dash is placed on tie wing corresponding to particular quadrant to which bracket belongs, ie, dots should always orient brackets as they are on upper tie wings, right denoting upper right

Figure 7-6 continued

quadrant, left denoting upper left quadrant. Correspondingly, dashes always orient their brackets such that they appear on lower tie wing; right for lower right quadrant, left for lower left quadrant. Upper central brackets are largest, therefore easily determined. Laterals are smaller and detectable from the cuspid brackets because of increased slot tip (11°) and extra size and curvature of cuspid bracket base. Upper bicuspid brackets are distinguishable from one another by simple addition of + to remaining tie wing adjacent to tie wing with dot. Thus +. signifies upper left second bicuspid bracket and .+ indicates upper right. Lower brackets follow similar patterns. Lower central and lateral brackets are identical in tip, torque and in/out angulations, therefore only right and left members must be distinguished with appropriate dash placement on lower tie wings. Lower cuspid brackets are distinguishable by their larger size, and lower first and second bicuspid brackets follow similar dash and + sign identification patterns as those of the uppers: −+, lower right second bicuspid; +−, lower left. Bicuspid brackets for lower are larger than lower central and lateral brackets but not as large as those for lower cuspid. Other preangulated bracket manufacturers use their own identification systems.

Figure 7-7 To properly move teeth with fixed appliances into bicuspid extraction sites, the two teeth on either side of site must be translated into position. This means bodily movement of teeth with no change in tip, torque, or in/out positioning en route. If teeth would be tipped into extraction site crown first, then uprighting them to bring root tips to proper position by wire bends, certain portions of tooth root would be moved first forward then backward through same bone twice! This is inefficient because it allows for unwanted rotation to appear as tooth rolls into space and as a result unnecessarily lengthens treatment time. However, translating tooth bodily is difficult because bracket cannot be placed at center of resistance, which is about 9 mm up root of tooth from center of bracket. This problem is solved by use of the power arm. Its design obviates use of extra wire bends or repositioning brackets, slot angulations, etc. Ideally, to counteract a center of resistance 9 mm up from center of the bracket, a 9 mm lever arm is needed. Extraction bracket accomplishes this in two ways to make equivalent of 9-mm lever arm. Extraction bracket base is engineered with antitip and antirotation designed into its base to counteract rolling of tooth as it moves. The 4-mm-wide bracket base combines with force generated by deflection of wire as a result of bracket slot's antitip and antirotation to generate 4/9 of the countermovement needed to effect true translation. The 5-mm length of power arm makes up extra 5/9 countermovement needed to equal equivalent of 9-mm lever arm that has net result of putting forces of translation at center of resistance of tooth, 9 mm up from bracket's center. The antitip, antirotation of bracket slot and base, and length of power arm combine for maximum efficiency.

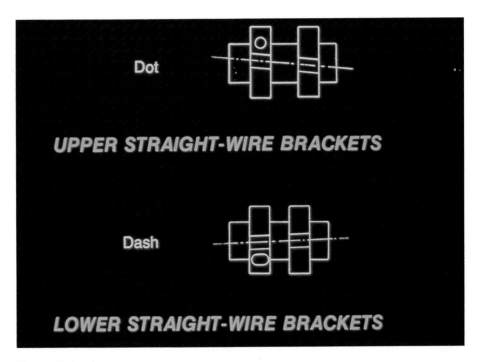

Figure 7-6

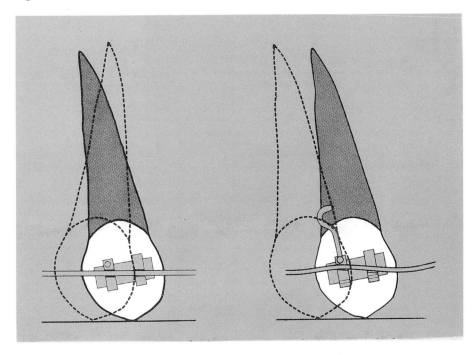

Figure 7-7

There are essentially two types of Straight Wire bracket systems. The first is the standard bracket system and is the one most commonly used when dealing with cases begun with functional appliances and active plates. It is designed primarily for cases in which all eight bicuspids are still present, a condition common to cases treated with FJOs, as this philosophy advocates extraction of second permanent molars, where indicated, as opposed to bicuspid extractions. Obviously, it is also the system of choice when no extractions at all are needed. Since little bodily movement and almost no translation of teeth are indicated in these types of cases, the standard bracket system uses all conventional Straight Wire design bases on all the brackets. There are no brackets with extra antitip or antirotation factors built into the bases of brackets to be used near bicuspid extraction sites as there are none.

The second type is the extraction bracket system, the first of which is the Roth setup. In this system certain brackets, namely the cuspid and bicuspid brackets, are manufactured with antirotation factors engineered into the bracket bases to compensate for the rotation effect exhibited by the teeth on either side of an extraction site as they are translated by elastic forces of one sort or another into the empty space left by the extracted bicuspid. Since extraction bracket systems imply bicuspid removal, the cuspid and bicuspid brackets are also produced with hooks or "power arms" cast right into the bracket base to help facilitate translation. The torque is increased for the upper centrals and laterals from 7 to 12 degrees on the centrals and 3 to 8 degrees on the laterals. Torque on the lower centrals and laterals remains the same. The tip on the upper cuspids is increased from 11 to 13 degrees and the torque from -7 to -2 degrees. Antirotation factors of 2, 4, or 6 degrees are also built into cuspid brackets depending on the size of the space closure to be effected. Torque remains the same for the lower cuspids at -11 degrees, but tip is increased from 5 to 7 degrees, and the same 2-, 4-, or 6-degree antirotation factors are available for lower cuspids. Torque also remains the same for the bicuspid brackets on the upper, but

Figure 7-8 **(A)** Standard nonextraction cuspid bracket is designed with 11° tip (no antitip). However, several "strengths" of extraction brackets are needed depending on distance tooth must be translated. **(B)** Minimum extraction bracket has 2° antitip, 2° antirotation, and is identified with one notch on occlusal edge. It is recommended for up to 2 mm of translation. **(C)** Medium extraction brackets have 3° antitip, 4° antirotation, and two notches. These are recommended for teeth to be translated 2 to 4 mm. **(D)** Heavyweights of extraction bracket guild are maximum extraction brackets. They are designed with 4° antitip, 6° antirotation, and three notches. They are recommended for teeth that must be translated more than 4 mm. Other similar compensating factors are figured into brackets for molars in event that they are ones to be translated. In case of molar brackets for translation, antitorque must be added also.

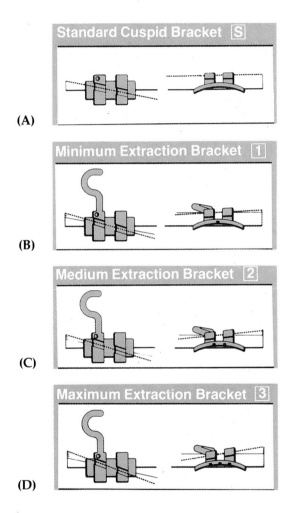

(A)

Standard Cuspid Bracket ⑤

(B)

Minimum Extraction Bracket ①

(C)

Medium Extraction Bracket ②

(D)

Maximum Extraction Bracket ③

again tip is changed from 2 to 0 degrees. Power arms are also added to the bicuspid brackets to assist in translation and space closure. Torque again remains the same on lower bicuspid brackets, but tip is changed from 2 to −1 degrees. Tip may be either 5 or 0 degrees and torque −9 degrees on standard first molar brackets on the upper, whereas in extraction bracket systems, upper first molar brackets are available in 0-, 2-, and 3-degree tip; and −9-, −13-, and −14-degree torque; and antirotation factors of 0, 12, and 14 degrees. Lower first molar brackets in the standard system have 2-degree tip and 26-degree torque universally, whereas in the extraction bracket system, lower first molar brackets come with 0-, −1-, or −2-degree tip and −26- or −31-degree torque, not to mention antirotation factors of 2, 4, or 6 degrees. Even stronger systems exist beyond this!

As can be surmised from the above, the extra tip and torque and anti-rotation factors built into an extraction bracket system are designed to compensate for the smaller, more compact arch that will result from extracting bicuspids in all four quadrants. These factors also combat the problems of teeth wanting to rotate while being translated by means of elastic forces in their path through the bone from their beginning pretreatment positions to their new locations in the now smaller arch which was made available by the missing or extracted teeth. The extraction bracket system has to make extra efforts to "cinch everything up a little" and add extra root torque and crown tip to keep the contacts correct and to help counteract the desire of teeth to relapse. Overcorrection is built into such systems so that once the appliance is removed, the teeth will settle into correct occlusion and anatomical relationships on their own.

But the main purpose for the entire extraction bracket system is for cases involving bicuspid extractions. In almost all cases treated by the FJO theme, when extractions are indicated, it is the second molars, not the bicuspids, that are sacrificed. Therefore the conventional standard bracket setup does perfectly well. All of the *original, ideal* tip, torque, and in-and-out anatomical relationships spawned from the Andrews study may be reproduced in cases so governed. Remember, none of the Andrews' 120 nonorthodontic normals, the standard that formed the basis for the original Straight Wire anatomical data, ever had missing bicuspids. The data were compiled for cases where all teeth were present!

THE ARCH WIRE

There are about as many different kinds of arch wires as there are fishing rods at the tackle shop. There are small companies whose sole purpose is the production of arch wires. However, a few have become standard fare in just about every "orthodontic tackle box."

There are essentially three types of arch wire which we shall discuss here which are used in the Straight Wire system—round, rectangular, and braided, which of themselves may be either round or rectangular. They come in various thicknesses and arch sizes.

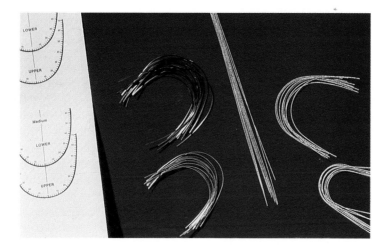

Figure 7-9

The braided wires are composed of three strands of wire twisted about themselves. Twisted wire offers the advantage of extreme flexibility and is therefore almost always the first wire used on a case where the amount of orthodontic deviation from the norm is greatest. Twisted wire is so flexible that it can be inserted at the beginning of treatment when it must follow a zigzag up-and-down, in-and-out path through all the variously positioned bracket slots. As it is ligated into all the brackets, it begins to exert its pressure on all the teeth at once and is excellent for "cracking things loose" and getting everything moving. It will start the process of leveling, aligning, and rotating the individual teeth and begin to approximate a better arch form to allow for the insertion of the stiffer round wires that will come after it. Twisted wire paves the way for the more rigid finishing wires by bringing the individual bracket slots into close enough anatomical harmony to allow insertion of the single-strand arch wires without distorting them from one bracket to the next such that bends would result in the arch wire which would negate their effectiveness. Twisted wire may be put through far more convolutions than single strand round wire without developing kinks. But even the twisted wires will kink or bend if forced into too sharp a bend. This is to be avoided as it destroys the effectiveness of the wire. If a discrepancy between one bracket on one tooth and the next bracket on the adjacent tooth is so great as to cause a bend to occur even in the highly flexible twisted wire during insertion into the bracket slots, one is far better off skipping the radically malposed tooth and waiting until the other teeth have been moved to a more favorable alignment relative to that tooth to permit engaging it with the arch wire, or supplemental mechanics must be used such as arch wire/elastic combinations, temporary repositioning of the bracket on the offending tooth, etc. One must never force an arch wire, twisted or otherwise, into a bracket slot such that it kinks the wire at that point of stress. If such occurs it is better to drop down to a smaller diameter, more flexible wire, or enlist supplemental mechanics as described above.

The round twisted wires come in four diameters: .015, .0175, .019, and .0215. The diameter is determined, not by measurement of the wire itself, but by the summation of the diameters of the three wires of which it is comprised. The higher the number, the more resilient and less flexible the wire. After about 1 month the wires might become fatigued and should be replaced. At replacement appointments, if the next size larger wire may be engaged in all the bracket slots without kinking or "popping off" the bracket, such may be done. Otherwise, remain in the same size until "stepping up" to the next-size bigger wire is possible. There is only one slight drawback to the twisted wire. Its rough braided texture does allow for the accumulation of a certain amount of plaque and fine food debris. But careful hygiene with soft brushes and oral rinses usually is all that is needed to keep the wire clean and new looking.

Twisted wire may be ordered in either straight blanks or preformed arches. Either works well. The straight blanks have a tendency to flare the anteriors forward slightly when engaged in the brackets and also exert slight lateral pressures posteriorly.

Round Wire

Round arch wires are made from preheated treated alloys that have a workable combination of elastic spring and memory with an increased resistance to fracturing. They may be used after the arch has had preliminary preparation with the twisted wire series. By virtue of their roundness, they "roll around" in the rectangular bracket slot, which greatly facilitates movement of the tooth back and forth along the arch wire but does absolutely nothing with respect to crown torque. But it certainly does well on everything else. Like the twisted wires, round wires should not be bent sharply or kinked in order to be made to fit the bracket slot. This destroys the total action of the arch wire in the system. (There are specific and deliberate exceptions such as distal tip backs, toe-ins, utility arches, etc, to be discussed later.) They are available in three sizes of arch forms: small, medium, and large; upper and lower; and four different wire diameter sizes listed in the Table 7-1.

Table 7-1
Round Wire Sizes

Diameter (mm)	Arch Forms
.014	Small, Medium, Large
.016	Small, Medium, Large
.018	Small, Medium, Large
.020	Small, Medium, Large

Rectangular Wire

Sometimes referred to as finishing arches, the rectangular arch wires serve to import crown torque to the teeth in the arch at the finishing stages of treatment by virtue of ligating the rectangular wire flush in the rectangular slot of the bracket. Thus if the tooth is not of sufficient or correct torque with respect to the long axis of the crown, the action of twisting the rectangular wire about its long axis during ligation to the bracket to bring it flush with the bracket slot causes the resultant force vectors to be transmitted to the tooth as the wire seeks to regain its original pretorque shape, which in turn moves the root of the tooth until the correct root torque or inclination is realized. This is a result of the torque that is built into the bracket slot base. The primary forces of rectangular wires are generated by this twisting along the long axis of the wire. This implies that the wire be firmly ligated to the bracket to ensure that the wire fits flat against the flat surfaces of the bracket slot. Sometimes, in cases where a tooth needs a lot of inclination correction, the firmer binding effects of wire ligatures may be needed at first rather than the standard elastic ligature. Rectangular wires may in fact tolerate only the very slightest amounts of in-and-out and up-and-down variance in the bracket slots of the teeth in the arch, but their main function is torque finishing. This is comprised of stabilizing the arch as a sort of fixed retainer and obtaining proper crown torque in the process. Rectangular wires come in small, medium, and large arch sizes for upper and lower arches listed in Table 7-2. The .018 × .025 is by far the most common; it is the size that most closely fits into the common .022 × .028 straight wire bracket slot.

Nitinol

There are many adjuncts to the basic tenets of the Straight Wire methodology that for the sake of brevity could not be discussed in detail. Entire other texts could be devoted to them, and probably will be. One of the most obvious examples is that of the subject of Nitinol—"the wonder wire." Its development for orthodontic arch wire purposes is an excellent

Table 7-2
Rectangular Wire Sizes

Dimensions (mm)	Arch Forms
.016 × .016	Small, Medium, Large
.016 × .022	Small, Medium, Large
.017 × .025	Small, Medium, Large
.018 × .025	Small, Medium, Large
.019 × .025	Small, Medium, Large
.021 × .025	Small, Medium, Large
.0215 × .025	Small, Medium, Large

example of the kind of progress a creative and questioning mind that is not bound by pedantic rigidity can accomplish. The very name of the wire itself bears witness to its unusual origins. The name "Nitinol" is derived from the two base metals from which it is constructed: "Ni" for nickel, "ti" from titanium, and "nol" from the Naval Ordinance Laboratory (NOL) (now the Naval Surface Weapons Laboratory) where the alloy was first developed (no doubt for reasons only less than humanitarian)! In 1968 in an article in the scientific section of a common weekly news magazine, the director of the NOL, William Buehler, reported a discovery of a "miracle" metal alloy with the most astounding elasticity and "memory" qualities. This event may easily have gone unnoticed except for the keen eye and incisively creative genius of one Dr George Andreasen, a dental educator at the University of Iowa.[22] Seeing the potential for the use of such an elastic and resilient metal in the construction of arch wires, Andreasen, in conjunction with the Department of the Navy, other government agencies, and Unitek Corporation, developed the use of the metal into arch wires with incredible properties. Though research is presently continuing on Nitinol, the arch wires are now available in both round and rectangular varieties and have been in clinical use since 1972. These arch wires have an extremely high resistance to deformation. This allows slightly heavier wires to be inserted sooner without kinking or "taking a set" when placed in the excessively misaligned brackets of the more severely malposed teeth in the arch. The wire will retain its memory in such instances and exert continued steady and gentle forces on the teeth for more efficient tooth movement. One Nitinol arch wire, say an .016 or .018 round, may be inserted and left alone to do a job that a whole series of arch wires of the twisted and round variety might be needed to accomplish. They are so resilient, some practitioners advocate sterilizing them once they are removed and using them over again on subsequent patients. This may also be the product of a consideration for their expense. But the wire also has other attributes that make it different from the standard stainless steel wires. Nitinol may *not* be soldered to, and it is recommended not to attempt to weld to it. It may *not* be electropolished or stress-relieved. Nor may teeth be translated along the wire by means of elastic forces. Also, its incredibly high resilience makes it mandatory to *always* cut the wire with a safety-hold distal end-cutting–type pliers, as once it is cut, the short free end is discharged at an extremely high velocity which may prove dangerous to nearby personnel. (Maybe that's a carryover from its ordinance beginnings!) When changing the shape of the arch wire to fit a given patient's arch, a three-pronged pliers or a specially designed Nitinol-wire bending pliers may be used. When using the three-pronged pliers, the thicker part of the base of the prongs are used, never the tips. To widen the anterior portion of the arch wire, place the middle beak on the labial side of the wire, and with a series of gentle constrictions of the beaks *en suite*, gradually widen the anterior portion as desired. Then, reversing the pliers so the single beak is on the lingual and starting at the cuspid area and working distally, continue the process until the desired arch form is attained. Using the specially designed Nitinol pliers, the technique is the same with the single concaved working surface side replacing the middle single beak of the three-pronged variety.

This brief excursion into the field of arch wires has by no means divulged all the types of wires available on the market today. There are even companies whose sole livelihood is derived from the design, manufacture, and marketing of arch wires. What are shown here are the most commonly used wires in the Straight Wire system. With these wires alone, one may perform functions that range from simple leveling, alignment, and rotation all the way to advanced mechanics such as opening the bite, tooth translation into extraction sites, increasing vertical with accentuated recurvatures, distal driving upper molars, and conventional Class II mechanics. Again, Straight Wire mechanics has revolutionized the orthodontic world with its accuracy, reproducibility, dependability, simplicity, and ease of operation. It has also put advanced orthodontic mechanics easily into the hands of the general practitioner.

BRACKET APPLICATION

There are two basic methods of bracket application, direct and indirect. In the direct method the bracket is placed on each tooth by hand; whereas in the indirect method, the brackets may be put on in groups by means of silicone trays. In this method all the brackets are sticky-waxed onto an accurate model of the case to be receiving the Straight Wire appliance. The brackets are placed in the ideal position on each tooth on the model, over which a streamlined silicone tray is processed. Once set, it is removed, and the wax removed from the bracket bases and the tray is ready to be transferred to the mouth, where the brackets are bonded to the teeth by placing the tray, or sectioned parts of it, in the properly prepared mouth.

But before either method may be initiated, the clinician must decide how he wishes to bracket the molars. Molar brackets may be acid-etched and bonded into place, but retaining a totally dry field that far back in the mouth for a sufficiently long enough time to permit correct bonding techniques may prove difficult at times. Also, the strength of the bracket-enamel bond in this method is at times, due to the stresses that may have to be exerted on the molars during treatment, considered by some to be suspect. These problems are eliminated by the use of bracketed molar bands.

Placement of banded brackets on molars follows the conventional techniques of molar banding. First, the contacts must be opened. Separating elastics snapped through the contacts using a forceps designed specifically for the job is a common method. Another easy way is by use of brass-separating loops. The one end of the loop is flattened to facilitate slipping it under the contact. Once pushed through, both ends are twisted about each other by grasping them with a Mathieu needle holder. The brass loop is twisted until the patient feels some slight discomfort of the wire tightening into the interproximal contact area. The brass loop method allows placement of the bands on the same day. If the loops are placed in the morning, the teeth will have become separated enough by that same afternoon to permit fitting of the bands. The brass loop is then untwisted, cut, and removed.

Most Straight Wire molar bands have brackets with buccal tubes (for use with advanced molar distalizing techniques like internal Class II labial bows or other molar distalizing mechanics) and Class III hooks on uppers or Class II hooks on lowers for the attachment of inter- or intra-arch elastics. Some have convertible buccal tubes, which allow the face metal covering

---

Figure 7-10   Direct bonding. Prior to molar band placement, teeth must be separated to permit bands to slip through contacts. Separating elastic rings may be placed using special forceps designed for that purpose. Snapping one part of ring through contact allows contraction of elastic ring to separate teeth. Three to five hours effect adequate separation in children, overnight for adult dentition. However, if contacts are too tight, brass separating rings are preferred. **(A)** Brass ring is slipped under interproximal contact and **(B)** twisted until patient feels slight amount of discomfort from tightness of wire. **(C)** It is then cut and **(D)** bent up into interproximal contact area to avoid irritation of cheek. **(E)** Once separation has been effected (which may only take four to six hours), the separating wires are **(F)** untwisted, cut, and smooth portion pulled through contact. Bands are selected that are as tight-fitting as possible, festooned to protect interproximal tissues, and cemented into place using masking tape loop to help keep cement off fingers of operator. **(G) (H) (I)** Once bands are properly seated and leveled with respect to long axis of tooth, other teeth may be prepared for direct (or indirect) bracket bonding. **(J)** Either dry laboratory pumice or special acid etch cleaning pastes are used with contra-angle brushes to clean teeth prior to etching. (Rubber cups are not advisable because oils used to process rubber may contaminate enamel, thus weakening bond. **(K)** Some clinicians may mark teeth to assure exact location of center of clinical crown. **(L)** Gel acids offer precise control of placement of etching material and easier visualization. **(M)** After etching for period of time prescribed by particular agent's manufacturer, area is thoroughly flushed with water and air dried so that definite chalky appearance may be easily seen **(N)** denoting etched area. **(O)** Composite-type self-curing bonding agents may be used, and once mixed only small amounts need be placed **(P)** on back sides of brackets. Bracket placement is on center of clinical crown of tooth **(Q)** so that bracket sides are parallel to long axis of tooth. **(R)** Anterior teeth may be bracketed either center of bracket on center of crown or by formula method previously described. **(S)** Elastic ligatures are used to ligate wire to bracket slots. Excess wire that protrudes through end of last molar brackets is cut flush with distal end of bracket with spring safety distal end cutter. **(T)** Case of maxillary dentition "strapped up" in appliance. (*Courtesy of Unitek Corp, Monrovia, CA.*)

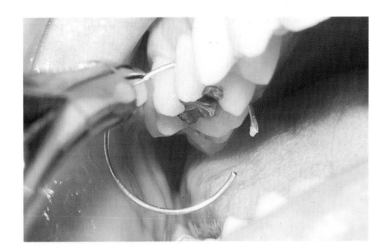

(A)

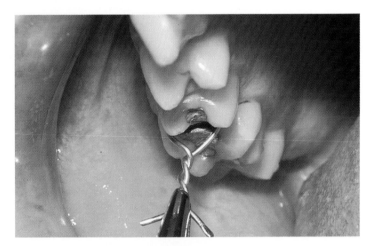

(B)

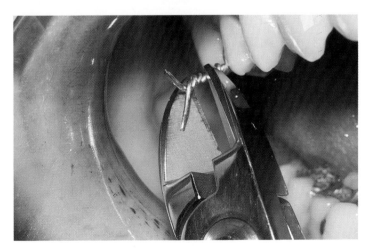

(C)

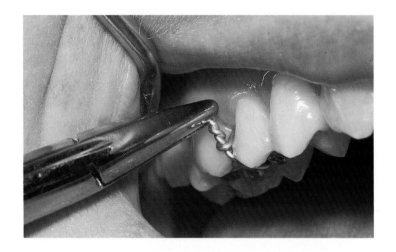

(D)

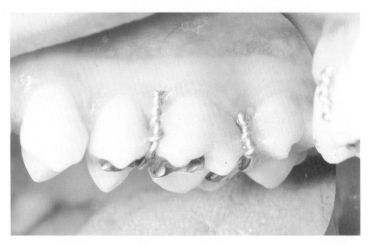

(E)

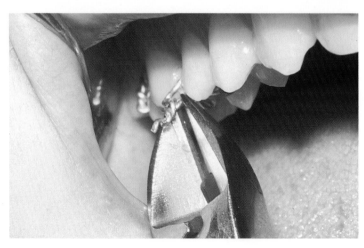

(F)

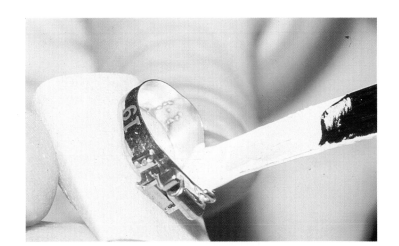

(G)

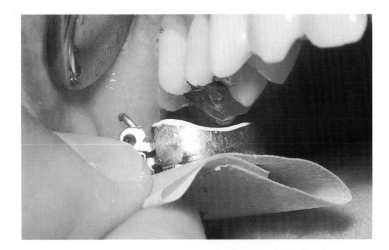

(H)

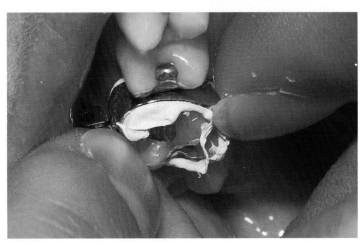

(I)

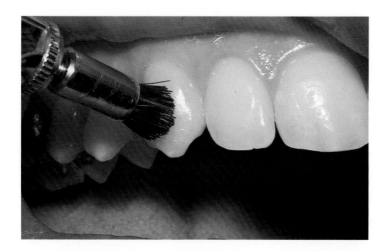

(J)

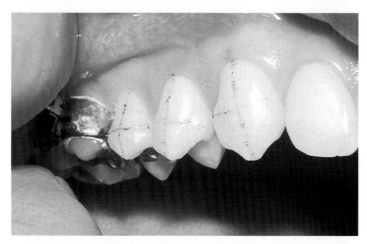

(K)

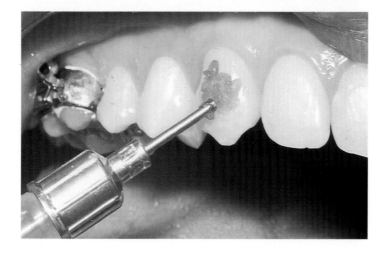

(L)

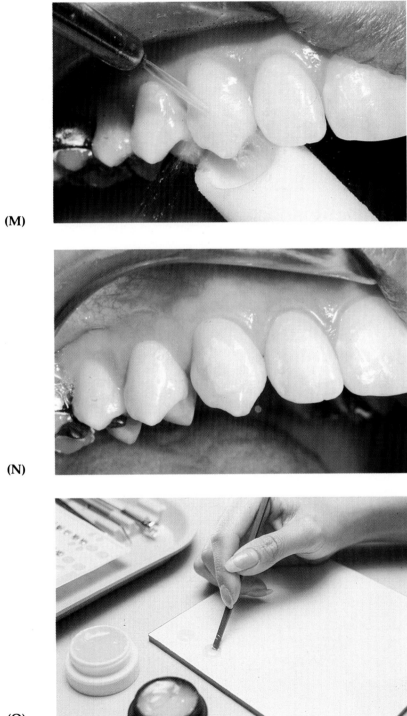

(M)

(N)

(O)

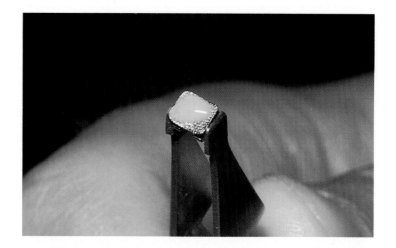

(P)

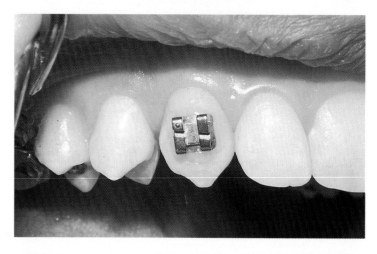

(Q)

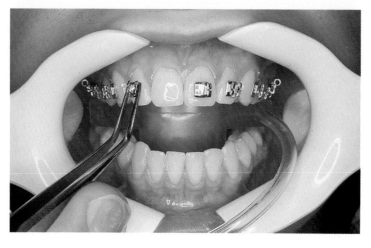

(R)

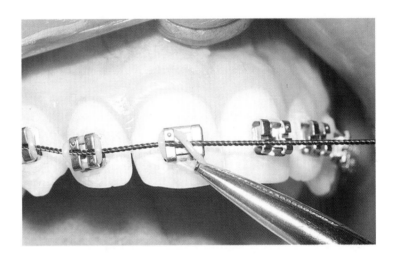

(S)

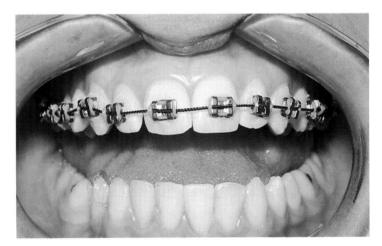

(T)

over the wire slot to be peeled off with a pliers to convert the slot from a closed to an open system. This facilitates passing the wire through the slot of the banded first molar into the slot of the banded second molar, which remains covered, if the two teeth are out of alignment enough to make passing a wire through both brackets difficult if both slots are covered by face metal. The lower bands should be seated such that the bracket aligns with the middle third of the clinical crown with equal positions of both mesiobuccal and distobuccal cusps showing above the edge of the band. Sometimes this requires festooning interproximally to allow proper seating. Upper molar bands should also be so aligned, but less of the distobuccal cusp should show above the upper margin of the band compared to the mesiobuccal cusp, which should be more prominent.

Placing the correctly sized band on the tooth first before putting cement in it allows the doctor to check the fit and crimp the edges. The band should be as tight as possible. The clinician should festoon the bands interproximally for the sake of the interdental col area. Also the interproximal portions should not extend up over the marginal ridges as this results in the band coming loose due to occlusal abuse. Once the band is ready for cementation, it may be placed on the sticky side of a small piece of masking tape. Mixed cement is flowed into a thick collar around the inside of the band. The masking tape not only keeps the cement neatly in place but also makes an easy handle for manipulating the bands into the mouth. The clinician may then press the band to place initially using the fleshy surface of thumb or finger, while the nonsticky surface of the tape protects same from the messiness of the cement. The band is seated first on the lingual, then to the buccal, squeezing cement out ahead of it as it goes. Band-seating instruments, such as a band biter, band seater, or common 3:4 plugger, may be used to drive the band home. Final adjustment may be made quickly before the cement sets with a How pliers grasping the band by its bracket.

The practitioner will either have to keep a fairly extensive inventory of brackets and bracketed molar bands or obtain them on an individual case-by-case basis from laboratories. Major orthodontic manufacturing firms that produce Straight Wire brackets, etc, all have kits available with sufficient numbers of bands and brackets of correct size and technique extraction or nonextraction (and this, of course, means bicuspids, not second molars).

Once molars are correctly banded, the patient is ready to receive the brackets. Teeth should be cleaned with common laboratory pumice and latch type contra-angle brushes.[23] It is felt by some that the oils in rubber cups or commercial "prophy" pastes act as a contaminant. Special care should be taken to get the facial surfaces of the bicuspids cleaned thoroughly of plaque, as these are the brackets that pop off most frequently, usually because these teeth accumulate plaque more readily than other areas like centrals, laterals, etc.

At this point, some practitioners using the direct method will make a light pencil line across the midline vertical height of contour of the tooth as well as a line horizontally at right angles to it through the center of the clinical crown vertically to help isolate the exact center of the tooth. Once etched, it is this point on the tooth, the exact dead center of the clinical crown, over which the slot of the bracket is placed. Brackets are placed such that the horizontal pencil line is parallel with the bracket base, *not* the bracket slot.

Another popular system of bracket positioning on the teeth is by means of the formula method. It does not govern the horizontal positioning of the bracket but merely the vertical position. Simply measure up to the center of the facial surface of the maxillary lateral from the incisal edge. Mark the spot and measure it in millimeters. (This is the same as one half its total clinical crown length.) Then measure the same distance up from the incisal edges of the upper centrals and the other lateral. This will place all four anterior incisors at the same level, which gives excellent esthetics and proper protection of the occlusion during disclusion. Add 1.0 mm to this value for the cuspid; then subtract 0.5 mm from that value sequentially for each tooth distal to the cuspid. For example purposes, let us say this value is 4.0 mm. So if the center of the clinical crown of the maxillary lateral is 4.0 mm, which we shall represent by CL, the position of the bracket for the maxillary cuspid should be CL + 1.0 mm or 5 mm. Then subtract 0.5 mm from the cuspid value CL + 1.0 mm for each tooth sequentially distal to the cuspid. (Always use CL as the value for the *upper* lateral.) Measure up 5 mm from the incisal edge of the cuspid, 4.5 mm for the first bicuspid, 4.0 mm for the second bicuspid, and 3.5 mm for the first molar, and a mere 3.0 mm for the maxillary second molar, if present. Aligning the slot on the bracket with the measured mark on the tooth aligns the brackets such that the marginal ridges will come out quite closely matched, once all the various arch wires have had their way. Of course, all cases will "settle in" a little to the final occlusion once the appliance is removed. The above formula may also be used on the lower teeth in similar fashion. Measure down from the incisal edge of the mandibular central or lateral incisor to the exact center of the clinical crown (one half its total length). Add 1.0 mm for the distance down from the incisal edge of the cuspid (CL + 1.0 mm) and 0.5 mm less on each tooth back to the second molar, if present. Again, mark these spots with a pencil on the tooth if bonding direct or on the model if using the indirect silicone tray method. Align the bracket slots even with these points measured from the formula. Where the bracket slot is, there the wire will be, and where the wire will be is where the tooth will eventually reside once the final wire rests passively.

Preparing the teeth with etching acids depends on the type used. Most commercially produced etching kits contain an acid that is either in liquid or gel form and is used for one to two minutes on each tooth. Bonding also is a product of the type of kit used.[24-32] Some bonding agents are mixed and placed on the bracket, which is in turn then placed on the tooth with a specialized bracket holding pliers, though common cotton pliers may be used. These types of bonding agents are of the conventional powder and liquid form. This method works well with the individual direct bonding process where brackets are placed one at a time but is a bit impractical for the silicone tray indirect method, as the composite material usually sets before a group of brackets may be covered and that particular section of the tray inserted. When direct bonding, the brackets are held in place for about one minute until the composite reaches an initial set. Some reach this initial set quicker than others. For the silicone tray or indirect method, contact setting composites work far better, as the composite setting reaction doesn't start until the catalyst makes contact with the base material. Since one is placed on the bracket and the other on the tooth, unlimited working time is available. In the tray method, expediency is enhanced by cutting the tray in three sections with a No. 11 Bard-Parker blade usually making the sections at the distal of the cuspids. Maintaining a totally dry field for the entire mouth all at once may be difficult, although the newer retraction-ejection devices now available from major orthodontic supply houses greatly facilitate this method. Cutting the tray in halves or thirds just makes it easier to manipulate. Accurately and thoroughly following the instructions of the respec-

---

Figure 7-11 Indirect bonding. Indirect *v* direct bonding process has been likened by some as "precision *v* approximation." In indirect bonding process, exact center of clinical crown of tooth is much more easily determined on study cast than in mouth. **(A)** Once teeth on plaster model have been properly marked, Straight Wire-type brackets may be easily and accurately sticky-waxed into place (with water-soluble adhesive waxes) **(B)**. Then special silicone elastic rubber trays are processed onto model **(C)** so that silicone tray material completely envelops not only teeth but also brackets. Once set, silicone "tray" may be removed **(D)**, taking brackets with it. Hot water baths remove sticky wax adhesive leaving the **(E)** tray holding bare brackets ready for bonding. **(F)** Orthodontic supply houses provide handy kits with all necessary material for obtaining dry field and bonding indirectly in mouth. **(G)** Again teeth are prepared in appropriate manner. **(H)** Field is isolated with buccal pads or cotton rolls **(I)**, bite blocks that simultaneously retract tongue are also handy. **(J)** Once totally isolated, teeth are easily kept dry for etching and bonding. Teeth may be etched with liquid or gel etching agents. **(K)** After appropriate etching times as per particular manufacturer's instructions, teeth are thoroughly rinsed **(L)** and chalky appearance of dried teeth **(M)** indicates proper etching of enamel that is ready for bonding. Sectioning tray into thirds **(N)** often expedites application of brackets. **(O)** Surface contact or slow-acting mix-type bonding agents are preferred in indirect technique because of extra time required to place bonding agents on multiple teeth and/or brackets. **(P)** With tray in place, gentle finger pressure is often helpful in acquiring good surface-to-surface contact between bracket and enamel. Once set (again as per instructions of manufacturer, which vary from three to seven minutes), trays may be removed **(Q) (R) (S)** exposing brackets bonded to teeth and ready for wire ligation **(T)**.

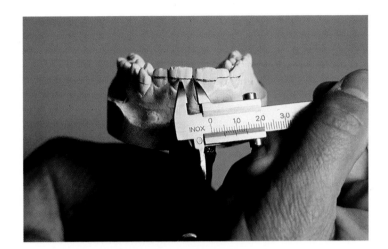

(A)

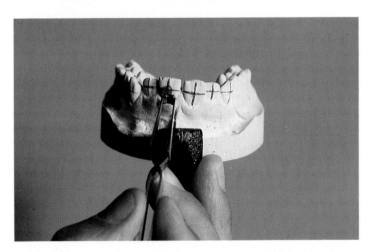

(B)

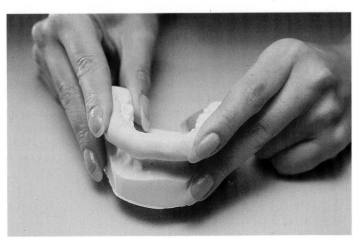

(C)

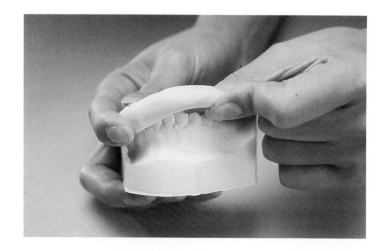

(D)

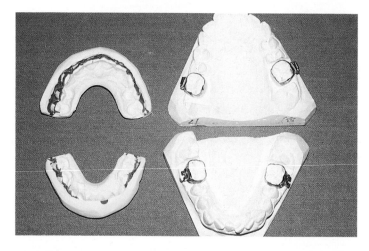

(E)

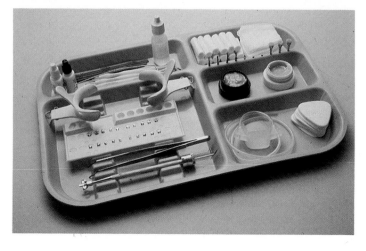

(F)

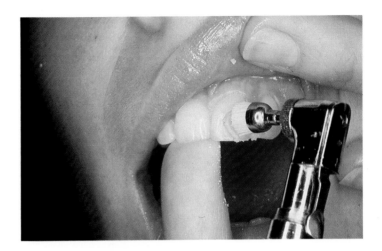

(G)

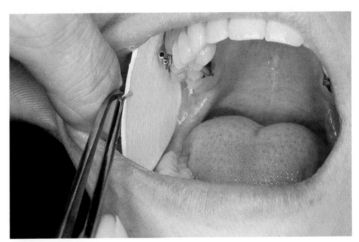

(H)

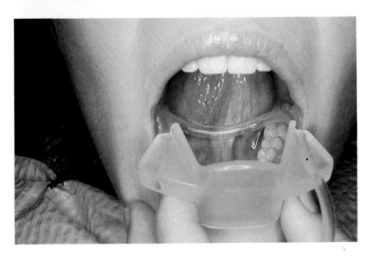

(I)

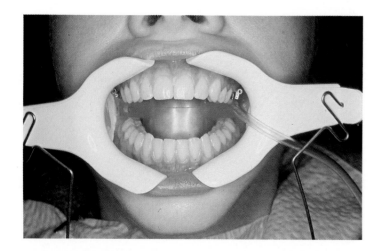

(J)

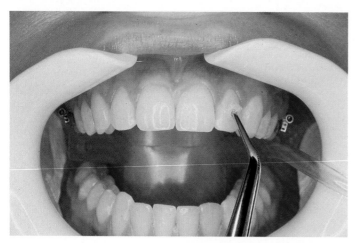

(K)

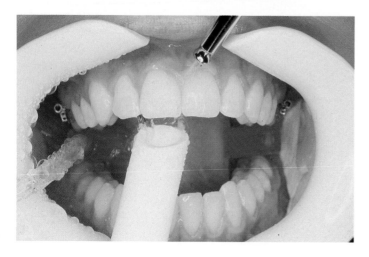

(L)

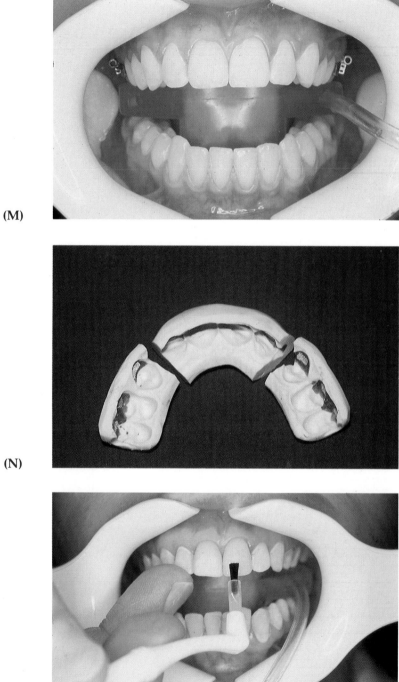

(M)

(N)

(O)

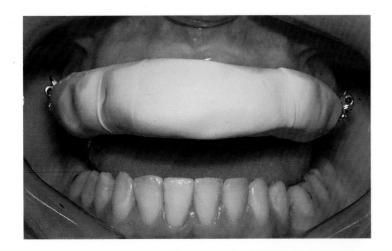

(P)

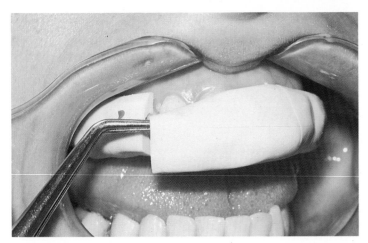

(Q)

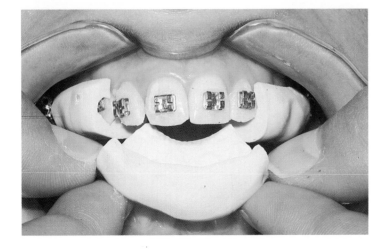

(R)

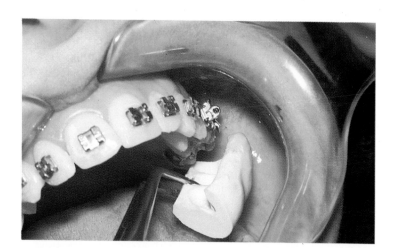

(S)

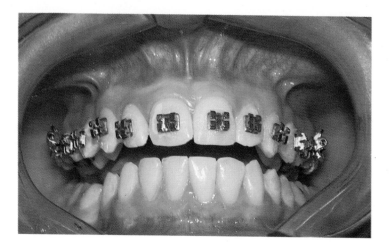

(T)

tive bonding composite kits used ensures correct bonding. Once the individually placed brackets are cured in place, or after curing once the silicone tray is removed, the case is ready to be wired.

PLACEMENT, ADJUSTMENT, AND SEQUENCING OF ARCH WIRES

The first arch wires that are placed are either the .015 or the .0175 twisted wire. In cases where the amount of fluctuation between one bracket slot on one tooth and the bracket slot on the tooth next to it is extreme, the clinician may have to resort to the extremely flexible .015 twisted or coaxial wire. But in most cases he may start with the traditional .0175 twisted wire to initially get everything moving. The first wire used is sometimes referred to as a "psychological wire" as it allows the patient time to adapt to the wearing of a fixed appliance by virtue of its very gentle forces. It is used at the beginning of treatment to obtain initial movements and begin minor leveling, alignment, and rotation motions. Teeth needing rotation might also get the extra help needed for this type of movement from the application of rotation wedges to the one set of tie wings, either mesial or distal, that the arch wire should *push against* to obtain the correct direction of rotation.

The wires may be ligated into place with small rubber elastic ligatures and the use of a small specialized Mathieu needle holder that has a special hooked beak ideal for grasping, stretching, and applying rubber elastic ligatures. After about 1 month the wire sometimes fatigues to the point where it should be replaced. If it is removed, the next larger size twisted wire should be tried in to see if it may be fully seated in all the bracket slots without kinking or pulling off a bracket (usually a sign of improper bonding technique). If it will go into place, move up to that wire; if not, stay in the present smaller, more flexible wire. After placing the wire and ligating it to all the brackets, the ends that protrude past the distal portion of the buccal tube of the last banded molar are cut flush with the end of the bracket tube with a distal end cutter. That is a pliers with a wire spring bar on the one cutting blade that holds the cut free end of the arch wire firmly in place against the base of the pliers while the excess piece of wire protruding from the distal of the bracket tube is being cut. This pliers prevents the free cut end of the wire from shooting down the patient's throat or penetrating intraoral soft tissues.

In some cases of Class I crowding, the case has been so well prepared by the active plates or functional appliances that preceded the placing of the Straight Wire appliance, that the case is brought to perfection with the use of the twisted wire alone or the use of the twisted wire followed by a short stint with the finishing rectangular wire. Others cases may require more involved Straight Wire finishing mechanics.

Once the series of twisted wires has been gone through, the arch is ready for the round wire series. Round wires that are most often used are the .014, .016, .018, and .020 with the .016 and .018 being the most commonly used. The .014 is quite resilient and after several months of the twisted wire series, especially if one ends in a .019 or .021 twisted, the teeth have usually been aligned, leveled, and rotated to the point where the insertion of the flexible .014 turns out to be redundant. Often one may progress directly from the .019 twisted to the .016 round or even the .018!

Once the patient is ready for the round wire series, the clinician must first choose not only the diameter of wire to be used, but also the size of the arch. Since not all arches are the same size, the preformed arch wires come in three sizes of arch shape: small, medium, and large. Even then, the arch wire may have to be reshaped slightly to coincide with the patient's particular arch size. This is done by means of the use of the wax bite template. Since most clinicians are too busy to bother with taking and pouring an alginate impression of the patient's mouth just to shape an arch wire to an ideal shape relative to that particular arch, the problem is expeditiously solved by use of a wax template. Heat a precut template of beeswax, common base plate wax, or bite registration wax of sufficient thickness in a water bath to permit placing in the mouth in flat sheet form and "impressioning" the teeth up to the level of the brackets so the brackets may just be seen in the wax. After removing and chilling the wax template in cool water to preserve shape, the arch wire to be used is laid over the template and gently shaped with the fingers or appropriate wire-bending or shaping pliers of choice until it coincides with the shape of the actual proposed individual ideal arch shape as closely as possible. This not only facilitates insertion, but also helps hold the arch shape produced orthopedically by the active plates and functional appliances that may have preceded Straight Wire therapy.

However, prior to this, one may wish to better prepare the arches for the full arch-engaging series of finishing wires by first accomplishing certain highly desirable tooth movements with a device that has greatly enhanced the use of the Straight Wire type of technique, the Brehm Utility Arch. The principle behind this type of technique is that the Brehm Utility Arch wire engages only the first molars and the four permanent anterior teeth. It may be used in either the upper and lower arches, and since it is designed to attach to only the first molars and four anteriors, it is ideal for use in the mixed dentition. By its ability to act on the two key portions of the arch from an orthodontic standpoint, the first molars and the anteriors, it allows the notions of interceptive orthodontics in the mixed dentition levels to come into full sway from a fixed appliance standpoint. Now, not only can the clinician rely on Straight Wire type of appliances to help perfect the positions of the teeth in the finishing of his cases *after* the active plate and functional appliance usage, but he may also enlist the aid of fixed-type mechanics to greatly aid and expedite the actions of removable appliances *prior* to their insertion. The Utility Arch may also be used where desired in the full adult dentition if the actions it effects are desired on the teeth it engages. However, its main forte lies in its use in the mixed dentition. It, like full-arch Straight Wire techniques, may be used first in the round wire form for more rudimentary leveling, aligning, and rotating of the six teeth in the arch to which it is attached; or if such is already adequate enough to permit, it can also be used in the rectangular wire form where its full powers and potential may finally be realized. The round wire type is primarily used to align the bracket slots of the six teeth sufficiently to permit the insertion of the rectangular wire model. (The Brehm Utility Arch will be discussed in further detail subsequently.)

Not only are the round wires good for the continuation of the leveling, aligning, and rotating process, but they also serve as guides for the retraction of teeth where necessary by the use of arch-condensing elastic forces and obtaining of arch symmetry. Obviously, one does not reshape the arch wire on the template of an asymmetrical or irregular arch to the point where these imperfections are repeated in the arch wire. It is these stiffer wires that help obtain the classical arch symmetry we are looking for and for which the previous steps have all been employed.

Numerous techniques are available with the insertion of the round wire series. Translation and tooth relocations are usually carried out on the .018. Open coil springs may be cut to 2 mm longer than the interbracket space of two teeth on either side of a blocked-in tooth to spread the teeth apart just enough to allow the retrieval of the crowded tooth by means of rubber retraction thread or other means. Closed coil springs may be placed on the arch wire to hold a space from closing between two brackets. The number of procedures possible are too extensive and varied to be mentioned here, but the principle behind why these techniques exist is that the bracket may *slide* along the round arch wire when necessary. The only thing impossible to perform with a round wire in a rectangular bracket slot is root torque. A round wire just naturally "rolls around" about its long axis in a square bracket slot.

By the time the round .016 and .018 wires have had their say, the case is usually nearly complete. The only thing that remains is for the insertion of the rectangular or finishing arches for stabilization and/or root torque if any is needed. Often it is! Again, the .018 × .025 rectangular finishing arches are shaped on the aforementioned wax template which has been stored as a part of the patient's records. Accentuated recurvatures may wish to be placed in the arch wires as a form of compensating curve throughout the series of round and rectangular wires. If an accentuated recurvature or compensating curve is used on a rectangular wire, this will torque the wire lingually about its long axis and it must be "anti-torqued" so the ends remain flat with the original horizontal plane. Holding the wire down firmly on a glass slab with an edge of a tongue blade or metal mixing spatula (if long enough) will usually divulge if the arch wire has been anti-torqued enough following the placing of accentuated recurvatures. Quite frankly, some clinicians feel if the case is good enough and little or no root torque appears to be needed, they merely use the .018 or .020 as a finishing or holding wire and proceed from there right to a retainer. However, this is a risky shortcut as most cases require some degree of root torquing by means of rectangular finishing arch wires to aid in attaining stability. After the initial work of arch preparation and alignment is completed by the active plates and functional appliances, finishing cases often consists of merely letting the Straight Wire appliance with its fully sequenced series of arch wires do its job.

"A man should keep his little brain attic stocked with all the furniture he is likely to use, and the rest he can put away in the lumber-room of his library where he can get it if he wants it."

Sherlock Holmes to Dr Watson
"The Five Orange Pips"
Sir Arthur Conan Doyle

Straight Wire Usage in the Mixed Dentition— The Utility Arch

If the total overall concept of Straight Wire mechanics were not a great enough boon to the practice of orthodontics in its own right, the modern concepts of its use in the mixed dentition add even more to its laurels. For years many felt that orthodontics utilizing fixed appliances was predicated on the existence of a complete or nearly complete set of adult teeth being present in the mouth. The lack of substantial deciduous root structure in an actual osseous functional matrix always precluded the banding of deciduous teeth. Often, patients 7 to 10 years of age who exhibited developing malocclusions were told that they could "have braces as soon as all the permanent teeth came in." This often meant postponing treatment until the patient was 12 to 14 years old. Until that time many a child was placed in a holding pattern of observed neglect, steadily worsening in the effects brought about by the maloccluding teeth, improperly developing bones, and most importantly, improper muscle function until treatment could be initiated in the early teens.

However, there were those of concerned insight who felt that while the permanent dentition was beginning to erupt in the early stages of the mixed dentition, if proper overbite, overjet, molar support, and lip seal could be established, the case would function reasonably normally. This normal function in turn, it was felt, would allow the forces of the tongue and other factors to exert and become major positive factors in developing the growth of the dental arches properly. This concept of "guided eruption" in the mixed dentition, if applied early enough in a developing malocclusion, helps eliminate the chances of more severe orthodontic as well as orthopedic complications from developing later on.

Now it is true that some of these mixed dentition problems can be very nicely taken care of with the proper use of functional appliances and/or active plates where indicated. But there is one knotty little problem that is very difficult for such types of removable appliance techniques to correct—

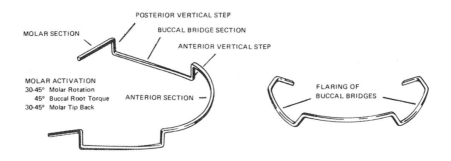

Figure 7-12   Standard Utility Arch (*Courtesy of Rocky Mountain/Orthodontics.*)

molar rotations! The upper and lower first permanent molars may well be in perfect axial position in a given dental arch, but when they are not and any rotation about their long axes is present, it almost universally is present in the form of mesiorotation. This can bring on a host of problems. One problem is that rotated teeth in the posterior quadrants take up more than their normal allotment of space or arch length (which is the opposite of what takes place in the anterior segments where rotation gives up arch length). This can increase the amount of crowding that may already be present anteriorly, expecially in the lower arch, or could also potentially contribute to such problems as other permanent teeth erupt. Another problem that may result is that the mesial rotation of the upper first molars, if severe enough, can alter the entire class of the case both dentally and skeletally. As the mesiobuccal cusp of the upper first permanent molar rotates mesially it moves forward over the occlusobuccal surface of the lower molar, sometimes enough so as to change the status of the relationship of the two from Class I to one-half or full Class II. This in turn brings the huge mesiolingual cusp of the upper first molar distally, which by virtue of the inclined plane action of the upper cusps on the lower molar help hold the entire mandible back slightly in a locking disto-occlusion. This can contribute to structural Class II problems, especially in the presence of Division 2 or retroclined angulations of the maxillary anteriors farther forward. It is also common knowledge that arches with crowded teeth usually exhibit some form of orthopedic underdevelopment. A great deal could be gained for the patient with such conditions if the aforementioned and highly desirable attributes of proper overbite, overjet, molar support, and lip seal could be obtained to bring the patient to a reasonable level of "normalcy" to unlock the potential for natural development. It would also be of great service if a method were available that could deliver such things consistently, predictably, and with a penchant for directly addressing that particularly difficult problem of molar rotation. Such an appliance exists in the form of that ingenious little device known as the Utility Arch. It was originally designed in the late 1950s by Ricketts et al[33] as a means of coping with molar tilting and second bicuspid intrusion problems during space closure in extraction cases. Grad-

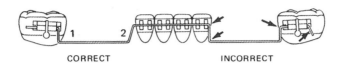

CORRECT   INCORRECT

Figure 7-13 The posterior step-up bend (1) should be made flush with mesial of buccal tube of bracket on molar band, whereas anterior step-down bend (2) should have leeway of 2 to 3 mm distal to lateral bracket. Distal extension is bent over only in Division 1 anterior arch retraction situations.

ually its multiplicity of uses became apparent. One of the first to modify its use from conventional Ricketts' methods and to alter its construction features while at the same time becoming one of its chief proponents was the "master Straight Wire clinician," Dr Waldemar Brehm of Encinitas, California. The Utility Arch allows the practitioner the advantage of "getting into" the mixed dentition early with a precisely positioning, rotation-controlling fixed appliance of consummate simplicity.

These at first odd-appearing and distinctively bent rectangular arch wires not only level, align, and rotate the two permanent molars and four anterior teeth to which they are customarily initially attached, but also may be used to retract or advance, intrude, or torque the four anteriors, open the bite, maintain or regain space, develop the dental arches, and assist in the correction from Class II to Class I. The unique appearance of these arch wires is due to their characteristic step-down bend that occurs in the wire between the distal of the lateral and the mesial of the first molar. This section of the arch wire is stepped down and flared buccally slightly to avoid interfering with the exfoliating deciduous or erupting permanent dentitions. Being that the arch wire must remain unattached across the cuspid and bicuspid area (brackets are never attached to deciduous teeth), the wire would be unsupported and interfere with normal function, especially the all-important function of the tongue during the period the deciduous teeth have exfoliated but before the permanent teeth have erupted. If not cleverly stepped down out of the way, the exposed and unsupported straight section of the arch wire under such circumstances would also be subject to bending or breakage during mastication. By virtue of not being attached through the cuspid and bicuspid area, the arch wire also has the ability due to bends at the molar area to exert tremendous forces on the molars while at the same time exerting forces of only one tenth the magnitude in the anterior area where much less energy is required to move teeth.

Utility Arches may be made individually from conventional arch wire blanks or obtained in the preformed "one-size-fits-all" variety that makes use of a male/female sliding rectangular tube arrangement through the step-down bend, referred to as the buccal bridge, which is individually adjustable to the patient's particular arch length from the distal of their laterals to the mesial of their first molars in either arch.

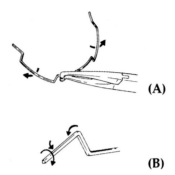

(A)

(B)

Figure 7-14 **(A)** To clear buccal bridge from impingement on muco-gingival tissues, torque it buccally at anterior step-down bend.
(B) However, when using rectangular wire it must be remembered that this will also torque distal leg that goes into molar bracket slot. Therefore, this distal section must also be countertorqued to compensate for movement of buccal bridge away from gingiva and allow untorqued level insertion into molar bracket once again.

Construction of the Individual Utility Arch

The standard mixed dentition Utility Arch is formed out of a .016 round or a .016 × .016 square arch wire. The common .016 round wire Utility Arch is most often the first wire used for the purposes of merely leveling, aligning, and rotating the teeth, and securing sufficient bracket slot alignment to permit reasonably unobstructed insertion of the .016 × .016 rectangular wire Utility Arch, commonly referred to as an activated wire. It should be initially cut to a length about 3 mm longer than the approximate area of the second permanent molars. This allows for the extra wire needed for the step-down sections or buccal bridges. First permanent molars are banded in the conventional manner and the four anteriors are given standard Straight Wire–bonded brackets. After observing the center of the arch wire by means of its midline mark and aligning that mark with the relative center space between the two central incisors, place a 3 mm anterior step-down bend 3 mm distal to the lateral incisor. Place the corresponding posterior step-up bend of equal amount just mesial to the buccal tube on the bracket of the banded first molar. Before the posterior step-up bend is placed, one may choose to place a cut piece of plastic tubing the approximate length of the buccal bridge on the wire to act as a guard against impingement of the wire in the gingival tissues during flexion of the arch wire as the activated forces of the Utility Arch express themselves during the movement of the teeth. Though the plastic tubing is handy, it is merely a nicety, not a necessity. Prior to insertion, the buccal bridges may be flared out away from the crest of the alveolar ridge to avoid tissue impingement by grasping the Utility Arch at the anterior step-down bend with a flat-on-flat pliers. Grasping the anterior portion of the arch wire with the opposite hand to the bridge sec-

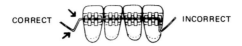

CORRECT   INCORRECT

Figure 7-14C

tion, torque the wire gently to produce the desired angular flare. Once complete, check for arch symmetry and arch wire flatness by laying the arch wire on a flat surface, flipping it over to check flatness from both sides. Once the arch wire has been prepared in this manner, it is still considered passive until activated prior to insertion. The only difficulty that might be encountered in making these Utility Arches by hand from arch wire blanks is that the distal step-up bend must be exactly flush with the mesial part of the buccal tube on the bracket of the first molars. There must also be a certain amount of clearance of the anterior step-down bend from the bracket on the lateral. This is taken care of by the 3-mm leeway space distal to the lateral. It should be checked so as not to bend down too close to the bracket as this will bind the tooth during its movement labially.

The alternative to making your own Utility Arches is the employment of the Brehm Preformed Adjustable Utility Arch. These arches come in one size for the lower and two sizes for the upper depending on the size of the patient's arches.

To customize the Preformed Utility Arch for an individual patient's needs, flare the buccal bridges laterally slightly to clear the gingivae and the height of contour represented by the alveolar crests; then place the distal ends of the arch wire in the buccal tubes of the first molar brackets. Next, place the anterior section of the arch wire into the slots of the anterior incisor brackets such that the midline mark of the arch wire is positioned between the central incisor brackets. It may be temporarily ligated into place with one elastic around the tie wings of one of the brackets to free up the hands. Of course, the buccal bridges always defer to the gingival, either upper or lower. The arch wire may then be lengthened as necessary by sliding the posterior step-up bend distally until it is flush with the mesial part of the molar bracket buccal tube. Care should be exercised so as not to puncture the patient's soft tissues with any excess free end of the arch wire as it is pushed through the buccal tube. This is permitted by the male/female sliding rectangular sleeve in the buccal bridges of the Preformed Arch wire. After double-checking to make sure the midline mark of the arch wire is still centered between the central brackets and both distal step-up bends have been extended fully to their respective molar brackets, carefully remove the arch wire taking off the single elastic ligature and taking care not to alter the length of the buccal bridges. Once removed, crimp the outer covering of the rectangular sleeve of the buccal bridge to permanently set the length of those sections by means of the special notch in the hinge area of the Brehm Utility Arch pliers. This prevents the sleeve from sliding on the wire. Excess free end wire that protrudes out the back end of the distal tube is left uncut (unless it penetrates the soft tissues) to facilitate insertion of the prepared arch wire once it has been activated. Once ligated to place, the excess protruding past the end of the buccal tube is cut with a distal end cutter, leaving a short 3- to 4-mm extension which is bent over flush with the distal end of the buccal bracket slot, but only if proclined Division 1 anteriors are to be retracted. This, in effect, acts as a tieback to keep the dogleg from pulling out of the buccal bracket wire slot as the forces of the bent wire express themselves and begin moving teeth. With the distal end thus bent over or "cinched back," the wire cannot pull out of the molar bracket slot as the toe-in bend rotates the molar distally. The arch wire therefore exerts maximum retracting effect on Division 1 anteriors. Cinch bends (or tiebacks) of the distal end are contraindicated if the anteriors are to be left unretracted as in the case of freshly advanced former Division 2 anteriors. In these cases not only is the distal end left straight but a 1- to 2-mm clearance should be left between the anterior bridge and the anterior brackets as a safety buffer zone against possible unwanted retraction.

Utility Arch Activation

Other than the aforementioned adjustment of the Preformed Utility Arch wire to fit individual cases, there are essentially four ways to adjust or activate the Utility Arch wire. They are:

1. Toe-in of the distal extension
2. Overexpansion and flattening of the anterior bridge of arch wire to expand the wire's width buccally
3. Tip-back of distal extension (usually lower arch only)
4. Flattening anterior step to increase arch length

As may be seen from the above, this is one of the few times that bends other than stops or accentuated recurvatures or compensating recurvatures are placed in the arch wire in the Straight Wire methodology. Before any of the following activation adjustments may be made to the arch wire, it should be shaped to rest passively adjacent to, but not necessarily in, the brackets of the teeth in the dental arch.

Buccal expansion of the arch wire.   The adjustments of the Utility Arch with respect to arch width are made to enhance the lateral development of the dental arches and are almost always used in conjunction with either toe-in or distal tip-back bends of the distal extension of the arch wire. The overex-

---

Figure 7-15 **(A)** Dr Waldemar Brehm. **(B)** Passive Brehm adjustable Utility Arch wire. **(C)** Activated arch wire exhibiting toe-in bends, used for distal rotation of first molars and buccal flaring of posterior bridges of arch wire. This assists in lateral development of case, if needed, while arch wire is being worn.

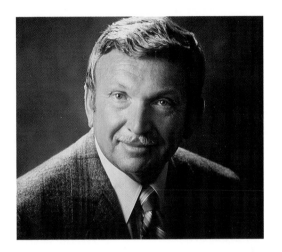

(A)

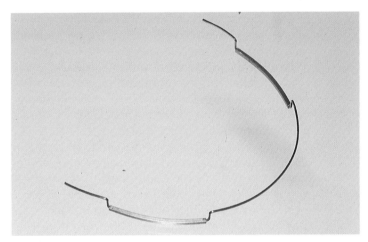

(B)

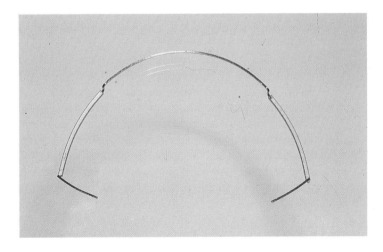

(C)

pansion of the Utility Arch is customarily made with a 5-mm space between the wire and the buccal tubes of the banded molar brackets on both sides when the distal rotating toe-in bends are used. This aids in the distal rotation and expansion of the molars laterally as the forces of the wire express themselves. Most cases requiring the interceptive use of the Utility Arch are in possession of some component of lateral underdevelopment contributing to the orthodontically crowded dental arch. On the other hand, when the tip-back bend is used in the distal extension of the wire to upright molars, a 3-mm expansion of the wire is used on both sides of the arch. This aids in distalizing the molars slightly along with uprighting them. Usually the expansion of the Utility Arch to 3 or 5 mm past the location of the buccal molar brackets bilaterally can be easily performed with finger pressure as the wire bends laterally in the anterior section easily without the need for pliers use. This is usually adequate for the lower arch, but sometimes the upper requires more than 5 mm with the tip-back bend. But it must also be remembered that the lateral forces exerted on the dental arch

---

Figure 7-16 **(A)** Activated Brehm Utility Arch wire is attached to anterior brackets and exhibits presence of both toe-in bends of distal extensions prior to insertion into molar bracket slots, used to distally rotate molars, and buccal flaring of posterior bridge section of appliance. This flaring is easily produced by simply flattening anterior bridge portion of appliance. This action aids in lateral development of arch when needed. (Note that to more clearly illustrate the principle of distal rotation of molars, toe-in bends were slightly exaggerated for the sake of this photograph.) **(B)** Once arch wire is inserted into molar brackets of teeth of typodont (hard plastic teeth set in synthetic artificial gum tissue of soft rubber-based material), action of toe-in bends may be seen to have an immediate effect on molars, as some distal rotation may be readily observed (permitted by elasticity of rubber-based material). **(C)** Action of cinched-back, toed-in, buccally flared Utility Arch is demonstrated here. Cinch back or tie back of arch wire consists of bending distal extension over slightly as it exits distal end of molar bracket slot. This locks distal extension into bracket slot and prevents it from pulling out (as during distal rotation). Net effect of arch wire so adjusted is to distally rotate and expand molars, and in so doing the anterior bridge is drawn lingually (helped by cinch back of the now locked in distal extension) and anterior teeth are retracted. Cinch back bends are not used in Division 2 anterior angulation situations. Here, distal rotation only may be accomplished by using a non–cinched-back toe-in bend; for as the molar is distally rotated by toe-in bend, straight unbent distal extension may slip forward slightly in buccal molar bracket slot as molar rotates. This helps prevent arch wire from being pulled lingually and exerting a retraction force on anteriors as toe-in bend expresses itself distally rotating the molar. This is desired in Division 2 cases, where anterior retraction is contraindicated.

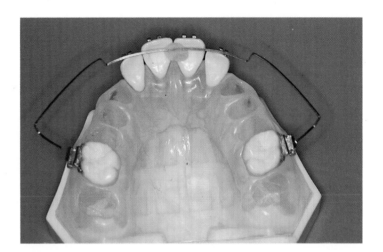

(A)

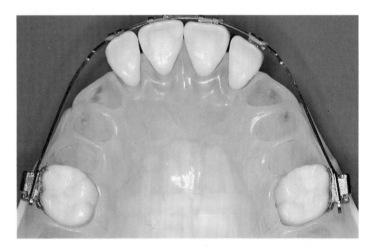

(B)

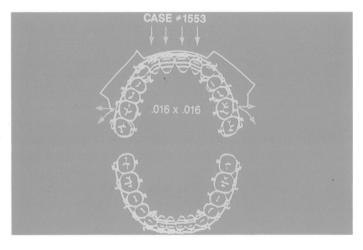

(C)

by the widened arch wire are slight, and if major development laterally is required, it is best performed with active plates such as the Schwarz which are more suited for such purposes. The clinically observed and generally accepted average limit for lateral development with Straight Wire only seems to be about 5 mm. When more lateral development than that is required to obtain proper arch form, active plates should be called upon first.

Toe-in bends of the distal extension.   One of the major uses of the Utility Arch wire in the mixed dentition is for the distal rotation of mesially rotated first permanent maxillary molars. Only occasionally do lower first molars require distal rotation. In order to obtain truly proper Roman arch form of the dental arches, the mesiobuccal cusp of the first molars, both upper and lower, should occupy the widest laterally measurable part of the dental arch. This is impossible if the molars are mesially rotated. Mesial rotation of a first molar also very importantly occupies more than its fair share of the arch length, and correcting the rotation, due to the tooth's rhomboidal occlusal outline, creates more space in the arch in which to realign other teeth, sometimes as much as 2 mm per quadrant! The toe-in bend accomplishes this maneuver to perfection and it does so easily, gently, and in as little time as 2 to 3 months. To activate the distal extension of the arch wire, a toe-in bend is placed such that the distal extension passes directly from the posterior step-up bend to a point approximately over or a little mesial to the distolingual cusp tip of the upper first molar. This places the distal extension at about a 65-degree angle to the buccal bridge. Once the toe-in bend is placed, the arch wire is flared away from the molars by the appropriate amount. In the mandible, much less of a toe-in angle is used; usually only 15 to 30 degrees is all that is necessary depending on the severity of the molar rotation.

As the toe-in bend expresses itself, it does more than correct the rotational aspect of the molar orthodontically, it also has far-reaching orthopedic effects. As the combined action of the toe-in bends and lateral overexpansion of the width of the arch wire exert their forces, the upper first molars rotate distally *and* move laterally slightly. This widens the arch laterally and in conjunction with the increase in arch length obtained by the rhomboidal effects of the rotated molar correction, leads toward an all-around larger and less crowded dental arch. But the mandible shows a slight change in position also. As the upper first molar rotates distally, the huge mesiolingual cusp of the tooth in effect moves forward mesially, and in so doing, the inclined plane action of its cusp slopes in contact with the lower first molar causes the mandible to close in an arc progressively further forward to maintain proper occlusion and interdigitation of the cusp slopes of the two large adult teeth. This aids in advancing the mandible forward from its skeletally Class II pretreatment position. This along with the movement of the mesiobuccal cusp of the upper first molar distally is all that is often necessary to effect the change from mild Class II or one-half Class II to Class I. The bite also has a tendency to open as the molars rotate and expand laterally. This may obviate the need for use of the Bionator altogether when Class II dental and skeletal discrepancies are borderline or not too severe.

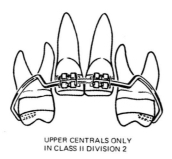

UPPER CENTRALS ONLY
IN CLASS II DIVISION 2

Figure 7-17

But the toe-in bend also has some very profound effects on the four teeth to which the arch wire is attached anteriorly. As the molars rotate distally, the net effect of the arch wire is to shorten itself anteroposteriorly and this of course retracts the four anteriors by imparting lingual crown torque and bodily retraction forces to these teeth. This may be easily seen by holding a prepared and activated arch wire with 65-degree toe-in bends in it by the fingers and attempting to straighten out the wire as it would be if inserted in the mouth. Holding the wire in this tensed position, one will observe how the anterior section of the wire is bowed forward slightly. By gradually releasing tension in the distal extensions and allowing them to assume their 65-degree angulation again, one will observe the arch wire shortening itself anteroposteriorly which in effect is the same as the anterior bridge retracting lingually. Such actions as these make this type of adjustment of the Utility Arch ideal for correction of Class II, Division 1, cases in the mixed dentition. This factor must also be compensated for in Class II, Division 2, cases where the movement of the upper centrals labially is desired. In such instances the round Utility Arch wire is adjusted so as to pull the crowns of the offending anteriors labially by flattening the anterior step-down bend slightly, just enough to keep the anterior bridge of the arch wire 2 mm out and away from the anterior brackets of the teeth to be torqued. This distance must be maintained throughout the course of treatment, which means that the anterior bridge must be steadily advanced as the molars rotate to maintain the 2-mm distance. Usually only the two upper centrals are bracketed and engaged with the arch wire until they are flush with the laterals at which time all four anteriors are ligated to the arch wire. Wire ligatures prove best for such purposes, as elastic ligatures may possess too much elasticity in these cases which prevents them from keeping the wire tightly engaged in the bracket slot.

Tip-back bend of distal extension. The distal tip-back bend of the distal extension is a bend designed to upright molars that are tilted forward and also intrude or advance the anteriors, depending on how the anterior bridge is adjusted, thus flattening out the curve of Spee. Toe-in bends and tip-back bends are never used at the same time. Toe-in distal rotations are usually accomplished first. Once the rotations are complete, the toe-in bend is taken out of the distal extension by straightening it out again and then the tip-back bend may be placed. The distal extension is bent gingivally to 30 to 45 degrees depending on the severity of the mesial tilt of the molar (usually the lowers) and the depth of the curve of Spee. This action of molar uprighting and anterior intrusion or advancement is ideal for increasing the vertical and opening the bite in closed bite situations. A slight increase in arch length will also be realized as the uprighting forces of the tip-back bend also tend to distalize the molars. Generally a 45-degree tip-back will generate about 100 to 120 g of force of an intrusive nature forward in the anterior area on the upper arch which is still at a very safe level biologically. Eighty to one hundred grams is the preferred limit to intrusive forces in the lower arch. It must also be remembered to utilize about a 3-mm expansion laterally on both sides of the arch of the distal extensions away from the molar brackets. This is easily done by finger pressure in the anterior bridge section as previously described. As the tip-back bend expresses itself, it also exerts a lingualizing force on the lower anteriors when the distal extension of the wire past the end of the buccal tube is properly cinched back, as with the toe-in bends also.

Flattening step-down bends to advance anteriors.   There are some occasions when it is desirable to bodily translate the entire tooth, root and all, labially. This is commonly done in the case of a blocked-in anterior where the apex of the root as well as the crown of the tooth are situated too far lingually. To advance teeth anteriorly by means of translation, the distance between the anterior bridge section of the wire and the bracket slots of the teeth to be translated is opened up by 1 to 2 mm. This is easily accomplished by opening up the 90-degree step-down-bend angles reciprocally by grasping the vertical step section of wire with a flat-on-flat pliers, and with gentle finger pressure bending the anterior and buccal bridge sections slightly

---

Figure 7-18 Tip-back bends of distal extension. After distal rotation and expansion of molars laterally with toe-in bend of distal extension, take toe-in bend out by straightening distal extension once again and place tip-back bend in it if needed. **(A)** This will act to open bite as it uprights and slightly distalizes molars and advances and intrudes anteriors. **(B)** Placing from 30° to 45° tip-back bend only produces 75 to 120 g force on anteriors **(C)** because of flexibility of arch wire and length of lever arm from buccal bracket on molar to brackets on anterior teeth. A tip-back bend that is tightly cinched back will exert lingualizing force on anteriors as molar uprights. This cinching back of distal extension consists of bending 3 to 4 mm of the wire protruding past distal end of buccal molar slot down over its edge. Thus distal extension is firmly locked in bracket slot and may not pull out during any form of tooth movement. **(D)** Tip-back bend of maxillary Utility Arch prior to engaging anterior brackets. **(E)** Tip back bend of mandibular Utility Arch prior to engaging anterior brackets.

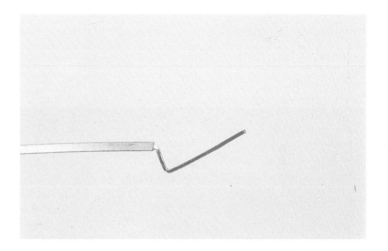

(A)

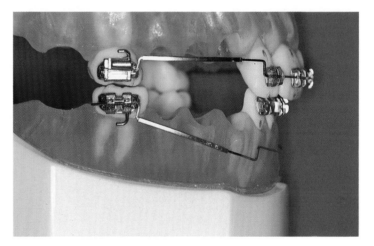

(B)

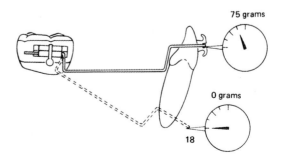

(C)

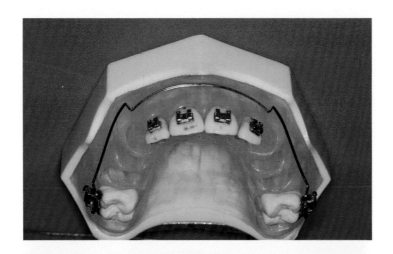

(D)

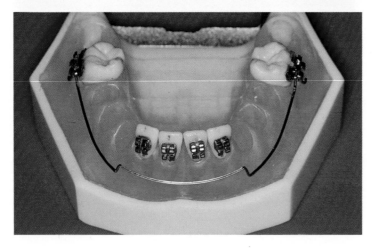

(E)

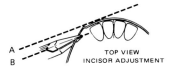

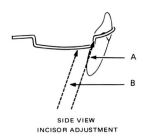

A   Activation on anterior step keeps activation parallel to anterior section.

B   Activation along buccal bridge near anterior step should come in slightly from behind and be kept parallel to anterior section of arch. Anterior section has contour so action is to the teeth on each particular side.

Figure 7-19(A)

CROWN TORQUE OR LABIAL ADVANCEMENT

CROWN TORQUE OR LINGUAL RETRACTION
(Turn plier over)

PLACEMENT OF PLIER

PLACEMENT OF PLIER

CRIMPING ANTERIOR END OF BUCCAL BRIDGE

CRIMPING ANTERIOR END OF BUCCAL BRIDGE

CRIMPING ANTERIOR VERTICAL STEP

ACTIVATION PRODUCES CROWN TORQUE ON THE INCISORS

OR

CRIMPING ANTERIOR VERTICAL STEP

LABIAL ADVANCES

LINGUAL RETRACTS

To advance the incisors or to effect labial crown torque, the intra-oral adjustments are made as illustrated above. The arch wire being deflected inward advances the incisor teeth, and places labial crown torque.

To retract the incisors or to effect lingual crown torque, the intra-oral adjustments are made as illustrated above. The arch wire being deflected outward retracts the incisor teeth, and places lingual crown torque.

Figure 7-19(B) Intra-oral adjustments.

away from the pliers that acts as a vise holding the vertical step section, slightly opening the two 90-degree right angle bends obtusely by an equal amount. This keeps the anterior and buccal bridges still parallel with each other while advancing the anterior bridge labially beyond the bracket slots by the desired amount. Once engaged and ligated to place, the combination of torque-free anterior pull of the overexpanded arch wire with its all-important rectangular wire–rectangular bracket slot effect brings about the bodily translation of the entire tooth and root labially. The slack is absorbed by the bowing out of the buccal bridge sections of wire, the same action that acts as an energy source, via the wire, to effect the translation anteriorly.

Again, it must be remembered that these techniques are predicated upon the effects of a rectangular wire in a rectangular bracket slot. One cannot expect these effects to occur with the use of a round wire in a rectangular bracket slot. (If round wire is used, the vertical step flattening will only produce a labial crown tip.) These effects may be taken advantage of if desired, but their principles must be clearly understood and delineated from rectangular arch wire adjustments.

As with any form of Straight Wire therapy, if the teeth to be bracketed are too irregular in position as to preclude immediate insertion of the .016 × .016, a lighter, more flexible, simple round arch wire might have to be used just to level, align, and rotate the teeth enough to permit the insertion of the less forgiving rectangular Utility Arch.

Another indication for the very light forces of the more flexible wires is in the very early mixed dentition. At this stage of the child's development, the apices of the roots are often still not quite completely formed and if orthodontic movement of such teeth is to be carried out, it should be done so in a very gentle fashion. This is where the construction of a .014 round wire utility arch is ideal. It delivers enough of a force to easily effect orthodontic movement of the teeth through the very young and "green" highly bioplastic alveolar bone without damaging the highly sensitive Hertwig's Sheath of the "blunderbuss" apices of the roots.

Sequential Adjustment

To avoid confusion (and poor results) as to the order of use of the various adjustments possible in the use of the Utility Arch, it may be handy for the operator to keep several rules of thumb in mind:

1. Always level and align the four anteriors as much as possible with .016 round Utility Arch wire prior to use of the activated .016 × .016 rectangular version. This means not only leveling, aligning, and rotating the four anteriors but also advancing the Division 2 anteriors to proper interincisal

---

Figure 7-20 Distal rotation and expansion. **(A) (B)** Note how molars have been distally rotated and expanded. This is more clearly seen in before-and-after study models of case. **(C) (D)** Notice how not only have molars distally rotated and expanded laterally but also Division 1 anteriors have been retracted to produce wider, more rounded Roman-type arch form. **(E)** As a consequence of this, the Class II mandible that has previously been locked in distoclusion because of former restrictions of narrow maxillary arch form is now free to develop naturally as it is guided by improved inclined plane action of teeth to normal Class I relationships **(F)** with proper overbite and overjet of arches. (*Courtesy of Dr Waldemar Brehm, Encinitas, CA.*)

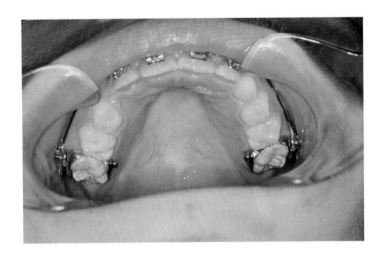

(A)

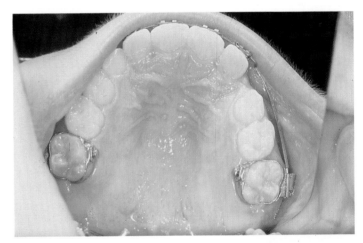

(B)

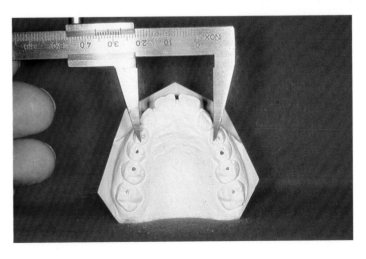

(C)

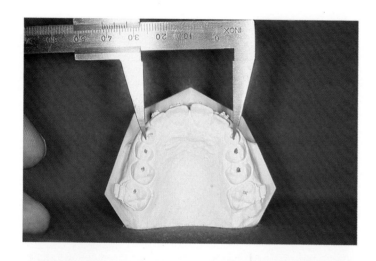

(D)

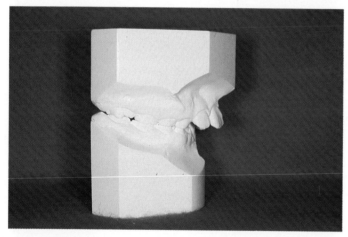

(E)

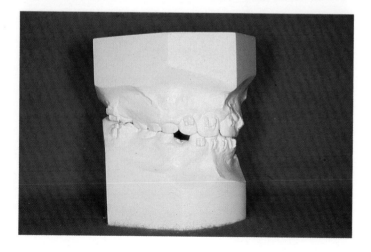

(F)

angulation prior to any use of toe-in or tip-back bends. Not only should such retroclined anteriors be corrected first (by activating the anterior step-down bends of the Utility Arch) but overcorrection to 2 to 3 mm past their final end-of-treatment position, or until multiple spacing appears between the teeth, is an entirely appropriate treatment action. Sometimes the upper centrals are so retroclined that only these two teeth may be ligated to the .016 round Utility Arch wire until they have been advanced enough to permit ligation to the laterals. Again, this is done prior to the use of any form of toe-in, tip-back, or lateral expansion adjustments of the arch wire.

2. Never place toe-in and tip-back bends into the distal extension at the same time.

3. Toe-in bends to rotate molars distally are placed first. Once completed they are taken out and tip-backs may be placed if needed.

4. Cinch-back or tie-back bends of the distal end of the arch wire over the distal end of the molar bracket, thus locking it in place, are used only when the toe-in bends used to rotate the molar distally are to be taken advantage of to retract proclined Division 1 anteriors. When such retraction is not desired the distal end is left straight along with a 1- to 2-mm "buffer" between the anterior bridge and the anterior brackets (prior to ligation).

5. You cannot efficiently rotate molars distally and advance anteriors at the same time.

CEPHALOMETRIC CROWDING—DETERMINATION OF ARCH CROWDING IN MILLIMETERS

The use of cephalometrics (described subsequently) provides the diagnostician with an important and extensive source of diagnostic data upon which to construct his treatment plan. Yet, even before analyzing the cephalogram by any one of a number of the cephalometric analysis systems available, an enormous amount of information may be obtained by simply measuring models!

Mixed dentition analysis has already been described and is handy for determining the needs for development of the dental arches to accommodate the prospective eruption of adult teeth once they arrive.

Schwarz' or Pont's analyses may also be performed in the mixed dentition, even if the first permanent bicuspids have not erupted yet, by merely substituting the location of the distal pits of the deciduous first molars (or "D") and adding 2 mm as an approximation for the future location of the permanent replacements. This, in conjunction with the use of the symmetroscope in the three-dimensional model analysis, can divulge a great deal of information to the treating clinician. Simple crossbites or arch width deficiencies may be treated with removable Schwarz plates, either upper or lower. And regaining lost E-space with Sagittal appliances has also been described. Yet there may still be some instances where dental crowding exists in the late mixed dentition stage where the arches are already near or on Schwarz' or Pont's indices of adequate arch width and the orthopedic and orthodontic alignments are close to or completely within Class I category. In such cases, orthopedic arch widening (overdevelopment), or molar distalization techniques may be totally contraindicated (improper upper or lower incisor angulation is the key to the differential diagnosis here). In these types of situations, all that is needed to relieve the dental crowding is the simple "straightening" of teeth to proper inclinations, and angulations, and that means Straight Wire!

Determining which way to develop an already adequate upper arch, either anteriorly or posteriorly, requires the advanced understanding of cephalometric interpretation. But treating the lower arch to relieve crowding involves only the simplest excursions into cephalometrics. Hence it will be

---

Figure 7-21   Case study. In this Class II, Division 2 deep bite malocclusion in mixed dentition, note large diastema **(A)** between maxillary centrals, deep overbite and lack of vertical **(B)**, and radiographic evidence of future blocked-out cuspids **(C)**. Study casts reveal **(D)** mesially rotated molars and **(E)** Class II, Division 2 angulation of anteriors and molar alignment as well as **(F)** blocked-out lower right cuspid (and potentially lower left cuspid) because of lingual inclination of Division 2 lower anteriors. Case needs arch development, advancement of incisors in form of labial crown torque, and increased vertical to aid in correction of Class II to Class I. Case is begun with upper and lower Utility Arches in .016 round wire to aid in torquing the incisor crowns forward. After this is accomplished, initial distal molar rotation may be initiated. The .016 round wire Utility Arches are then given classic tip-back bends to upright molars, continue advancement of anteriors, and increase vertical **(G) (H) (I)**. In addition, elastic power chain is run across four maxillary anterior brackets to condense open spaces and thereby gain increased arch length. (Note: Had overjet been too tight to permit immediate bracketing of lower arch, upper arch would have to be advanced for brief period first to move upper anteriors forward enough to allow bracketing of lowers. Because enough space in form of overjet existed at beginning of treatment, both arches could be bracketed simultaneously.) After initial period of Utility Arch usage, note how vertical has increased **(J) (K) (L)**, along with condensation of open spaces between upper anteriors. At this point, lower .016 round Utility Arch was replaced with .016 × .016 Brehm Preformed Utility Arch. Upper round version was also replaced with .016 × .016 Standard Utility Arch. Note how up to this point all photos show bowing of buccal bridges indicative of activation anteriorly of step-down bends confluent with Division 2 technique. Note how individual step-down bends are opened up to more obtuse angle necessary to impart advancing or labial-type forces to anteriors. Once anteriors are advanced to more acceptable interincisal angle and vertical has been increased, (*continued*)

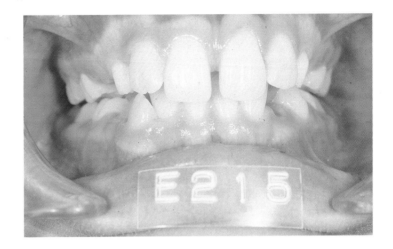

(A)

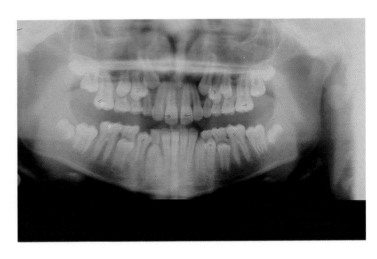

(B)

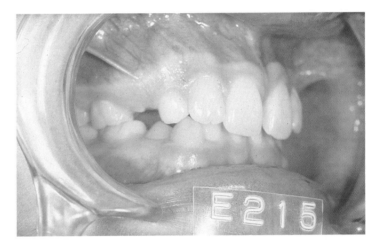

(C)

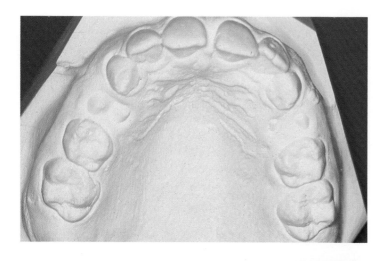

(D)

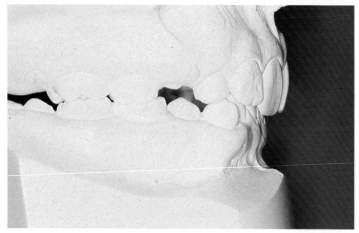

(E)

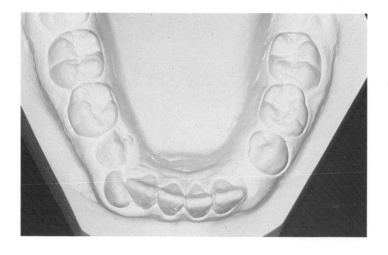

(F)

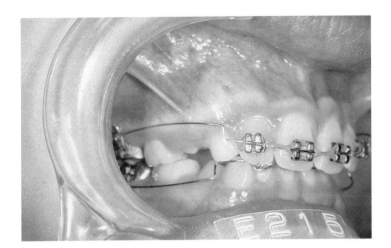

(G)

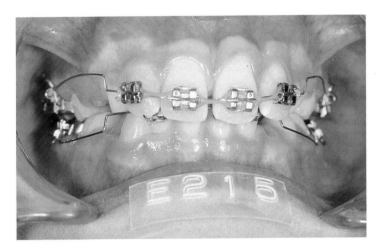

(H)

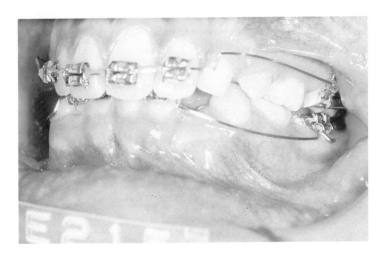

(I)

discussed in this section, as the Utility Arch is the appliance of choice to relieve major mandibular orthodontic crowding in the mixed dentition. In fact, the process even derives its name from the information made available from the type of x-ray used in the determination of "cephalometric crowding."

By determining the amount of cephalometric crowding anteriorly, one can determine if molar distalization techniques will be required posteriorly. So it must be remembered that the entire process is predicated upon arches that are not in need of major lateral development. This is always carried out prior to any other forms of treatment to relieve crowding.

Figure 7-21 continued

arches begin to develop nicely. At this point, Utility Arches may be removed in favor of more conventional Straight Wire-type methods **(M) (N) (O)** even though not all of permanent teeth have arrived yet (such as permanent cuspids). A variety of wires may be used here from braided or twisted to round. Here .016 round is used because of degree of levelness and alignment already present, a product of Utility Arches that preceded it. Once cuspids do arrive, they may be bracketed **(P) (Q) (R)** and brought into place provided not too much kink is required so as to permanently distort the somewhat rigid .016 wire, as in case of upper left cuspid. Once cuspids have been brought in and progressively heavier wire series has been gone through, case is ready for final tip, torque, and bite opening, which consists of use of conventional Class II elastics. For such purposes, rectangular arch wires are fitted with soldered posts distal to all four laterals **(S) (T) (U)** cut to the appropriate length and bent over. These serve as hooks for Class II elastics in case of upper arch wire and Pletcher springs for sake of stabilization of both arches. Class II elastics are placed **(V) (W) (X)** from Class II hooks on buccal brackets of lower first molar to hooks on maxillary arch wire distal to laterals. Using Dontrix gram gauge to measure amount of stretch supplied by any one of variety of combinations of size and/or length of elastics, force of 400 to 500 g per side is used to obtain final tip, torque, and bite opening. Pletcher springs, custom made merely for length relative to each case, are used in all four quadrants during finishing tip, torque, and bite opening procedures. In maxillary arch, they are placed with prefabricated spring-loop portion on buccal Class III hook of most distal banded maxillary molar bracket to soldered hook distal to maxillary lateral. They are placed in upper arch to help stabilize anteriors and provide protective, counteractive force to undesired vectors of Class II elastic forces on upper anteriors. In lower arch, Pletcher springs help prevent lower anterior arch from being "dumped forward" slightly as result of undesired vectors of Class II elastic forces in this region. In mandibular arch, they run from buccal Class II hooks of most distal banded mandibular molar bracket to
(*continued*)

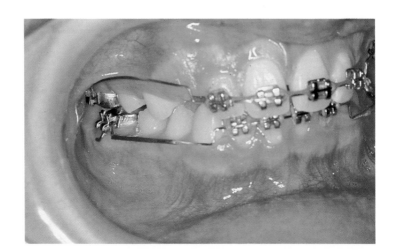

(J)

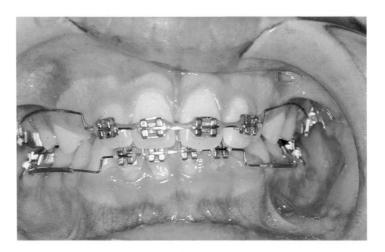

(K)

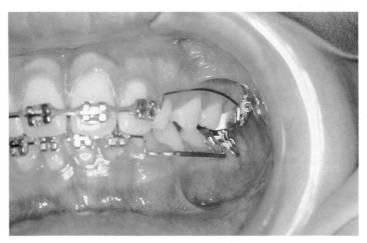

(L)

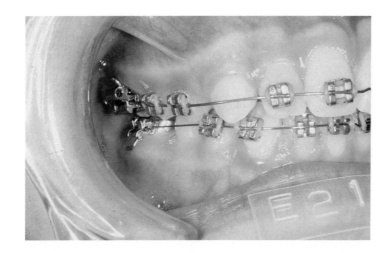

(M)

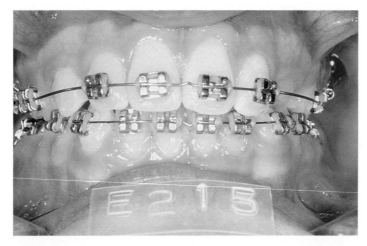

(N)

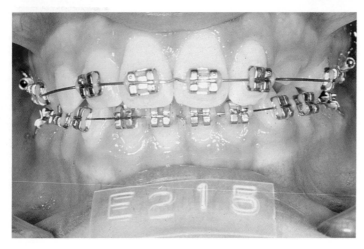

(O)

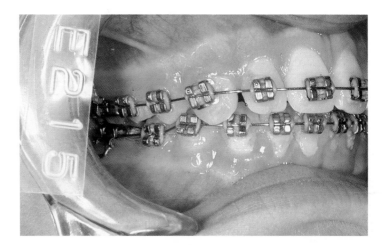

(P)

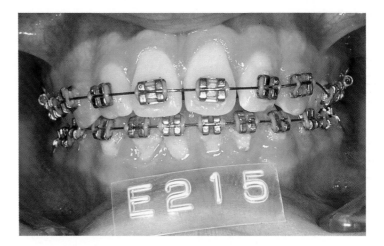

(Q)

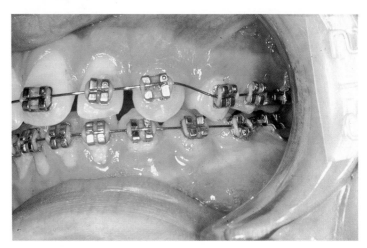

(R)

The basic truism upon which the technique is based is that for every millimeter the lower centrals are tipped forward, a full 2 millimeters of arch length is gained throughout the arch. Conversely, for every millimeter the lower central incisors are tipped lingually, a full two millimeters of arch length is used up, or will be required, throughout the arch. For example, if a lower arch exhibits 4 mm of total arch crowding, by merely torquing the lower incisors' facial surfaces 2 mm more labially, enough space will be made available throughout the arch in which to align the remaining teeth. The questions then arise as to how to measure the arch to determine the amount of crowding present (in millimeters) and once that value is known, how far does one safely advance or retract the lower incisors? And if the lowers are to be advanced to some sort of limit, how far, in fact, may they be torqued labially before molar distalization must be called upon to relieve the crowding that might still remain?

Figure 7-21 continued
soldered hook distal to lower lateral. They should exert force of 50 g per spring. This is product of their being made to customized length as per dictates of each case. They should be made 1 to 2 mm shorter than distance from their attachment at molar hook to soldered hook on arch wire. This is easily done by placing loop of prefabricated spring on molar hook and kinking free end wire at post on arch wire. Grasping kink (after removing spring from mouth) with bird beak or Jarabak-type pliers, wire arm is spun about, pliers tip in direction of spring end until newly formed anterior attachment loop is about 2 mm shorter than distance between hooks (about 2 to 3 twists). Excess free end is snipped at base of loop and the customized Pletcher spring, 2 mm shorter than distance between its attachment hooks when passive, is ready for use. Placing prefabricated end on molar bracket hook and pulling loop end up over soldered arch wire hook stretches spring just about enough to produce desired 50-g force. This process of cinching everything up a little during phase of obtaining final tip torque and bite opening is form of slight overcorrection common to most fixed-appliance-oriented regimens of treatment and is usually accomplished in 1 to 3 months. A common scenario is to employ 400 to 500 g of Class II elastics for 24 hours per day for 1 month, then 8 to 12 hours per day for 1 month. Once slight overcorrection in above manner is complete, appliances may be removed and case may be allowed to settle in. **(Y) (Z) (AA)** Final case shows excellent results. A lower 4 × 4 retainer was employed for 12 months to allow muscles to adapt to new dental environment. Upper Hawley retainer was also used. Serial cephalograms **(BB) (CC) (DD)** reveal development of case through unlocking of Class II, Division 2 malocclusion to final correction to both skeletal and dental Class I. (*Courtesy of Dr Waldemar Brehm, Encinitas, CA.*)

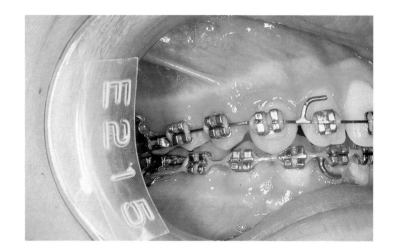

(S)

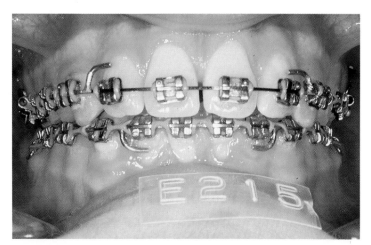

(T)

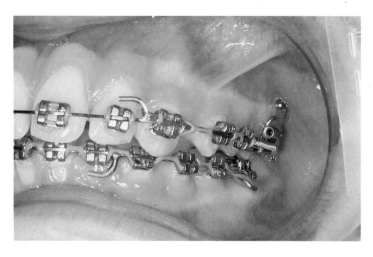

(U)

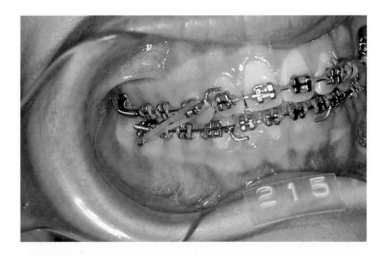

(V)

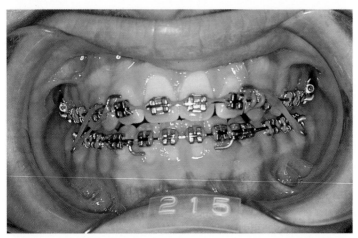

(W)

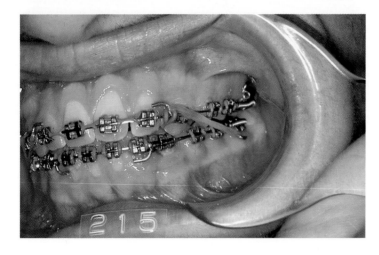

(X)

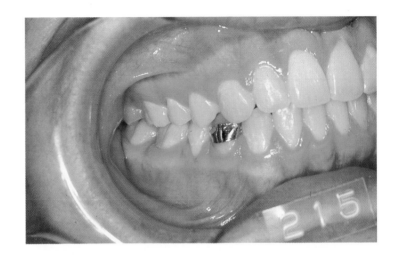

(Y)

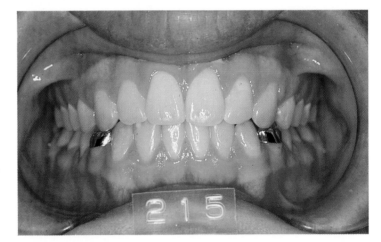

(Z)

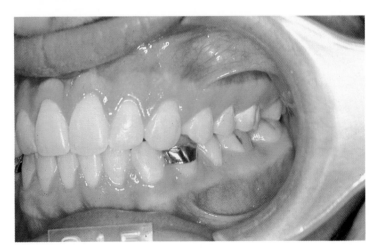

(AA)

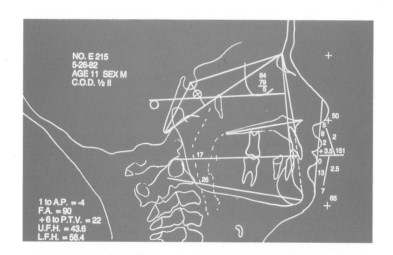

(BB)

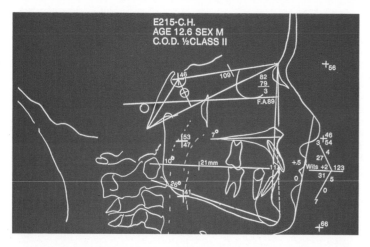

(CC)

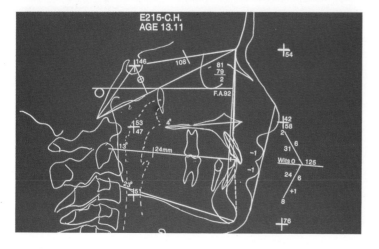

(DD)

Model Measurement in the Determination of Crowding

The process of determining the amount of crowding present in the lower arch as defined in millimeters is essentially a simple concept. Merely measure the length of the dental arch as an unbroken line over the center of the crest of the alveolar ridge. Then measure and add the sum total of the mesiodistal widths of all the adult teeth mesial to the molars, and then subtract the difference.

Alveolar Arch Length − *Mesio-Distal width Total* = crowding in millimeters

AAL − MDT = amount of crowding (mm)

It is obvious that for an arch to exhibit crowding, the result of the above equation would have to be a negative number, although it is never referred to as such. It is merely referred to as 4-mm crowding, 8-mm crowding, etc.

To determine the mesiodistal width of the adult teeth in the arch (molars are not counted), either measure them directly from a study cast, or if unerupted, use the average widths from the table below.

Mandibular cuspid...6.6
Mandibular first bicuspid...7.0
Mandibular second bicuspid...7.0

Now the summation of the mesiodistal widths of the teeth in the lower arch is easy enough, but the determination of the alveolar arch length requires a bit of poetic, or in this case, orthodontic "license." The alveolar arch length represents the length from the mesial of the one first permanent molar around the arch to the mesial of the opposite first molar. This is easily accomplished with the use of a fine jewelery chain and a somewhat discerning eye. Holding the study cast vertically with the lower incisors point down, hold the chain against the mesial of the first permanent molar and let it hang down so its path of arc travels over the centermost part of the alveolar ridge, regardless of where the incisor teeth lie, with the other end of the chain on the mesial of the other first molar. The length of the chain is adjusted manually until the crest of its arc falls directly over the crest of the ridge. This is where the diagnostician must attempt to "see through" what might be the distracting incisal edges of the lower incisors to where the center of the crest of the alveolar trough should be. The length of the chain from mesial first molar to mesial first molar in this position represents the alveolar arch length.

Once the amount of crowding in millimeters has been determined for the lower arch, the problem that then faces the clinician is how much, if any, of the crowding may be relieved by torquing the lower anteriors forward. Two cephalometric lines serve as limits against which the status of the position of the lower central incisors may be judged. They are the A-P line and the N-B line. The A-P line represents a line drawn on the lateral cephalogram from the A-point in the maxilla to the pogonion in the mandible. The N-B line represents a line drawn on the lateral cephalogram from the nasion at the bridge of the nose to the B-point in the mandible. The facial surface of the lower central incisor should lie 2 to 3 mm anterior to the A-P line, whereas it should be 4 mm anterior to the N-B line.

Now may be seen the value of these simple measurements and calculations. Remembering that for every millimeter that the central incisor's facial surface moves forward, two millimeters of total arch length is gained posteriorly; with one cephalometric x-ray tracing the practitioner immediately knows whether or not extractions will be indicated or not. For example, let us assume a given lower arch exhibits 8 mm of measured crowding. If the lower incisors prove to be 4 mm lingual to the N-B line, by moving them (usually torquing the crowns labially) 4 mm forward to the N-B line, the arch will gain a total of 8 mm, enough to relieve the crowding throughout the arch. However, if the same 8 mm of crowding is exhibited in an arch where the facial surfaces of the lower central incisors prove to be only 2 mm short of the N-B line, moving them forward the 2 mm until they are cephalometrically correct, only 4 mm of total arch length will be gained for the whole lower arch leaving the arch still in possession of 4 mm of crowding. At this point one would be remiss to overdevelop the lower anterior excessively past the generally accepted cephalometric limits. And since the case is already adequately wide enough, extra arch length cannot be gained by overexpansion laterally past Schwarz' or Pont's indices. In times past, and unfortunately too often in the present, this led the practitioner to extract bicuspids to gain the space necessary to relieve the rest of the crowding. With the application of FJO principles, extractions are likewise indicated in such circumstances, but it is not the bicuspid that is removed but rather the second molar that is merely replaced.

The Moon is a Moon still,
Whether it shine or not.

Eighteenth century proverb

Class II Incognito

Upon careful reflection, one may easily see why second molar replacement is a logical choice for such circumstances as those described above. Once the cephalometric crowding has been relieved anteriorly, remembering

Figure 7-22 **(A)** Prototype devices used to measure arch length take advantage of fine chain that may be held by gravity over crest of ridge **(B)** then measured for total linear length. This then may be compared to total of mesiodistal widths of all teeth anterior to first molars. **(C)** Modified Boley gauge with chain may be held over model then **(D)** extended to easily read total arch length.

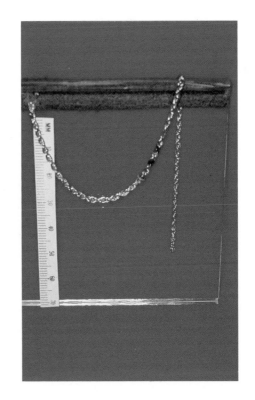

(A)

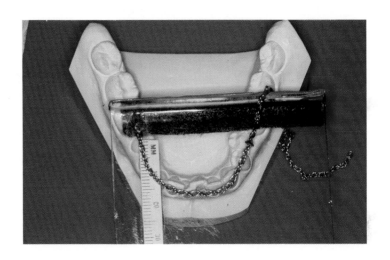

(B)

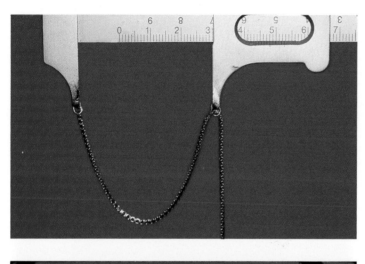

(C)

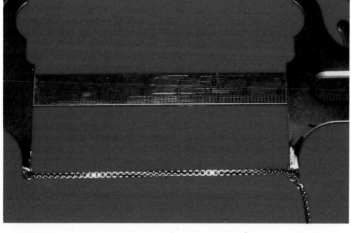

(D)

that the case is already on Schwarz' or Pont's, the only way crowding may still exist is if the cuspids, bicuspids, and first molars have drifted forward anteriorly. Once the four lower anteriors are in their cephalometrically correct positions and the arch is wide enough, they themselves cannot possibly be crowded as all rotations and angulation deficiencies have necessarily been eliminated. Therefore, any further crowding or foreshortening of the dental arch will by default have to appear in the bicuspid and cuspid area. This occurs because these teeth have drifted forward mesially. Reversing this process is the natural and correct resolution of such problems. This is predicated upon second molar removal and mandibular Sagittal I technique. This may be done with impunity even if it converts the case from a dental Class I to a dental Class II. In the age of the Bionator, once such a case has been distalized in the lower arch to dental Class II, the mandible, and its whole lower dental arch may be easily translated forward to Class I again. This is not as unusual as it may at first appear to those unfamiliar with Bionator technique. Advanced cephalometric analysis of such a case will reveal that it is one of two types. If the case proves to be skeletal Class II, the distalization of the lower molar out of dental Class I to the dental Class II relationship merely removes the "mask" from the case which at first appears Class I due to the forward drifting of the lower molars but is in reality a Class II in "dental disguise." Thus distalizing posterior quadrants to relieve the remainder of the crowding in such a lower arch obtains proper arch form and paves the way for the "arch-aligning appliance" that will necessarily follow: the Bionator.

Alternatively, the other type of cephalometric revelation that might possibly occur is that the case is not skeletal Class II, but in fact a true skeletal Class I. In this case the only way the upper molars could remain in pretreatment dental Class I, with the lower molars (and bicuspids and even cuspids) drifted forward, is for the upper posterior quadrants to be crowded forward by the same amount. Thus not only will lower Sagittal I technique be taking place in the mandible, but it will also be needed in the maxilla to the corresponding degree.

It might be thought that in the crowded mandibular arch, Sagittal II technique might serve just as well as the lower Utility Arch. Not so. The lower Sagittal II, anchoring itself against the intact second molars for its forward thrust, is excellent for torquing the four lower incisor crowns labially. It has no ability to rotate and expand molars distally, nor level, align, or rotate any of the four lower anteriors, which is often needed in cases where such teeth have been crowded in lingually.

Thus it may be seen that once cephalometric crowding has been relieved to its maximum degree anteriorly, any remaining crowding is actually posterior quadrant crowding and may be relieved by distalizing posterior quadrants with Sagittal I technique with all the amenities of second molar replacement! The upper arch will either be treated the same way or left alone and the Bionator called upon to realign the difference.

THE CONCEPT OF "SERIAL GUIDANCE"

Another interesting and exotic concept developed by Brehm and his associates is that of the principle of "serial guidance."[34] It is a theory quite different from the basic premise of the removable appliances such as the Bionator. For the functional appliances to effect their change, they guide the bones and muscles to normalcy by virtue of their inherent design characteristics, and the teeth, mere passengers in the alveolar trough, follow suit. In the concept of serial guidance, on the other hand, the principles of "guided eruption," carefully timed extractions of deciduous teeth, reliance on naturally occurring muscle function, and the space-holding properties of the Brehm Utility Arch wire combine to effect a process whereby the teeth are guided to normalcy and the bone and muscle follow suit—at least to a certain limited degree. Many times in the mixed dentition, that is all that is needed! However, this revolutionary new concept is totally predicated on proper overbite, overjet, and lip seal.

When the Utility Arch is placed in the mouth, it is activated to rotate molars distally and expand the molars laterally. Anterior teeth are leveled, aligned, rotated, and usually torqued or translated labially to some degree. As the teeth move outward in all directions from the center of the mouth, the alveolar bone follows along with it due to function on the teeth during their movement. This makes for a naturally larger dentoalveolar arch. To this is added the extra arch-enlarging stimuli of that very most powerful of muscles, the tongue. The force of the tongue is brought to bear on the alveolar process through the serial guidance of eruption of the permanent teeth. Once the roots of the permanent teeth have been determined through radiographic survey to be better than half-formed, the deciduous teeth above them are extracted,[35] an initially startling notion! However, since the Utility Arch is already present, no spaces are closed in by posterior tooth migration. Quite the contrary, the surrounding teeth are expanding out and away from the center of the mouth due to the ever-aggressive invading action of the tongue while the arch wire rests passively. This leaves the forces of the tongue in these situations to manifest themselves to their most beneficial degree. The tongue is an aggressive muscle complex that is always *hungry to occupy space*. It oftentimes will eagerly take what it can get. With the Utility Arch holding the permanent teeth to which it is attached in place like a sophisticated full-arch space maintainer, the fresh extraction sites created by the removal serially of various deciduous teeth allows a newfound space

Figure 7-23   Serial Guidance. **(A) (B)** When Utility Arches are being used they may serve as glorified space maintainers to permit earlier extraction of remaining deciduous teeth. This allows tongue to exert arch development forces on highly formative erupting teeth.

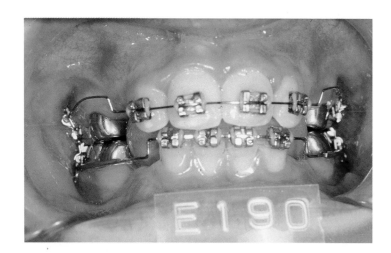

(A)

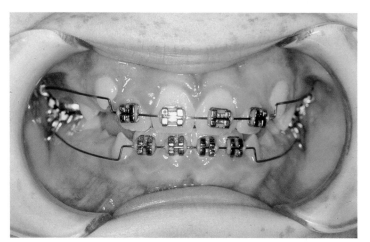

(B)

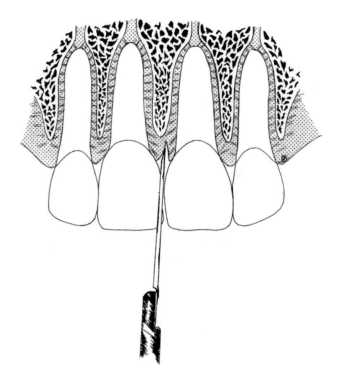

Figure 7-24 Edwards technique: the circumferential transseptal fibrotomy.

for the tongue to push itself into.[36] This, in fact, it does. And in so doing, the tongue applies a constant suboptimal force to not only the alveolar process of the extraction sites, but also to the erupting permanent teeth once they arrive. In the time before the arrival of the permanent teeth, the tongue has become well accustomed to occupying the space of the extraction sites and has begun to exert its "expanding" influences on the alveolar process of that area already by the time the permanent teeth finally erupt. A tooth is highly sensitive to forces placed on its externally during its eruption sequence[37,38] and therefore responds to the forces placed on it by the tongue in an "outward" direction as it erupts in the mouth. The bioplastic nature of the "green" alveolar bone also responds to such forces and the entire dentoalveolar arch is developed to a slightly larger size by this entire tandem process of arch wire–tongue combination. The limits of arch development by this process of mixed dentition–guided eruption seems to hover around 4 to 5 mm of lateral expansion, the generally accepted limits for lateral development in either the mixed or adult dentition for Straight Wire only. Arch width deficiencies greater than that should be corrected first on a more orthopedic basis by the old standby arch-widening appliances designed specifically for that purpose such as the Schwarz plate.

Summary

If a single word were to be selected to describe the characteristics and position of the Utility Arch in the broad field of orthodontics or the more restrictive field of mixed dentition orthodontics, it would have to be versatility. The Utility Arch allows the clinician to divorce himself from the services of the orthodontically less specific active plates when such would be only the second appliance of choice in the treatment of mixed dentition malocclusions. Sometimes the removable appliances are the primary indicated treatment devices of choice by virtue of the specific needs of the patient coinciding exactly with what the removable appliances have to offer. Yet, at other times the demands of a case are for a more exacting and dentally individualized form of treatment, one which demands what the Utility Arch in turn has to offer. By means of its ability to rotate molars distally and advance occlusions to a certain degree from mild or a one-half Class II to a Class I relationship, the Utility Arch also frees the practitioner from "forcing the case with a Bionator" to correct mild Class II problems when in fact the case might already be in a skeletal Class I with a mere one-half Class II dental relationship. Thus it is an appliance and technique that fits in perfectly well with the other appliances and techniques of the FJO System. It allows one more instance where the best possible form of treatment is made available for the patient's sake in answering the ever-present therapeutic question, "What are the patient's needs?" The FJO system is not married to a given appliance or technique, but rather is dedicated to employing whatever is necessary to assure the best possible results of balanced temporomandibular joints, balanced faces, and balanced stable functional occlusions.

EDWARDS TECHNIQUE

At this final stage of treatment one may wish to employ the pericoronal transeptal fibrotomy or Edwards technique. The transeptal fibers of the pericoronal gingiva have an exceedingly long elastic memory, especially about rotation. Often teeth that have been given any sort of orthodontic rotation whatsoever would benefit from the extra help that might come from the Edwards technique.[39-50] Local or intra-ligamentary anesthesia is at first administered and then a No. 11 scapel blade is inserted into the depth of the gingival sulcus and the transeptal fibers are carefully sectioned circularly around the gingival sulcus of the tooth with care being exercised so as not to press the sharp tip of the blade so far into the depth of the sulcus as to possibly snap off a tip of the blade. An excellent modification of this technique is to leave a small portion of the labial sulcus uncut. It is felt that this avoids the possible development of Stillman's clefts on the facial surfaces of the ginviva. This is referred to as a modified Edwards procedure. The transeptal fibers soon reattach in a healthy mouth, but with their elastic memory put into permanent "'surgical amnesia,'" the chances for relapse of the tooth to its former rotated position are minimal. Every little bit helps.

Bracket Removal and Retention

Once the case is complete and the rectangular wire, most commonly a .018 × .025, has had its full way for at least several months with the bracket slots giving the case its final torque, the bands and brackets may be removed and impressions made for final retainers. Many clinicians feel that cases in which second molars have been removed will be so stable by the time the tandem treatment of active plate/functional appliance/Straight Wire is complete that no retainers will be necessary. However, whenever any rotations of more than the slightest amount are present in the case prior to treatment or if there has been a moderate to considerable amount of tooth movement by the Straight Wire component of the regimen late in the treatment time-line, it is wise to seriously consider active retention as a safeguard against any posttreatment minor tooth movements that would be considered more than just the normally acceptable "settling in" of the case. A simple rule of thumb is: "Rotations require retention."

Removing bonded brackets requires the use of either the Unitek or Ortho Organizers bracket-removing pliers. The cutting edges of the Unitek are placed at the mesial and distal edges of the bracket base and the pliers

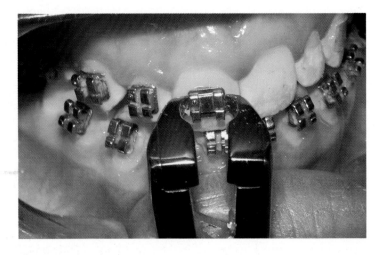

(A)

Figure 7-25 Bracket removal. **(A)** Placing beaks of pliers at interface between bracket base and enamel surface, pliers handles are gently squeezed together, pliers beaks are driven under bracket base, and **(B)** bracket snaps off. **(C)** Once removed, excess composite may be removed either with fine finishing burs (type that cut composite but not enamel) and light pressure or **(D)** conventional discs used to trim and polish composite material as per standard composite technique. (Note: take care to avoid generation of heat during composite reduction with either burs or discs, as this may damage pulp.)

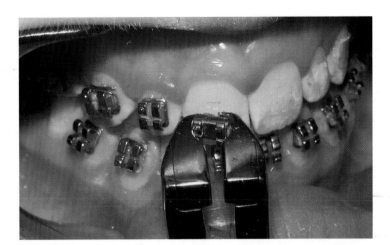

(B)

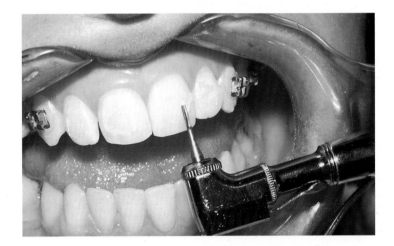

(C)

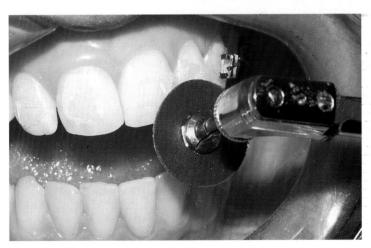

(D)

is squeezed firmly but gently until the bracket pops off. Covering it with the fingertip of the free hand prevents the bracket from becoming lost.

Removing posterior bands may be done with posterior band-removing pliers or common crown pullers. When using the common crown pullers, place the notched end of the shaft over the gingival lip of the buccal tube and give the weight a stroke to the end and the band usually comes nearly completely off the first time. Disks of the garnet variety or high-speed finishing burs that will remove composite but not cut enamel may be used to get rid of excess and leftover bonding material similar to removal of "flash" in common Class III and V operative techniques involving composite restorative materials.

SIMPLE RETENTION APPLIANCES

As the art of moving teeth became more sophisticated with the advent of the fixed appliances of E. H. Angle, it became increasingly obvious that after the method of moving teeth had been completed, a method had to be employed that would keep them there once all fixed appliances were removed.[51-55] This post–fixed appliance area of treatment soon became the standard domain of the retentive devices introduced during the World War I era by C. A. Hawley.[56-58] They have been among the most widely used retentive appliances for nearly half a century. They are simple to construct, moderate of design, moderate of cost, moderate in appearance, and unfortunately also only moderate in efficiency. The acrylic palate on the upper

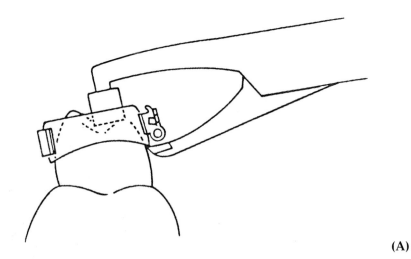

(A)

Figure 7-26 (A) Posterior bands may be removed with conventional band-removing pliers or **(B) (C)** by use of common crown pullers, placing working end of crown-puller tip over buccal molar band bracket.

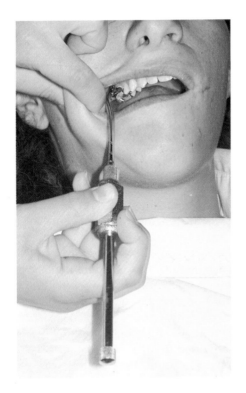

(B)

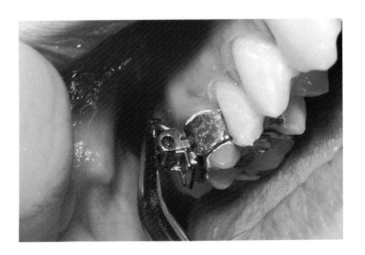

(C)

is effective in holding arch form, but the single bare wire running across the labial surface of the maxillary anteriors is less than noteworthy at holding rotations.

The spring-retainer represents a vast improvement over the standard Hawley in that an acrylic band is used to increase holding power fortified by a loop of wire formed to encircle the six anteriors. This acrylic and wire band is fashioned to come in close proximity to both the labial and lingual surfaces of the anterior teeth, either upper or lower. The wire loop that rises up over the distal contacts of the cuspids to complete its circular path is enveloped with a clear band of acrylic processed directly against a model of the teeth themselves approximately half as wide as the facial surfaces of the anterior teeth, a little less so lingually. Thus if a tooth wishes to rotate back to its pretreatment position, or drift in any direction for that matter, it feels the opposing forces of the broad surface area of contact of the acrylic that fits flush against its facial and lingual surfaces. The retentive force of the surface area of contact of the acrylic band is intensified by the springiness of the wire loop where the wire crosses over the distal contact of the cuspids labial to lingual. This is where tension may be increased by discreet adjustments of the bend in the wire with appropriate pliers. Teeth slightly out of position may be moved into ideal position (tipped actually) and even rotated slightly, provided space exists for them to be moved into, by processing the retainer on a model where the teeth have been sliced off and repositioned to ideal "setups" in wax. The addition of a small isthmus of two wires to connect this circular wire and acrylic affair to a standard Hawley palate gives the clinician the "best of both worlds": palate-holding/arch-holding acrylic for retention of arch form, and the more precise broad surface area contact tooth-holding effects of a wire-fortified processed acrylic labiolingual band. Extensions may be added to the lowers to aid in the stability of their being worn in the mouth.

Figure 7-27   Full-tooth surface contact retention (the Tru-tain). **(A)** Upper and lower case models with properly trimmed Tru-tain retainers in place. **(B)** Upper and lower retainers trimmed in conventional manner. **(C)** Retainers in place in mouth: Note how much more esthetic these retainers are than conventional Hawley type **(D)**. **(E)** Upper case model properly trimmed on model trimmer to facilitate correct vacuum forming of conventional upper retainer. Note thinness of plaster base. **(F)** Model for use in construction of retainer to be used after correction of Division 2-type problems where possible lingual relapse of upper anteriors is to be resisted. Trimming of retainer to leave palatal portion intact aids in resisting arch collapse. Even though palatal portion is not trimmed off model as in **(E)**, it is still left as thin as possible to aid in vacuum forming. Similar designs are used to reinforce retention in cases that have had any form of lateral development.

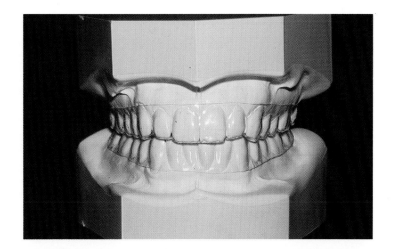

(A)

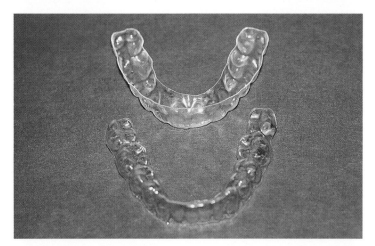

(B)

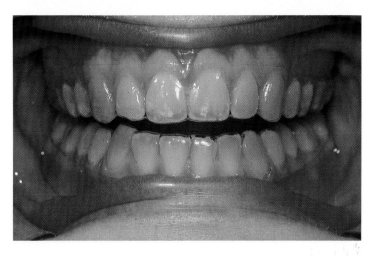

(C)

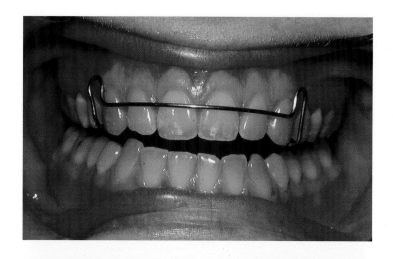

(D)

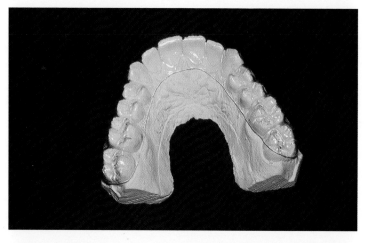

(E)

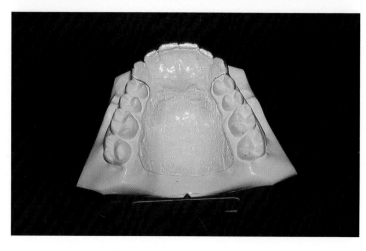

(F)

Most retention regimens, following fixed appliance usage (especially those involving the correction of that old orthodontic thorn, rotations), involve a standard 6-month active/6-month passive–type program, subject of course to individual variations and needs. "Active" means nearly 24 hours per day wear, and "passive" implies night wear only.

"Things well-fitted abide."

Jacula Prudentum
G. Herbert, Ed., 1651

FULL-TOOTH SURFACE CONTACT RETENTION: THE "TRU-TAIN"

The advent of the spring-retainer represented a great improvement in retention appliances over the old Hawley type. The secret was in the greatly increased surface area of contact of the directly processed acrylic "band" with the facial and lingual enamel surfaces of the anterior teeth. This provided much more force per area of contact for retentive purposes over the naked wire of the Hawley. The addition of the spring-type tension of the wire loop of the spring-retainer proved extremely advantageous in keeping teeth in place, especially rotations. However, in practical applications the spring-retainer by virtue of this very same acrylic and wire band is also a bit unsightly, as the rather obvious tract of acrylic running across the anterior teeth is quite noticeable to the eye. Recently a new type of retainer has been developed with the advantage of providing even greater surface area of contact between the teeth and the appliance. It also appears to be the all-time hands-down winner as far as esthetics is concerned, since from a distance of more than 2 ft it is for all intents and purposes completely invisible. This new "superretainer" is the vacuum-formed clear plastic, ultrathin, full-tooth surface contact elastic retainer developed by Dr Lloyd Truax of Rochester, Minnesota.[59]

As one of the founding fathers of the Orthodontic Department at the Dental School of the Mayo Clinic, Dr Truax was well familiar with the problems of keeping teeth in place with conventional retainers once fixed appliances were removed, especially those teeth that had been either greatly translated and/or rotated. The fact that this was in the "pre-second molar replacement era" also made the need for suitable retentive appliances paramount. Over about a 3-year period in the early 1970s, taking a cue from the original designs of Nahoum, Dr Truax developed an appliance that offers the maximum tooth surface retentive contact. This appliance also has the qualities of durability, minimal size, extremely high levels of comfort and esthetic appearance, and is constructed out of a hypoallergenic, economical material that is incredibly easy to work with. The plastic is a crystal-clear, polychloro-based polymer that is initially produced in thin sheets that appear similar to the material used for little toy windows in children's dollhouses. The material is heated to a pliable, soft consistency in vacuum-formers especially designed for this process. It is then vacuum-formed down over a plaster model of a maxillary or mandibular arch. (The models are poured up without bases to aid in the vacuum-forming of the plastic over the stone model.) Once formed, the plastic takes on the most astounding properties. It remains crystal-clear, rigid enough to provide firm retention, and yet flexible enough that the appliance can be easily bent or twisted without breaking. Its elastic memory is superb and it will quickly regain its vacuum-formed shape. Since the term "full-tooth surface contact clear plastic retainer" is impractical, these types of devices are simply referred to among members of the profession by their brand name "Tru-Tain." They may be quickly and easily constructed as follows:

Impressions are poured up with stone and without a base (both maxillary mandibular). A U-shaped model is preferred so the plastic can be properly vacuumed down more easily over the model.

The Sta-Vac heater, the only type that may be used in this process other than the Pro-form, is turned on to heat (five to six minutes) while the bottom or gingival portion of the model is leveled on the cast trimmer.

Place the plastic in the heater frame and heat 1.5 to two minutes. The plastic is pliable to the touch, and little bubbles will just start to form in the plastic. These are a result of trace amounts of chlorine that are released by heating the polychloro-based polymer plastic. It is very important to heat the plastic in the machine properly, or it will not form correctly over the model. Overheating the plastic (until the plastic sags below the frame) will result in a retainer that is too thin and may have creases.

The vacuum motor must be turned on first, then the heater frame with the plastic may be brought down over the model. The vacuum is left on until the plastic is closely adapted to the model (about 5 seconds).

The excess plastic may be trimmed from around the edges of the model with a large scissors.

A scalpel is used to trim the plastic from 1.5 to 2.0 mm below the gingival crest all around the labial, buccal, and lingual of the model.

A How pliers may then be used to pull the excess trimmed plastic from the model. The model is saved, usually by the patient, for possible future use should the appliance become lost or otherwise need replacing. Should such an occasion arise, the patient need only bring in the original model, and a new retainer may be constructed in approximately five to seven minutes!

Remove the retainer from the model and trim it more with a crown and bridge scissors. It is not necessary to buff the edge of this material. In fact, buffing will make it ragged. Edges are made smooth simply by cutting them evenly with the scissors. Once the edges are cut smooth to desired length, the retainer is finished and ready to place. The plastic is clear, thin, resilient, and very tough. Minor movements of teeth can even be made by altering positions of teeth on the model before vacuum-forming the plastic. The thinness of the plastic allows for flexibility, resiliency, and stability without excessive rigidity.

What is possibly most astounding about these little retainers is the regimen under which the patient wears them.

1. *Placing the retainer for a growing child.* After bands and/or brackets have been removed and the retainer constructed, have the child place the retainer night and day for three days, removing it only to eat and brush. Then have the child wear his retainer every night for 6 months (active phase). If need be, retention may be discontinued gradually, ie, twice a week for 6 months, once a week for 6 months, then discontinued completely (active phase). If along the way the retainer becomes tight, the patient may have to back up a step and place it once again every other night or every night again until stability appears to have been achieved. Of course, second molar replacement techniques *greatly* facilitate retention stability.

2. *Placing the retainer for an adult.* Instruct the adult patient to place his retainer night and day for three days, then every night for 12 straight months. Then proceed to the passive stage of retention following a regimen that is the same as for a growing child.

3. *Placing the retainer after repositioning teeth.* To help the retainer move a tooth that has been slightly repositioned on the model prior to vacuum-forming, place the retainer night and day for 2 months removing only to eat and brush, then nights only for 6 months, then as per above instructions.

The patient may be checked at 6-month intervals. If there are holes worn in the occlusal surface, the retainer is fine; but if it has started to crack up the sides, a new retainer is indicated. Some patients are reported to have had the same retainers 4 to 5 years and never need a new one. On the average one retainer should last through the course of the retentive period. Instruct patients to brush their retainers at least once a day with toothpaste or soap, or some sort of effervescent soaking-type denture cleaner. They should never run the retainer under hot water, but use room temperature or cool water as the material is thermoplastic. At the checking appointments, these retainers may be cleaned in an ultrasonic device that will restore them to nearly new condition. As a result of the above, the retainers are extremely popular with both patient and doctor alike. The days of the far less esthetic, less efficient, less economical, bulky acrylic and wire retention devices appear to be numbered.

"Thus at the flaming forge of Life,
Our fortunes must be wrought,
Thus on its sounding anvil shaped,
Each burning deed and thought."

"The Village Blacksmith"
Henry Wadsworth Longfellow
1807–1882

ARMAMENTARIUM

Nationally known orthodontic supply houses and manufacturing companies all have highly trained representatives located throughout the country available either by phone or in person to assist the clinician in filling his professional needs relative to his orthodontic armamentarium. There are essentially three areas of materials utilized: arch wires, brackets and bands, and the hand instruments to get the appliances on and off (sometimes referred to as a support system). One may want to add to this a miscellaneous fourth category of force systems such as rubber elastics, springs, wires, etc. These all act to add extra forces in one direction or another to the bracketed teeth.

Most companies have arch wires available in kits with their own holders or will assist the doctor in ordering wires in individual packets, usually of 50. Arch wire–holders are very handy as a way of storing and organizing the many various types of arch wires a practitioner may accumulate.

The same is true of bands and brackets. Most major companies have package deals available which include all the various sized bands and the one-size-fits-all brackets sufficient for a specified number of cases available with their own organized storage cases which again are extremely handy. The initial cost of such kits is usually substantial, not because of the number of brackets, but because of the number of bracketed bands that must be made available. Direct bonded brackets fit any size tooth, but unless the clinician wishes to use direct bond brackets on all molars (a situation not wholly advisable for durability reasons) a large number of molar bands with brackets processed on them of a variety of sizes must be kept on hand to fit the various sizes of molars an individual case may present. A kit with enough direct bond brackets for ten cases will by necessity have to have far more than 40 molar banded brackets. The kits usually come with an average assortment of molar bands for both right and left, upper and lower, with greater numbers of the more common sizes most often used.

Of course, individual cases may be done by sending accurate models to professional orthodontic laboratories for band selection and bracket setup. The laboratories will even include the necessary arch wires needed to complete the entire case. But for the practitioner doing a large number of cases, this is a little less economical both financially and timewise.

As supplies of arch wires and brackets and bands are diminished, they may be replenished by ordering the specific replacements for those which have been used. Hence, though the initial investment for this particular section of the armamentarium is high, maintenance of the components becomes more economically feasible.

One thing about which there can be no dispute is the types of hand instruments needed to support the work done on the appliances. A clinician may or may not have an adequate stock of bands and brackets on hand, but there is no substitute for having the right hand instruments for the right job available when needed. At first the number of instruments necessary may seem extensive but in actuality it is not. Like a set of golf clubs, once around the course and it will be obvious why each one is needed and what its specific design capabilities are. The following is a description of the minimum number of instruments needed to attach and adjust Straight Wire appliances.

Direct bond bracket-holder. This is a handy little reverse-action tweezers which has beaks designed and serrated specifically for holding brackets of any size for direct bonding techniques. This allows the operator to place the beaks of the tweezers on the bracket and merely hold the tweezers while placing the bracket without having to squeeze it at the same time as the spring tension of the tweezers holds the bracket firmly in the beaks. Once positioned on the tooth correctly with the bonding material in place, squeezing the tweezers releases the bracket. This type is useful on anterior teeth but difficult to use on posteriors.

Posterior direct bond bracket-holder. This bracket-holder is a spring-loaded affair that distantly resembles a form of Cavitron tip. It is offset 90 degrees and has a small head and small serrated tips to allow a better field of vision for direct bonding of posterior teeth.

Band-biter. This is a little plastic handled instrument that has a hardened stainless steel little square peg projecting from the end of it at a 90-degree angle. The handle serves as a bite stick. As the band is put to place with the cement, the corner of the square peg is placed over a section of the occlusal surface of the band offering resistance to proper seating and the patient is instructed to slowly bite on the instrument, which helps seat the band in a tight spot correctly. They are not absolutely necessary, but they are so inexpensive that they are certainly worth having in the orthodontic kit.

Schure band-seater. Another band-seating instrument is the Schure bandseater. It has one end with an offset and highly serrated tip for engaging bands by direct friction. This end resembles the common 3/4 amalgam plugger, but the serrations are much coarser and extend on all four sides of the working end up to the straight shaft. The other end has a heavy-duty scalertype tip handy for the removal of excess cement.

Ligature director. This little instrument is used to help place wire ligatures around brackets. One end is an offset hatchet-shaped working end with a small notch in the blade and the other end is a straight shaft with a notch. These are handy for tucking the cut twisted ends of wire ligatures under the tie wings of the brackets and keeping them out of the way for the sake of the patient's comfort.

Elastic removers. These are similar to common explorers and therefore not really necessary. Though they work well, so do the common explorers.

Mathieu needle-holder. There are two types of these forceps, and both are extremely valuable to the operator. Borrowed from the field of surgery, the Mathieu needle-holder has the standard needle-holder working end, but the handles are pear-shaped and meet at their ends, which have positive locking ratchet-type ends. When gently squeezed together in the palm of the hand, the spring in the handles allows the individual locking serrated ends to engage, thus holding the instrument closed. Squeezing it further pushes these ratchet handle ends past their point of engagement and they unlock from each other and the device springs open. This allows instant opening and closing without the awkward action of putting the operator's fingers through the rings of the ends of common needle-holders. There are two sizes of Mathieu needle-holders. The larger standard size has the conventional heavy-duty beaks that are handy for placing brass separating wires. The smaller-sized instrument has a notched tip with a tiny bird beak 90-degree offset tongue-and-groove beak that is extremely handy for grasping and placing elastic ligatures. (A similar working end arrangement is available in a tempered notched mosquito forceps for those who prefer standard thumb and finger ring handles.)

Anterior band remover. This pliers has a broad flat beak with a transverse groove on the edge opposing a longer tipped beak with a rubber cap on it. The rubber capped base beak is placed against the incisal edge of an anterior tooth while the grooved beak is engaged against the gingival edge of the band. The rubber cap protects the incisal edge of the tooth while the operator squeezes the handles of the pliers, putting the dislodging force to the band. It is also used by some in a similar manner to remove bonded brackets. But this techique may be a little jolting to the patient as the bracket is snapped off the surface of the tooth extremely securely. When the bracket is snapped free, it is driven into the rubber guard of the pliers which chews up the guard after a short time. Cut-off ends of plastic saliva ejectors may be used as an easy and economical replacement to the rubber protective cap (certain size ejectors only).

Direct bonded bracket-removing pliers. A slightly gentler way of removing direct bonded brackets is with the more efficient direct bonded bracket-removing pliers. The beaks are offset at 60 degrees to allow easy access to both anterior and posterior brackets. The "cutting" edge of each beak is placed on either side of the bracket at the base where the composite bonds it to the tooth and it is firmly but gently squeezed by the operator until the bracket pops off.

Posterior band-removing pliers. This pliers has a purchase end for engaging the gingival portion of the band and a bracing beak offset at 90 degrees with a protective nylon cushion tip, which is placed against the occlusal surface of the tooth. Replacement nylon tips are available. Quite frankly, a common sliding lug crown puller also works quite well in these instances. The notched end of the crown puller may be placed over the buccal tube of the band and gentle tapping usually removes the band easily.

How pliers. Either a How or a Weingardt pliers should be available in every rack for the purposes of grasping arch wires, for insertion of same into posterior buccal tubes, or for grasping the buccal tubes of posterior bands themselves for adjustment of the freshly seated band to the proper angulation before the cement dries. The How pliers has two little serrated pancakelike projections at the ends of straight tubular arms, ideal for grasping. A variation of this pliers is to have the arms offset halfway down their length, but the standard How pliers usually is sufficient.

Weingardt pliers. This is an all-purpose utility pliers with beaks that are offset in a gentle curve. It is very handy for inserting arch wires into buccal tubes and, again, for adjusting bands by grasping them by the buccal tubes before the cement hardens.

Distal end cutter. One of the most important instruments in the clinician's armamentarium, the distal end-cutting pliers, is a prerequisite for cutting arch wires that are already ligated to place intraorally. Its purpose is to cut the protruding excess wire sticking out the distal end of the buccal tube of the last banded molar flush with the end of that tube so that no projection of wire is left to irritate buccal tissues. But more importantly, this pliers has an ingenious little wire spring bar built into it that rides firmly just past the cutting end of one of the beaks. The cutting edges are offset at almost 90 degrees, and when the operator places the beaks flush against the distal end of the buccal tube and cuts the wire, the wire spring bar presses the free cut end of the arch wire firmly against a special flat surface of the opposing beak, thus preventing the scrap piece from flying into the tissue, or worse, down the patient's trachea! A masterpiece of cleverness in design, it is a must for all operators. It comes in a regular and small size. It is touted that the smaller pliers makes working in more compact areas of smaller mouths more accessible, but frankly, the standard pliers is plenty small enough for almost every situation, and having two would most likely prove redundant.

Wire cutters. Wire cutters are another story. There are two basic types. The first is a pin and ligature cutter. These pliers have fine beaks that are ideal for cutting wire ligatures that have been placed on brackets or small arch wires up to the .016 round. Do not try cutting anything larger with these fine pliers, especially the .018 × .025 rectangular. If attempted, it will only score the cutting edge of the pliers or ruin it altogether. This is where the second, heavy wire cutter comes into play. It is truly best to have one of each. Never try to force an instrument to do a job for which it was not designed. It usually winds up making twice the work plus the added expense of replacing original equipment.

Ribbon arch pliers. The ribbon arch pliers is used as a small hand vise with which to grasp rectangular arch wires. The opposing edges of the beaks are milled flat with radii on the edges to guard against scoring or marring the wire. These pliers are handy for putting accentuated recurve bends in rectangular arch wires in more advanced techniques as well as anti-torquing wires that have been so shaped. The width of the working surfaces is .060.

Hollow chop pliers. This pliers is used to form arch wires. It has a smooth rounded broad beak that fits into a flush fitting trough on the other beak. It can also be used to put recurve bends in round arch wires.

Three-prong clasp-adjusting pliers. This pliers is essential for the adjustment of labial bows and clasps on functional appliances and active plates, but it also has a variety of miscellaneous uses in Straight Wire technique for which it may be occasionally called upon.

Jarabak pliers. The Jarabak pliers has a fine round beak against a rounded flat. The fineness of the two ends is ideal for precise bending of small light wire, eg, the formation of attachment loops on the free ends of Pletcher springs.

Band-crimping pliers. These little pliers are helpful in reforming and crimping the edges of bands to assist in their adaption to the tooth.

Band-slitting pliers. This pliers is designed with specially hardened flush cutting edges for the purpose of cutting loose upper and lower bands with minimum trauma to the patient. It represents an alternative to pulling tight bands off in one piece with either a band-removing pliers or crown puller. Their availability is not absolutely essential, but they do offer the option of a different method of band removal.

Stop pliers. This pliers has a V-shaped notched pair of working beaks, which when placed over an arch wire and crimped down, form a 1-mm peak in the wire, which acts as a stop to prevent the wire from sliding through the bracket slot past that point (or conversely keeps the bracket and its tooth from sliding down the arch wire past that point).

Occulist pliers. Occulist pliers come in two sizes and are used primarily for adjusting the Crozat appliance. They can also be used for adjusting clasps and wires on active plates.

Brehm utility arch wire pliers. These pliers are used to construct the Brehm utility arch wires. The notch and groove arrangement is used to crimp the adjustable sleeve of the preformed Brehm utility arch wire.

Pliers rack. These simple white plastic containers are very helpful in providing a neat, compact, organized place to keep the various pliers necessary and readily accessible. They also have a drawerlike compartment for containing the various hand instruments that are used exclusively during Straight Wire techniques.

Figure 7-28 **(A)** Direct bond bracket-holder. **(B)** Posterior direct bond bracket-holder. **(C)** Band-biter. **(D)** Schure bind-seater. **(E)** Ligature director. **(F)** Elastic removers. **(G)** Mathieu needle-holder. **(H)** Anterior band remover. **(I)** Direct bonded bracket-removing pliers. **(J)** Posterior band-removing pliers. **(K)** How pliers. **(L)** Weingardt pliers. **(M)** Distal end cutter. **(N)** Wire cutters. **(O)** Ribbon arch pliers. **(P)** Hollow chop pliers. **(Q)** Three-prong clasp-adjusting pliers. **(R)** Jarabak pliers. **(S)** Band-crimping pliers. **(T)** Band-slitting pliers. **(U)** Stop pliers. **(V)** Occulist pliers. **(W)** Brehm utility arch wire pliers. **(X)** Pliers rack. (*Courtesy of European Orthodontic Products, St Paul, MN.*)

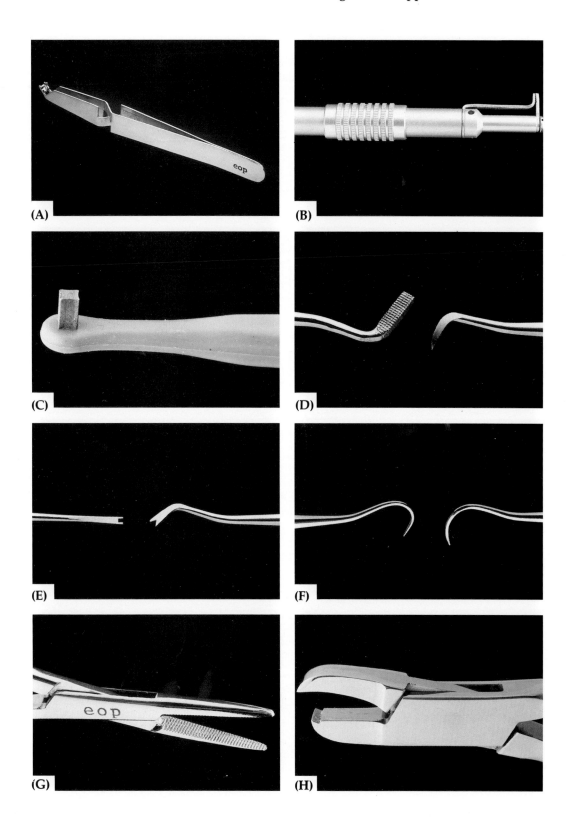

(A)

(B)

(C)

(D)

(E)

(F)

(G)

(H)

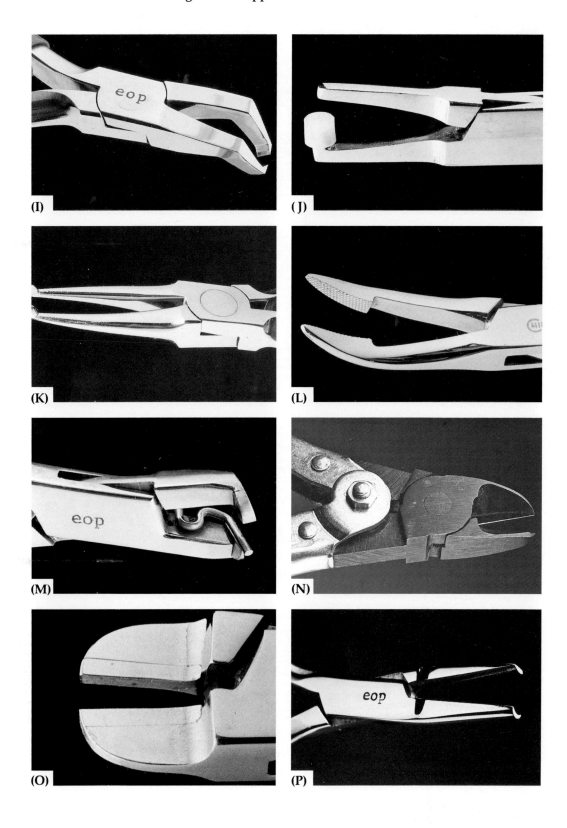

(I)

(J)

(K)

(L)

(M)

(N)

(O)

(P)

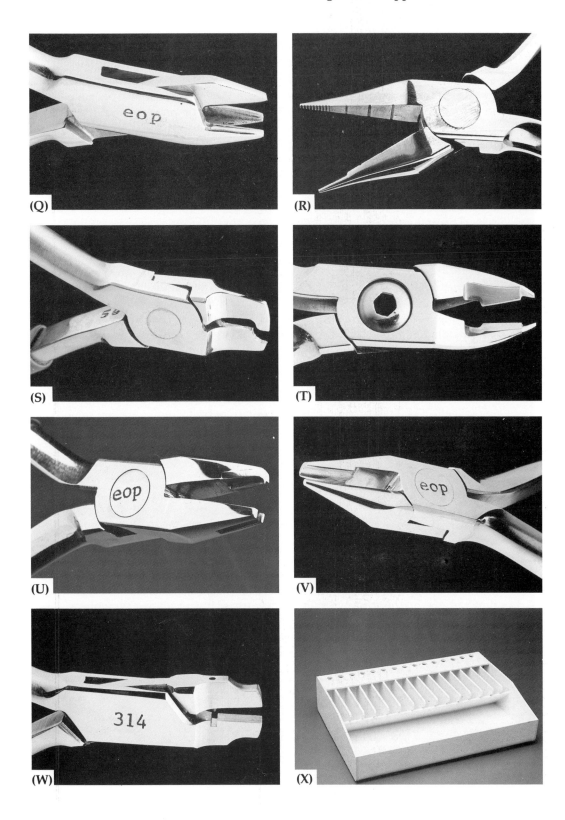

(Q)

(R)

(S)

(T)

(U)

(V)

(W)

(X)

Other various forms of paraphernalia also accompany every rack of arch wires and hand instruments in the Straight Wire armamentarium. These are the force systems, which provide external forces of one sort or another to assist in the movement and rotation of teeth. The primary source of energy in the appliance is, of course, the arch wire itself. But supplemental forces may be added to speed up a particular type of movement desired on an individual tooth or group of teeth.

Separators

The first group of extras are the separators. Before a case can even be "strapped up" in a Straight Wire appliance, the posterior teeth must be separated to allow the proper seating and cementation of the molar bands. The importance of separation of teeth prior to banding has always been recognized and was noted even as far back as Angle himself, who wrote of it in 1907. His method, which might still be the best to this day, consists of passing a brass ligature wire under the contact point of the two teeth to be separated and passing it over the occlusal surface of the marginal ridges where the two ends are twisted together about as tightly as the patient will reasonably tolerate. Angle also stated that sufficient space will occur as a result of the pressures generated by the interproximally tightened wires in a matter of a few hours. This is true. Brass ligatures so placed in the morning will effect enough separation of the teeth to permit banding by that same afternoon. These types of wire ligatures will open the contact on the average 0.01 inch, as described by Hoffman. This is twice the thickness of the metal of the molar band. Some practitioners feel the teeth are too sensitive to permit a comfortable banding session for the patient after they have worn the brass separators for only one day. But in Straight Wire technique, one is only banding the molars, not every tooth in the arch. Also, if the second molars have been removed, there is little difficulty in separating the solitary first molars enough to prevent banding that same day. If the separating ligatures are to be left on for more than a day for some reason, the operator should make sure the twisted cut ends are bent and tucked in the interproximal space in a manner so as to avoid possible tissue irritation. Upon removal, the operator untwists the ends with a How or similar type pliers, separates the ends, and cuts the end beneath the contact with a pin and ligature cutter. Care must be taken as to where the cut, free end wire piece will go. Placing the index fnger of the free hand over the piece as it is cut usually controls it nicely. Grasping the occlusal portion of the wire with again a How, Weingardt, or similar pliers, roll the ligature out of the interproximal space.

These types of brass separators are available in diameters 0.020 for use in the anterior region and 0.025 for use in the bicuspid and molar region. They come ring-shaped with one end flattened to facilitate slipping them easily under the contact. They are easy to see and manipulate by the clinician and difficult, if not impossible, for the patient to dislodge or lose. They accomplish all the separation they will ever obtain in about the first 24 hours, then simply maintain the space from then on. About their only drawbacks would be either the irritation of the soft tissure caused by the cut twisted ends, which can be easily prevented by proper installation, or their potential for poor hygiene maintenance. But considering the relatively short time they are in place, this becomes a moot point.

Elastic separators have also been devised that work well. The ring type looks like an oversized bracket elastic. A special elastic separator forceps has been designed to hold and spread the elastic "doughnut" taut so it may be snapped through the contact. As the elastic gradually constricts, it forces the teeth apart. Again, about 0.01 inch is opened up between the teeth in the first 24 hours. But unlike the brass separators, the elastic rings keep on separating the teeth at a somewhat reduced rate until they have moved the teeth so far apart they may be easily slipped out. But elastic separators tend to cause the teeth to become a bit more sensitive during separation than do brass ligatures, and the possibility exists of the separation occurring to such an extent that the elastic may become lost or even slip into the subgingival space of the interdental col area. If left undetected because the clinician considered it lost, the hiding elastic would act as a foreign body and cause obvious periodontal problems.

After several days of wear, any sensitivity of teeth that might exist due to separation will disappear regardless of the type of separators used. Separation should always be sufficient enough to allow reasonably unrestricted seating of bands. If a certain contact remains inadequately opened, the operator might be fooled into thinking the band fits tightly enough when in fact it does not. An inadequate interproximal opening causes the operator to use extra pressures to force the band through the tight contact. This increases the chances of problems relative to the patient's comfort and safety. A band should be tight on a tooth due to closeness of fit, not tightness of contact.

Rotation Wedges

Rotating teeth used to be one of the more frustrating and time consuming procedures in orthodontics. Now things are easier. The rotation wedge, used in conjunction with Straight Wire mechanics, makes rotating teeth a predictable and easily controlled process. There are two basic types of wedges. Both work equally well. The first is a single small bracket-sized barrel-shaped object made of rubber with a small rectangular flange on it running along its long axis. This flange has two square holes in it. These holes correspond to the tie wings on the bracket to which the wedge is attached. These rubber-type rotation wedges are placed on the brackets of teeth to be rotated *before* the arch wire is ligated to place. Grasping the main body of the wedge with the tips of a fine Mathieu needle-holder with the flange free, the operator engages the holes of the flange on the tie wings of the bracket such that the barrel of the wedge is parallel to the interproximal line angle. The wedge is always placed on either the mesial or distal tie wing relative to the direction of rotation desired. If the tooth is to be rotated in a mesial direction, the wedge is placed on the mesial tie wing. If the tooth is to be rotated in a distal direction, the wedge is placed on the distal tie wing. The wedge also possesses an inside and outside surface. The outside surface has two tiny projections on the barrel that are placed over one another vertically and act as guides for the arch wire. They help stabilize the wedge between the tooth and the arch wire and keep the arch wire from slipping off the wedge. As the arch wire passes through the bracket slot, it is ligated in place with an elastic ligature looped around the remaining free tie wing. Once so positioned, as the arch wire passes through the bracket slot and on its way to the next bracket, it must climb up over the bulging rubber body of the rotation wedge. This causes a distortion of the wire, which in turn puts pressure on the facial surface of the wedge. This pressure is then translated into a rotational force to either the mesial or distal, depending on which tie wing has the wedge attached to it. The wedges may remain on the bracket tie wings throughout treatment and are not affected by wire changes. All teeth needing rotational correction would benefit from the extra advantage of having rotation wedges placed on them to speed up their proper positioning in the dental arch. The sooner they arrive at that position, the longer they will have the opportunity to be retained there by the arch wire during the remaining course of treatment. This in turn maximizes their stability and minimizes their chances of relapse. It is also advisable to consider the possibility of performing a modified Edwards transeptal fibrotomy on all teeth that receive any appreciable amount of rotation once they have been correctly positioned.

The second type of rotation wedge looks only distantly related to the first. It consists of a similar-sized clear, hard latex bead fastened to the center of a common ligature wire. This type of rotation wedge is placed on the bracket *after* the arch wire has been ligated to place. It is positioned in a manner similar to the rubber wedge adjacent to the tie wing of the direction in which the tooth is to be rotated. The free ends of ligature wire are wrapped about the bracket and its opposite tie wing where they are twisted, cut, and tucked out of the way. If mesial rotation is desired, the bead is placed adjacent to the mesial tie wing under the arch wire while the free end wires are looped about the bracket and tied off at the gingiva of the distal tie wing, again under the arch wire. If distal rotation is desired, the opposite procedure is followed. The wedge is placed against the distal tie wing and tied off at the mesial. When using these types of rotation wedges, it is best to ligate the arch wire to the bracket with ligature wire rather than elastics as this allows a little tighter twisting of the cut ends of the wedge wire giving more rotational force.

Rotation wedges greatly speed up the correction of rotated teeth and may be routinely used on all bicuspid and anterior teeth. Their small size also allows them to be used on anterior teeth without creating an undue esthetic problem.

Direct Bond Lingual Buttons and Cleats

These small metal buttons and cleats have bases on them similar to direct bond brackets and may be bonded to the lingual surfaces of desired teeth in an identical manner. They provide attachment points for elastics or springs when such are needed as aids in solving rotation, extrusion, or retraction problems. Molar bands may come with or without these devices already welded in place on their lingual surfaces.

Elastics

There is an entire family of elastics from which the clinician may choose for the purposes of providing extra force for the rotation, extrusion, or bodily movement of teeth. Contrary to what some might think, the use of intra-oral elastics dates back well into the last century. Dr E. Maynard first described the use of elastics in orthodontic treatment in an article entitled, "Irregularity of the Superior Denture," published in 1843! (That was the year the first wagon train left from a small town named Elm Grove near Independence, Missouri, for Oregon! Also in 1843, President Tyler was told by Mexican General Santa Anna, that there would be war if the US Congress tried to annex the Republic of Texas. It did and there was.)

Near the turn of the century, Calvin Case lectured on the use of elastics on an intermaxillary basis, and in 1902 Henry A. Baker also discussed their use and is generally credited with being the first to really define their use on an intermaxillary level.[60,61] Since those days all sorts of elastic materials have been developed. They may be used on an interarch basis running from one arch to the other in an angulated or vertical direction, or they may be used on an intra-arch basis, running from tooth to tooth for the purposes of space closure, rotation, etc. The following are some of the more commonly used elastic materials.

Circular elastics.   These are generally used for intermaxillary elastic traction either in Class II or Class III mechanics. They come in three grades of elasticity: light, medium, and heavy. They may be obtained in a variety of sizes ranging from 1/8- to 3/8-inch diameter. These "rubber bands" are used more in the fixed appliance techniques for bite opening and attempts to take the opposing arches from Class II to Class I.

Elastic ligatures.   These tiny ringlets are used to ligate arch wires to brackets. They are slipped on corner by corner to the four tie wings of the bracket with an instrument such as a fine Mathieu needle-holder with the notched tip. They fatigue and lose their elasticity after being exposed to the fluids of the mouth for a while and should be changed whenever arch wires are changed or at routine checking appointments. Though they hold the arch wire in the bracket quite well, when it is desirable to cinch the wire into the slot as tightly as possible, as in root torquing procedures requiring extraordinary stresses, the more rigid conventional wire ligatures serve best.

Chain elastic.   Sometimes referred to as a "power chain," a chain elastic looks like a line of elastic ligatures all connected together. It is one of the most commonly used means of traction for the consolidation of spaces tooth to tooth or across an entire arch. A chain elastic may be attached to the hooks on molar brackets and the tie wings of the bonded brackets where it may double as an elastic ligature to hold the arch wire in the slot. It is always used on an intra-arch basis running from tooth to tooth in the same arch, never from one arch to the other. It, too, fatigues after exposure to the fluids of the mouth for some time and should be changed every 2 to 4 weeks. It comes wound on plastic spools from which it may be cut to the desired length.

Elastic thread.   A material designed for finer uses in areas that by their convolution or inaccessibility make the use of chain elastics or metal springs impractical, elastic thread has a variety of uses. It may be tied to a lingual button and slipped through the contact to be tied to the arch wire on a tooth that needs rotation, thereby assisting the arch wire and rotation wedge in bringing about the tooth. It may also be tied to a bonded bracket of a severely lingually placed tooth that is out of reach of the arch wire because of the proximity of the two teeth on either side of it. The elastic thread may be run from the bracket of that tooth to the arch wire where the combination of the elastic tension of the thread and the slightly lingually distorted arch wire to which it is tied bring the tooth far enough labially so that it may be ligated to the arch wire without causing a permanent distortion in the wire or popping off a bracket. There are two types of thread available. One is hollow and knots tied in it crush the lumen which prevents slippage. The other is solid.

K-modules.   These traction devices are a cross between circular elastics and a thick piece of straight elastic thread. They are more powerful than common elastic thread or power chain and consist of a straight piece of tubular elastic with a round attachment module at each end. But since they come in only several preformed sizes, their use is limited.

Stainless Steel Coil Springs

Metal coil springs are another "graybeard" of the orthodontic armamentarium. Prior to the introduction of stainless steel, the coil spring was made of precious metal. Its use dates back easily to the early 1800s and probably further. In 1854 T. W. Evans described a technique whereby he retracted protruding maxillary incisors. He anchored coil springs against the maxillary molars and attached their free ends to a wire that was attached to, and crossed over the protruding teeth. Stainless steel, first introduced by Simon in Europe, became available to the American orthodontic community in the mid-1930s, where it has been used for springs as well as every other type of intraoral device ever since. Both open and closed coil springs are used in specific tooth moving or retaining situations. The measurement of a spring size is denoted by the spacing of the coils and the lumen diameter.

Open coil springs. Open coil springs are cut to desired lengths from the spools in which they are packaged. They may be placed on arch wires for the purposes of exerting pressure between two brackets to drive the respective teeth apart along the path dictated by the arch wire. An example would be the case of a lingually blocked-in upper lateral incisor. Provided there is space for the crowding central and cuspid adjacent to this lateral to be moved into, a piece of open coil spring may be cut and placed on the arch wire between the cuspid and central brackets. As the compressed spring tries to expand, it drives these two teeth apart along the arch wire, thus creating the necessary space to allow the lingually blocked-in lateral to be brought forward with power thread tied between the lateral bracket and the arch wire. The amount of spring length cut is usually 2 mm greater than the distance along the arch wire between the two outer-edge brackets of the teeth to be thus separated. If a great deal of separation is required, consecutively longer pieces must be subsequently cut and replaced as former pieces of spring expand and lose their power. The use of open coil spring is almost exclusively relegated to placement on arch wires between the brackets of teeth to be separated. The most common size is 0.010×0.030.

Closed coil springs. Less frequently used, the closed coil springs have no spacing between their coils which are confluent. They are cut and placed on arch wires between the brackets of teeth, not to create space, but to maintain it. This may also be done by putting a stop in the arch wire with a stop pliers, but this inhibits the movement of the arch wire proper, which may not be desirable. On certain occasions the operator may wish to hold two adjacent teeth apart at a constant distance while keeping the arch wire free to move back and forth through the bracket slots of these teeth. Here closed coil springs, cut to the exact desired distance to be maintained between two brackets, may be placed on the arch wire between these two teeth to prevent the teeth from moving together while the arch wire freely slides through the lumen of the spring.

Pletcher springs. These little springs have a reverse loop at one end of their coil section for attachment to the hooks of molar brackets and a piece of straight uncoiled wire at the other end. The straight piece of wire is used to attach to the hooks or brackets of anterior teeth or arch wire sections. The attachment loop is made in this wire by grasping it as the desired location with a Jarabak pliers, spooling the straight piece of wire about the beaks of the Jarabak several times to form a loop, and cutting the excess free at the base of the newly formed loop. This custom-made spring is then placed with the coil end attached to the molar hook and the straight arm end attached to a hook soldered to the arch wire, usually in the cuspid region. In order to do this, however, the coil section of the spring must be stretched as the custom loop is always placed short of the attachment site when the spring is passive. Thus the stretched spring exerts its force to retract or more correctly anchor the entire arch wire. Pletcher springs are almost always used bilaterally and nearly exclusively for the bracing of the lower arch against the forces of Class II elastics to prevent these forces from "dumping" the lower anteriors forward during final tip, torque, and bite opening procedures.

Wire ligatures. Wire ligatures may either be made of plain ligature wire from a spool with the aid of a ligature-forming pliers or they may be obtained preformed. Wire ligatures are sometimes preferred over elastics when extremely positive forms of ligation of arch wires into bracket slots are required. A handy little variation of the above is the Kobiashi hook. This is nothing more than a wire ligature with a little loop soldered in it that acts as an attachment hook for a spring or elastic once the ligature is placed on the bracket. The loop may be squeezed shut to stiffen it prior to placement on the bracket. Once placed on the bracket over the arch wire and twisted down, it should be checked for tightness of fit by attempting to rotate it about the bracket with a small pliers or ligature holder since if it spins loose, the action of the elastic will be negated.

Once again, most major orthodontic supply houses and manufacturing firms have starter kits available with a variety of the most commonly used elastics, springs, ligatures, and accessories all packaged neatly in their own carrying and storage cases. This makes for ideal access and easy organization.

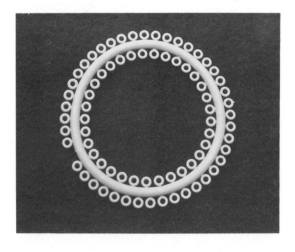

(A)

Figure 7-29   (A) Separating elastics. **(B)** Elastic separating forceps. **(C)** Rotation wedges. **(D)** Intraoral elastics and attachment/removal tools. **(E)** Elastic ligatures. **(F)** Chain elastics. **(G)** Tubular elastic thread. **(H)** Open coil spring. **(I)** Pletcher spring. (*Courtesy of European Orthodontic Products, St Paul, MN.*)

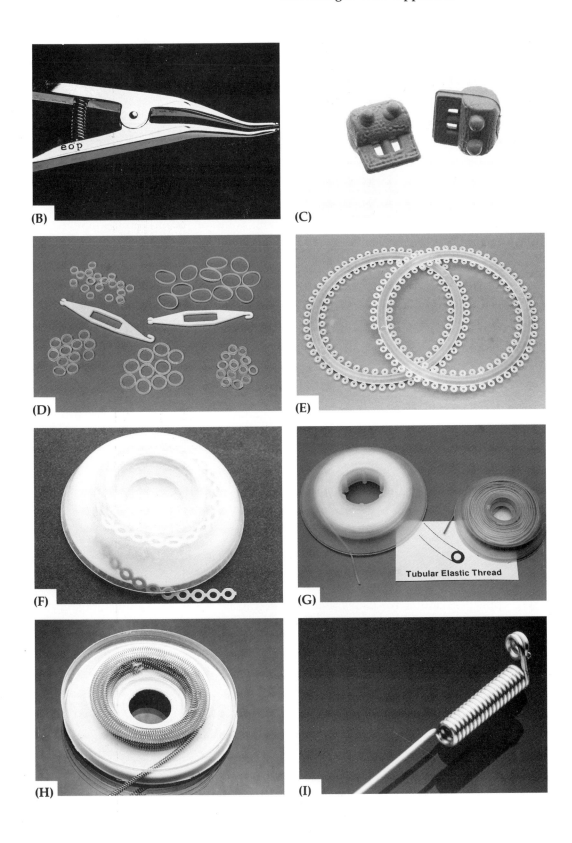

(B)

(C)

(D)

(E)

(F)

(G)

Tubular Elastic Thread

(H)

(I)

Non omnia possumus omnes
"We cannot do all things"

Virgil

FINISHING

What we have attempted to elucidate here are a few of the basic principles of the Straight Wire system of fixed orthodontics. We have discussed the philosophy of its inception, some of the procedures and techniques of its methodology, and part of its basic armamentarium. The purpose of this text is not, however, the discussion of all of the aspects of this system, but rather the clinical management of functional appliances and active plates in maxillofacial orthopedia. But the very old term "orthopedia" was chosen on purpose to denote a discipline that is neither purely orthodontic, nor purely orthopedic, but rather a logical combination of both. The Straight Wire appliance is the representative of the purest form of *orthodontic* component to this multidisciplined form of treatment just as the Bionator is the representative of the purest form of functional *orthopedic* treatment, or at least as close as we can come. No more will just pure fixed orthodontics or pure removable orthopedics be enough. In the future we will utilize both as one discipline. The union of the two to provide a total treatment modality for producing the best care possible for the patient is truly a marriage that must have been made in heaven; but remember, therein also lies the source of thunder and lightning!

It is beyond the scope of this text to purvey all the aspects of Straight Wire technique and the reader is referred to other sources for detailed information on a more extensive level. Straight Wire appliance–oriented texts of that genre may be likened to a ticker-tape parade up Fifth Avenue of New York City; whereas what we have done here is merely taken a leisurely stroll down a country lane on a summer's evening "filled with linnet's wings."

The Straight Wire appliance is an important sequence in the work laid down in the foundations of the maxillofacial complex by the functional appliances and active plates that preceded it. By virtue of the ingenious Brehm Utility Arch and its almost limitless capabilities, Straight Wire techniques can even be called upon to pave the way for functional appliances, first by preparing the mixed dentition properly on an orthodontic level so the removable-type appliances won't have to work quite so hard on an orthopedic level. Though not always needed, these simplified fixed appliance techniques are an extremely important tool to be able to fall back on where indicated. Without them, the clinician was seriously hampered in his ability to complete all cases to the level of perfection possible today. However, so much may be accomplished with modern-day removable appliances that a knowledge of Straight Wire technique even on the most basic of levels will serve to go a long way in assisting the clinician in finishing his cases to a high standard of excellence and lending credence to the old axiom, "Anyone can move a tooth."

REFERENCES

1. Angle EH: The latest and best orthodontic mechanism. *Dent Cosmos* 1928;70: 1143–1158.
2. Olwer OA, Wood CR: Lingual, labial appliances and guide plane. *Int J Orthod* 1932;18:1182–1190.
3. Johnson JE: A new orthodontic mechanism: the twin wire alignment appliance. *Int J Orthod* 1934;20:946–963.
4. Steiner CC: Power storage and delivery in orthodontic appliances. *Am J Orthod* 1953;39:859–880.
5. Begg PR: Differential force in orthodontic treatment. *Am J Orthod* 1952;42: 481–510.
6. Stoner MM: Force control in clinical practice. *Am J Orthod* 1960;46:163–186.
7. Jarabak JR: Development of a treatment plan in light of one's concept of treatment objectives. *Am J Orthod* 1960;46:481–514.
8. Storey E, Smith R: Force in orthodontics and its relation to tooth movement. *Aust J Dent* 1952;56:11–18.
9. Smith R, Storey E: The importance of force in orthodontics: The design of cuspids retraction springs. *Aust J Dent* 1952;56:291–304.
10. Jarabak JR, Fizell JA: *Technique and Treatment with Light Wire Appliances.* St Louis, CV Mosby Co, 1963, p 259.
11. Baumrind S: A reconsideration of the propriety of the "pressure-tension" hypothesis. *Am J Orthod* 1969;55:12–22.
12. Lee B: Relationships between tooth movement rate and estimated pressure applied. *J Dent Res* 1965;44:1053.
13. Weinstein S: Minimum forces in tooth movement. *Am J Orthod* 1967;53:881–903.
14. Reitan K: Some factors determining the evaluation of forces in orthodontics. *Am J Orthod* 1957;43:32–45.
15. Haldorsen H, Johns EE, Moyers R: The selection of forces for tooth movement. *Am J Orthod* 1953;39:25–35.
16. Hixon EH, Atikian H, Callow GE, et al: Optimal force, differential force and anchorage. *Am J Orthod* 1969;55:437–457.
17. Hixon EH, Aasen TO, Aranzo J, et al: On force and tooth movement. *Am J Orthod* 1970;57:476–489.
18. Nikolai RJ: On optimum orthodontic force theory as applied to canine retraction. *Am J Orthod* 1975;68:290–302.
19. Boester CH, Johnston LE: A clinical investigation of the concepts of differential and optimal force in canine retraction. *Angle Orthod* 1974;44:113–119.
20. Angle EH: The upper first molar as a basis of diagnosis in orthodontia. *Dent Items Interest* 1906;28:421–439.
21. Andrews LF: The six keys to normal occlusion. *Am J Orthod* 1972;62:296–309.
22. Winder A: The amazing story of nitinol and Dr. Andreasen. Iowa City, *The Iowa Alumni Review,* Feb/Mar 1977.
23. Sheykholeslam Z, Brandt S: Some factors affecting the bonding of orthodontic attachments to tooth surface. *J Clin Orthod* 1977;11:734–743.
24. Lee HI, Orlowski JA, Enage E, et al: In vitro and in vivo evaluation of direct-bonding orthodontic bracket systems. *J Clin Orthod* 1974;8:227–238.

25. Keizer S, ten Cate JM, Arends J: Direct bonding of orthodontic brackets. *Am J Orthod* 1976;69:318–327.

26. Reynolds IR, von Fraunhofer JA: Direct bonding of orthodontic attachments to teeth: The relation of adhesive bond strength to gauze mesh size. *Br J Orthod* 1976;3:91–95.

27. Reynolds IR, von Fraunhofer JA: Direct bonding in orthodontics: A comparison of attachments. *Br J Orthod* 1977;4:65–69.

28. Gorelick L: Bonding/The state of the art: A national survey. *J Clin Orthod* 1979; 13:39–53.

29. Gorelick L: Bonding metal brackets with a self-polymerizing sealant-composite. A 12 month assessment. *Am J Orthod* 1977;71:542–553.

30. Zachrisson BU, Brobakken BO: Clinical comparison of direct versus indirect bonding with different bracket types and adhesives. *Am J Orthod* 1978;74:62–78.

31. Dickinson PT, Powers JM: Evaluation of fourteen direct-bonding orthodontic bases. *Am J Orthod* 1980;78:630–639.

32. Demuth PR: Direct bonding with Lee Unique. *Br J Orthod* 1981;8:31–32.

33. Ricketts RM, Bench RW, Hilgers JJ: *Mandibular Utility Arch: The Basic Arch in the Light Wire Technique. Biomechanics of the Light Progressive Technique.* Rocky Mountain/Orthodontics 1972, No. 7, pp 17–22.

34. Brehm W: Personal communication, July 1984.

35. Fanning EA: Effect of extraction of deciduous molars on the formation and eruption of their successors. *Angle Orthod* 1962;32:44–53.

36. Breakspear EK: Further observations of the early loss of deciduous molars. *Dent Pract* 1961;11:233–252.

37. Brodie AG: The fourth dimension in orthodontics. *Angle Orthod* 1954;24:15–30.

38. Moyers RE: *Handbook of Orthodontics.* Chicago, Year Book Medical Publishers, 1958, pp 93–106.

39. Edwards JG: A surgical procedure to eliminate rotational relapse. *Am J Orthod* 1970;57:34–36.

40. Edwards JG: A study of the periodontium during orthodontic rotation of teeth. *Am J Orthod* 1968;54:441–461.

41. Skogsberg C: The use of septotomy in connection with orthodontic treatment. *Int J Orthod* 1932;18:659–682.

42. Erickson BE, Kaplan H, Ainsberg M: Orthodontics and transeptal fibers. *Am J Orthod Oral Surg* 1945;31:1–26.

43. Reitan K: Experiments on rotation of teeth and their subsequent retention. *Trans Eur Orthod Soc* 1958;124–140.

44. Reitan K: Retention and avoidance of post-treatment relapse. *Am J Orthod* 1969; 55:776–789.

45. Wiser GM: Resection of the supra-alveolar fibers and the retention of orthodontically rotated teeth. *Am J Orthod* 1966;52:855–856.

46. Strahan JD, Mills JRE: A preliminary report on the severing of gingival fibers following rotation of teeth. *Dent Pract* 1970;21:101–102.

47. Parker GR: Transeptal fibers and relapse following bodily retraction of teeth: a histologic study. *Am J Orthod* 1972;61:331–334.

48. Kaplan RG: Clinical experiments with circumferential supracestal fibrotomy. *Am J Orthod* 1976;70:147–153.

49. Pinson RR, Strahan JD: The effect on the relapse of orthodontically rotated teeth of surgical division of the gingival fibers: pericision. *Br J Orthod* 1973;1:87–91.

50. Ahrens DG, Shapira Y, Kuftinec MM: An approach to rotation of relapse. *Am J Orthod* 1981;80:83–91.

51. Dewey M: Some principles of retention. *Am Dent J* 1909;8:254–257.

52. Oppenheim A: The working retainer in the therapeutics of Class II. *Am J Orthodontist* 1911–1912;3:94–99.

53. Lischer BE: *Orthodontics.* Philadelphia, Lea & Febiger, 1912, 185.

54. Case CS: Principles of retention in orthdontia. *Int J Orthod Oral Surg* 1920;6:3–34.

55. Riedel RA: A review of the retention problem. *Angle Orthod* 1960;30:179–194.

56. Hawley CA: A removable retainer. *Int J Orthod* 1919;2:291–298.

57. Hawley CA: The principles and art of retention. *Int J Orthod* 1925;11:315–326.

58. Hawley CA: The removable retainer (exhibit). *Int J Orthod* 1928;14:167–168.

59. Truax L: Personal communication, October 1985.

60. Graber TM: *Orthodontics, Principles and Practice.* Philadelphia, WB Saunders Co, 1961, pp 443–445.

61. Angle EH: Further steps in the progress of orthodontia. *Dent Cosmos* 1916;58: 969–994.

CHAPTER 8
Why Continue?

After a brief consideration of the ideas presented in this text, it may readily be surmised that possibly at no other time in the history of this discipline has such a total and overwhelming assault been mounted on traditional orthodontic values and treatment methodologies. Although specific aspects of the overall concepts of FJO techniques appear in various forms throughout the more conventional orthodontic theater of operations, up until the recent decades the total program has never crystalized into such a movement so sweeping in its implications. Active plate usage, though not totally embraced by the American fixed appliance–oriented orthodontic community, was considered common knowledge and assumed a supporting role in the catalog of armamentarium. But the two key turning points in the forging of a new approach to orthodontic treatment philosophies that firmly established the new directions modern orthodontic therapeutics would take were the perfection of the arch-alignment capabilities of the Bionator and the arch-perfecting capabilities of the Straight Wire appliance. The orthopedic implications of the Bionator and its abilities at wholescale mandibular advancement and vertical-increasing capabilities in addition to the simplified techniques for fixed appliance usage brought on by the ingenious Straight Wire appliance opened up whole new vistas of possibilities not only as to what could be done in correcting the patient's malocclusion but also in the areas of who could perform it!

The emergence of the total scope of functional jaw orthopedics founded on the tandem regimens of active plate/functional appliance/Straight Wire combinations of treatment and staunchly fortified by the blessings of second molar replacement techniques where indicated, has changed the evolutionary course of orthodontics forever! Fortunately, it is a change for the better. It also is a timely change, as we have always known that malocclusions were problems of more than just "crooked teeth." We always knew there were orthopedic and myofunctional problems inherent in the malocclusion also. It is only fitting, proper, and logical that eventually various techniques would be developed that would directly and effectively address these other, until now somewhat neglected, etiological components of the malocclusion.

However, all change, even change for the better, cannot be effected without the risk of a certain amount of insecurity being felt by those participants involved. This is partly due to the fact that the individual often is merely unfamiliar with the common workings of a newer process and therefore feels a little threatened by them, or that the darkness and difficulties of uncharted areas must be confronted alone. We in the orthodontic discipline are not quite so taxed. One at first might think the only way to engage the new techniques is through the expression of a certain amount of faith in their promises. Such is not the case, however, with the active institution of FJO treatment principles. It only appears that way. The profession is fortunate in that it may draw on the lifetimes of experience of the "founding fathers" of some of the basic FJO tenets and cull the very best of their great achievements for its own purposes, distilling the knowledge and information they have accumulated down to the core truths that are best suited for its purposes. Taking the best of these truths and managing them wisely allows the profession to produce ever-better treatments for the patient.

Yet there is still a point at which each individual practitioner must take the first steps in the newer directions implied in the FJO techniques; and although this does not require so much as an act of faith, it does imply a certain amount of trust. Trust not only in the effectiveness of the particular appliance or technique but also trust in the patients and their response to it, and maybe most importantly, trust in the practitioner's own technical abilities and clinical judgment. The latter has, no doubt, served the practitioner suitably in developing to the present. With so much at stake, there is no reason to feel that it will not continue to do so again in the future. The practitioner is still ultimately in charge and therefore must continue to assume the responsibility for doing his or her own thinking. No treatment manifesto, technique prescription, or institutional dogma can do the thinking instead.

Neither can this text. This is why the discussions of the various merits of the appliances and techniques addressed have been on the most basic of levels. The appliances we have elucidated here are about as simple as they come. All sorts of modifications, additions, and augmentations to these basic appliances will no doubt appear throughout the evolution of the science. Yet the basic tenets of such fundamental appliances as the Bionator, Sagittal, Schwarz, or Straight Wire appliances are so profound that once these principle characters are understood and mastered, the amount of variation possible in both their design and usage combinations, either simultaneously in the same mouth or in their order of sequence of use, is limited only by the needs of the particular case and the individual clinician's own ingenuity. However, to obtain maximum benefit from the employment of these methods and to manage their use in the most efficient manner possible with respect to time and effort, a sound understanding of the true needs of the individual case is essential. This in turn relates the burden of responsibility for treatment sequencing to the very important process of comprehensive diagnosis.

Not only must the diagnosis of a given patient's particular needs be as accurate and comprehensive as possible, but the clinician must be able to understand how the diagnostic aids he now has at his disposal relate to the newer methods of treatment the FJO system presently represents. He must not only consider "What is?" but more importantly, "What is significant?" Due to the different approaches and capabilities of certain therapeutic aspects of the FJO system, this consideration is not always the same as it was under more restricted conventional forms of therapy. Therefore, the clinician is not only responsible for understanding the mechanics of newer treatment modalities, but he is also obliged to relate them properly to newer interpretations that may be inferred from his diagnostic process. This must be done in order to properly manage the far-reaching potentialities of the entire system. Therefore, continued effort in the pursuit of this knowledge must be initiated and maintained. Merely mastering the use of a newer appliance or a given technique here and there might not prove adequate. However, discussion of the significance of the use of FJO treatment methods and their relationship to traditional diagnostic and treatment-sequencing processes is, as might be surmised, a rather extensive issue. But a fundamental knowledge of basic appliance mechanics must come first, and it is to this end that we have assigned this particular volume.

We have come a long way since the early days in 1908 when a general practitioner named Viggo Andresen first devised a retentive- type appliance that would change the jaw-to-jaw relationship of his daughter's occlusion and hence also change the course of maxillofacial orthopedic appliance therapy forever. His "miracle" appliance may not seem so astounding to us in light of modern-day knowledge, but what *is* astounding is the results this evolutionary path has finally produced in composite modern-day therapy. For not only may we now more thoroughly address and correct malocclusions on an orthodontic, orthopedic, and myofunctional level; but presently the system is being called upon to ascend to one of its loftiest ends, the treatment of the individual suffering from occlusally and/or orthopedically induced temporomandibular joint pain, dysfunction, and malarthrosis. And in an incredible irony of ironies, the treatment regimen that will step forward to make heretofore the singular most important contribution to the effective, noninvasive treatment and correction of adult temporomandibular joint pain–dysfunction problems is the same system that can now be used in the treatment of malocclusions in the developing dentitions, and which most often prevents the inception of these retrusive condylar problems in the first place!

The FJO system of therapeutics has solved not only the problem of the correction of severe skeletal Class II mandibular retrusion, the bane of conventional fixed-appliance orthodontic therapy, but it is also prepared to assume the office of a major form of adult treatment for the patient whose retruded condylar positions are the etiological source of chronic TMJ problems. It may now be seen that both the clinician treating malocclusions in the developing child and the clinician treating temporomandibular joint problems in the adult have been blessed with a treatment modality that represents a true deliverance from one of the most critical and vexing therapeutic problems with which they are confronted on a daily basis. When the concepts that the FJO system represents are both grasped and accepted in their entirety, it might at once be discerned that the "miracle" alluded to by previous generations of orthodontic practitioners actually refers not to a single prototype appliance but rather to an entire treatment approach that is far more sweeping in its significance and is in fact presently about to be realized. The onus of carrying through with the present rests squarely on our shoulders as the ghosts of the past quietly look on from behind us.

We have awakened to the dawn of a new era in maxillofacial orthodontic and orthopedic treatment modalities, and it will only be a matter of time before their full impact is felt throughout the entire spectrum of the orthodontic community. This will be to the mutual benefit of not only the patient and the practitioner but also the profession as well. The nobility of each of these individual subjects should always remain before us. In their interest the therapeutic evolutionary process *must* continue, enabling the important earlier contributions, insights, and dreams of men like Kingsley, Andresen, Häupl, Angle, Andrews, Witzig, and numerous others, to elegantly and masterfully be carried on and to eventually come to fruition on the grandest of scales.

After generations of trial and error, success and failure, acceptance and rejection, a means has finally been delivered, an aggregate of the many that seems almost as if it were a gift for the future enshrined in a stunning and exalted heritage from the past. It asks only to be recognized and utilized for the maximum benefit of the direct objects of its concern—we humans. We now stand at a critical turning point in the development of our profession where we truly walk arm in arm with our own destinies while before us the path of evolutionary progress lies waiting. To an individual, we dare not fail in its ascent.

> *"But a miracle is a miracle—a sign of God.*
> *In a world of chaos we stand unprepared,*
> *When it suddenly shines in glory and*
> *might."*

> *"The Miracle"*
> The Poems of Dr Zhivago
> *Boris Pasternak 1890–1960*

INDEX

Page citations in italics refer to captions and accompanying illustrations.